ANALYTICAL AND QUANTITATIVE CARDIOLOGY

ADVANCES IN EXPERIMENTAL MEDICINE AND BIOLOGY

ANALYTICAL AND QUANTITATIVE CARDIOLOGY

Edited by

Samuel Sideman

and

Rafael Beyar

The Julius Silver Institute
Technion–Israel Institute of Technology
Haifa, Israel

PLENUM PRESS • NEW YORK AND LONDON

Library of Congress Cataloging-in-Publication Data

Analytical and quantitative cardiology / edited by Samuel Sideman and
   Rafael Beyar.
      p.   cm. -- (Advances in experimental medicine and biology : v.
   430)
    Includes bibliographical references and index.
    ISBN 0-306-45762-8
    1. Heart--Research--Methodology. 2. Heart--Physiology-
-Mathematical models.   I. Sideman, S.   II. Beyar, Rafael.
III. Series.
QP112.4.A53   1997
612.1'7--dc21   97-36238
                                                                     CIP

Proceedings of the 10th Goldberg Workshop on Analytical and Quantitative Cardiology: From Genetics to
Function, held December 2 – 5, 1996, in Haifa, Israel

ISBN 0-306-45762-8

© 1997 Plenum Press, New York
A Division of Plenum Publishing Corporation
233 Spring Street, New York, N. Y. 10013

http://www.plenum.com

10 9 8 7 6 5 4 3 2 1

Printed in the United States of America

Dedicated to

Enid "Dinny" Silver Winslow, daughter of Julius Silver, who established the Julius Silver Institute of Biomedical Engineering at the Technion–Israel Institute of Technology, Haifa, in 1968, was born on August 5, 1933, and left us on October 5, 1995. She graduated from Smith College, Columbia University, and the New York University School of Law.

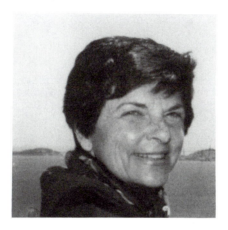

Dinny was an enthusiastic supporter of the Technion and a warm personal friend. Her vivacity, warmth, enthusiasm and intellectual curiosity made her a most respected and greatly loved friend of the Julius Silver Institute Family and all of us deeply miss her. It is with great sadness and much love that we decidate this book to her memory.

תנ צב"ה

The 10th Henry Goldberg Workshop
Analytical and Quantitative Cardiology:
From Genetics to Function
December 2–5, 1996
Haifa, Israel

Organizing Committee

Professor J. Bassingthwaighte
> Center of Biomedical Engineering, University of Washington, Seattle, WA, USA

Professor R. Beyar, Co–Chairman
> Department of Biomedical Engineering, Technion–Israel Institute of Technology, Haifa, Israel

Professor S. Sideman, Chairman
> Department of Biomedical Engineering, Technion–Israel Institute of Technology, Haifa, Israel

Professor R. Reneman
> Department of Physiology, University of Limburg, Rijksuniv, Limburg, The Netherlands

Professor E.L. Ritman
> Biodynamics Laboratory, Mayo Medical School, Roshester, MN, USA

Professor Y. Rudy
> Department of Biomedical Engineering, Case Western Reserve University, Cleveland, OH, USA

Scientific Advisory Committee

Professor W.M. Chilian
> Department of Physiology, Medical College of Wisconsin, Milwaukee, WI, USA

Professor M. Gotsman
> Cardiology Department, Hadassah Medical Organization, Jerusalem, Israel

Professor E. Kaplinski
> The Chaim Sheba Medical Center, and Tel Aviv University Sackler School of Medicine, Tel Hashomer, Israel

Professor E. Marban
> Department of Cardiology, Johns Hopkins University School of Medicine, Baltimore, MD, USA

Professor M. Morad
> Department of Pharmacology, Georgetown University, Washington, DC, USA

Professor G.W. Schmid–Schönbein
> Department of Biomedical Engineering, University of California, San Diego, La Jolla, CA, USA

The 10th Henry Goldberg Workshop on
ANALYTICAL AND QUANTITATIVE CARDIOLOGY:
FROM GENETICS TO FUNCTION
Haifa, Israel

Sponsored by

THE TECHNION–ISRAEL INSTITUTE OF TECHNOLOGY
MR. JULIUS SILVER, NEW YORK, USA
MR. HENRY (DECEASED) AND VIOLA GOLDBERG, NEW YORK, USA
THE ISRAEL CARDIOLOGY SOCIETY

PREFACE

The tenth Henry Goldberg Workshop is an excellent occasion to recall our goals and celebrate some of our humble achievements. Vision and love of our fellow man are combined here to: 1) Foster interdisciplinary interaction between leading world scientists and clinical cardiologists so as to identify missing knowledge and catalyze new research ideas; 2) relate basic microscale, molecular and subcellular phenomena to the global clinically manifested cardiac performance; 3) apply conceptual modelling and quantitative analysis to better explore, describe, and understand cardiac physiology; 4) interpret available clinical data and design new revealing experiments; and 5) enhance international cooperation in the endless search for the secrets of life and their implication on cardiac pathophysiology.

The first Goldberg Workshop, held in Haifa, in 1984, explored the interaction of mechanics, electrical activation, perfusion and metabolism, emphasizing imaging in the clinical environment. The second Workshop, in 1985, discussed the same parameters with a slant towards the control aspects. The third Goldberg Workshop, held in the USA at Rutgers University, in 1986, highlighted the transformation of the microscale activation phenomena to macroscale activity and performance, relating electrophysiology, energy metabolism and cardiac mechanics. The fourth Goldberg Workshop continued the effort to elucidate the various parameters affecting cardiac performance, with emphasis on the ischemic heart. The fifth Workshop concentrated on the effect of the inhomogeneity of the cardiac muscle on its performance. The sixth Workshop highlighted new imaging techniques which allow insight into the local and global cardiac performance. The seventh Goldberg Workshop was devoted to in-depth exploration of the basic micro-level phenomena that affect the cardiac system, with particular emphasis on the electrical activation. The eighth Workshop concentrated on analysis of the interactions between these phenomena and the development and application of new cardiac research and clinical practice. The ninth Goldberg Workshop, held in Haifa, in 1994, dwelt in-depth on the molecular and subcellular aspects of the cardiac system. This tenth Workshop is devoted to the analytical and quantitative analyses leading from basic genetics to cardiac function and is aimed to highlight the interface between structure and function at all levels of the cardiac system. The challenge is to combine the analytical system approach and engineering principles with the multiple molecular and/or genetic factors and stimuli, and the macroscale interactions which determine cardiac function.

No one walks alone, and the support and encouragement of friends along the way is greatfully acknowledged. First and foremost, we thank Henry (now deceased), and his wife Viola Goldberg who provided the means to pursue our goals, and Mr. Arthur Goldberg who contributed to our last Workshop. Special thanks are due to Mr. Julius Silver and his daughter Dinny (now deceased) whose support and trust through the years gave us the means to pursue excellence. Thanks are also due to the Women's Division of the American Technion Society as well as other Friends of the Technion in the USA and Canada who made this cardiac expedition a reality. Last, but not least, our thanks to our colleagues who served on the Advisory and Organizing Committees and to Ms. Deborah E. Shapiro, whose dedication and hard work has helped put these Workshops in the annals of science.

Samuel Sideman
Rafael Beyar

INTRODUCTORY REMARKS

It is a pleasure to see such a group of eminent scientists from all over the world sitting together and discussing the major issues of modern cardiology and cardiological sciences. The fact that this meeting is so unique goes hand in hand with the uniqueness of this wonderful person, Sam Sideman; "Shmulik" as we call him here. It is the spirit of this man which I have followed now for many years, which has created this center of biological, bioengineering, cardiological science here in Haifa. It is his energy, intelligence, initiative, and leadership that has done that. When you look at the group that works with Sam, and one of the most eminent is my dear friend Rafi Beyar, you realize that something wonderful has been established, and that stability and continuity in the future have been assured. I am a clinical cardiologist and when I look at the program of this Workshop, I feel that I may have made a mistake becoming Dean of the Faculty of Medicine at Tel Aviv University, which prevents me from staying throughout all the Workshop and enjoying modern science. But eventually, whatever comes out from you wonderful people working in laboratories, looking into the secrets of heart and blood vessels, will reach the clinicians' hands and save lives. The coronary care unit today, any cardiological institute, or a cardiac operating room, are testimonials to what modern science and technology have done to improve the present and future of our patients.

We are grateful to all of you for taking the time to join us here in Israel. Have a good productive meeting and enjoy yourselves. Finally, thank you, Shmulik, for what you have done and for what you are.

Professor Elieser Kaplinsky
Dean, Sackler School of Medicine
Tel Aviv University
Head of Cardiology
Tel Hashomer Hospital

CONTENTS

I. Molecular Signalling

II. The Contractile Mechanism and Engergetics

III. Cardiac Mechanics and Flow Dynamics

IV. Vascular Structure and Remodeling

V. Myocardial Structure and Function

VI. Electrical Activation and Propagation

VII. The Cardionome: Concepts in Modeling

I. MOLECULAR SIGNALLING

CHAPTER 1

CA^{2+}–SIGNALING IN CARDIAC MYOCYTES: EVIDENCE FROM EVOLUTIONARY AND TRANSGENIC MODELS

Martin Morad and Yuichiro J. Suzuki[1]

ABSTRACT

Cardiac contraction is regulated by a number of Ca^{2+}–mediated processes. Here we consider the effects of modification imposed on the Ca^{2+}–signalling mechanism by evolutionary developments and transgenic manipulations. Ca^{2+}–signalling appears to be mediated via influx of Ca^{2+} through the DHP receptor in preference to the Na^{+}–Ca^{2+} exchange protein, and activates the ryanodine receptor and the Ca^{2+} release from the SR. Here we report on functional consequences of overexpression of the Na^{+}–Ca^{2+} exchanger and calsequestrin. The data does not support a physiological role for the Na^{+}–Ca^{2+} exchanger in signalling Ca^{2+} release, but can serve to modify ionic currents which determine the duration of the action potential.

INTRODUCTION

The initiation of cardiac contraction in the mammalian heart appears to be regulated by a number of Ca^{2+}–mediated processes that include entry of Ca^{2+} through the L–type channel, release of Ca^{2+} from the ryanodine receptor of the sarcoplasmic reticulum (SR), reuptake of Ca^{2+} by Ca^{2+}–ATPase, and Ca^{2+}–binding to calsequestrin for storage in the SR. To keep cellular homeostatic Ca^{2+} balance, the Ca^{2+} that is not recirculated into the SR is extruded via another set of proteins identified as Na^{+}–Ca^{2+} exchanger and sarcolemmal Ca^{2+}–ATPase. The experimental evidence obtained over the past decade on the cellular

---

[1]Department of Pharmacology, Georgetown University Medical Center, 3900 Reservoir Road NW, Washington, DC 20007–2197 USA

Analytical and Quantitative Cardiology
Edited by Sideman and Beyar, Plenum Press, New York, 1997

level suggests the following sequence of events for the role of Ca^{2+} in excitation–contraction (E–C) coupling:

1. Membrane depolarization opens the L–type Ca^{2+} channel allowing Ca^{2+} influx;
2. Ca^{2+} entering via the Ca^{2+} channel binds to and opens the SR ryanodine receptors;
3. Ca^{2+} released via the ryanodine receptor activates the contractile filaments and in part inactivates the Ca^{2+} channel;
4. a fraction of Ca^{2+} is then sequestered from the myoplasmic space into the SR by Ca^{2+}–ATPase, while another fraction is extruded from the cell by Na^+–Ca^{2+} exchanger and sarcolemmal Ca^{2+}–ATPase; and
5. Ca^{2+} entering the SR is bound primarily to the Ca^{2+}–binding protein of the SR, calsequestrin and is primed for re–release.

Although a large body of literature exists for the above scheme and it is universally agreed that the above scheme is the primary Ca^{2+}–signaling pathway for cardiac E–C coupling, a number of questions remain not only as to the exact molecular mechanisms of the various steps in Ca^{2+}–signaling, but also as to the role of some of the Ca^{2+} proteins in regulation or triggering of contraction. For instance, what are the molecular mechanisms of Ca^{2+}–induced Ca^{2+} release and what molecular steps render the Ca^{2+} release mechanisms graded? What stops the release of Ca^{2+}? Does the Ca^{2+}–induced Ca^{2+} release accommodate or inactivate in the presence of high Ca^{2+} concentrations? Is the Na^+–Ca^{2+}exchanger directly involved in causing Ca^{2+} release under physiological conditions? What is the role of Na^+ and T–type Ca^{2+} channels in physiological release of Ca^{2+}? What role does Ca^{2+} content of SR or the level of expression of calsequestrin play in the release process?

Some of the questions posed here have been the subjects of numerous publications. There are essentially two opinions on the subject of Na^+–Ca^{2+} exchanger as a possible trigger for physiological release of Ca^{2+}. Morad and his colleagues [1–3] consistently find little support for such a mechanism under physiological conditions. Others [4–7] attribute a significant amount of physiological Ca^{2+} release to the Na^+–Ca^{2+} exchanger. In this respect, recent data on activation of Ca^{2+} sparks in isolated cardiac myocytes using confocal microscopy suggests absence of localized Ca^{2+} release (sparks) when the Na^+–Ca^{2+} exchanger is induced to operate in the Ca^{2+} influx mode [8, 9]. This finding is consistent with the observations of Adachi–Akahane et al. [3] which show that Ca^{2+} influx via the exchanger may be easily buffered in myocytes dialyzed with 0.4 mM EGTA, while the ability of Ca^{2+} influx through the Ca^{2+} channel in activation of Ca^{2+} release remains highly resistant to high concentrations of dialyzing Ca^{2+} buffers (14 mM EGTA + 2 mM Fura–2) or BAPTA. Such a finding suggests possible preferred accessibility of Ca^{2+}channel to the ryanodine receptors vis–a–vis the exchanger [2]. Here, we report on studies which attempt to examine modification imposed on the Ca^{2+}–signaling mechanism by evolutionary developments and transgenic manipulations.

FUNCTIONAL CONSEQUENCES OF OVEREXPRESSION OF Na^+–Ca^{2+} EXCHANGER

To measure and quantify the level of functional expression of the exchanger in ventricular myocytes, we measured I_{Na-Ca} activated by caffeine–induced Ca^{2+} release. There is significant species differences in the level of expression of Na^+–Ca^{2+} exchanger [10]. Table 1 compares the density of the exchanger current in a cardiac myocyte freshly isolated from the hearts of different mammalian species. While the density of I_{Na-Ca} varied over two to three–fold in different species (as measured by I_{Na-Ca} induced by caffeine–triggered Ca^{2+}

Table 1. I_{Na-Ca} activated by caffeine–induced Ca^{2+} release

Species	(n)	Ca$_i$–transients (nM)	I_{Na-Ca} (pA/pF)
Guinea pig	10	398 ± 35	1.84 ± 0.25
Hamster	11	412 ± 39	4.06 ± 0.45
Mouse	14	496 ± 0.63	1.61 ± 0.16
Rat	22	355 ± 29	0.81 ± 0.14
Human	4	229 ± 25	0.93 ± 0.18

I_{Na-Ca} was activated by rapid application of 5 or 10 mM caffeine to a myocyte dialyzed with 0.1 – 0.2 mM Fura–2 and voltage–clamped at –80 mV. Part of the data was obtained from Sham *et al.* [10].

release), the efficacy of Na$^+$–Ca^{2+} exchanger in triggering Ca^{2+} release at physiological potentials remained very low. That is, under whole cell–clamp conditions and Fura–2 dialyzing concentrations of 100 – 200 μM, Ca^{2+} influx through the Ca^{2+} channel at 0 to +20 mV was not only the primary but often the only mechanism mediating the release of Ca^{2+}. Thus, we found that blocking of the Ca^{2+} channel with the 100 μM Cd^{2+}, irrespective of species examined, consistently and completely abolished Ca^{2+} release from the SR as previously reported for the rat [1].

To examine whether the failure of the exchanger to release Ca^{2+} arises from low density of I_{Na-Ca} vs. I_{Ca} in cardiac myocytes, transgenic mice overexpressing the cardiac exchanger were developed [11]. The level of overexpression of the cardiac exchanger in transgenic mice was evaluated by western blot analysis, immunofluorescent antibody staining, Na$^+$–dependent ^{45}Ca uptake in sarcolemmal vesicles, and by direct electrophysiological measurements of I_{Na-Ca} in whole cell–clamped myocytes in response to caffeine–induced Ca^{2+} release. Table 2 shows a three to five–fold increase in the level of expression of the exchanger current in transgenic ventricular myocytes. With the exception of threefold larger I_{Na-Ca} in transgenic vs. the control myocytes, all other parameters such as cell size (capacitance), I_{Ca}, and Ca^{2+} release triggered by I_{Ca} or caffeine remained the same.

Figure 1 compares the magnitude and the time course of Ca$_i^{2+}$–transients and I_{Na-Ca} in transgenic myocytes and their non–transgenic littermates. Although caffeine–triggered Ca$_i$–transients appear to be similar in magnitude, the activated I_{Na-Ca} is about three times larger and decays faster than that of control myocytes. Figure 1C shows that Ni^{2+} blocked

Table 2. Properties of transgenic myocytes overexpressing Na$^+$–Ca^{2+} exchanger

	Control		Exchanger (+)	
Cell size (Cm)	192 ± 9 pF	(n=19)	204 ± 7 pF	(n=31)
I_{Ca}	2189 ± 207 pA	(n=19)	2129 ± 209 pA	(n=31)
Δ[Ca^{2+}]$_i$	364 ± 22 nM	(n=10)	337 ± 23 nM	(n=15)
$I_{Na/Ca}$, caffeine–induced	1.61 ± 0.16 pA/pF	(n=14)	4.96 ± 0.63 pA/pF	(n=16)
Δ[Ca^{2+}]$_i$, caffeine–triggered	410.3 ± 26.2 nM	(n=14)	437.4 ± 30.6 nM	(n=16)

Control and transgenic ventricular myocytes were dialyzed with 0.1 mM Fura–2. I_{Ca} was activated at 0 mV from holding potential of –60 mV. Caffeine–triggered Ca$_i$–transients and I_{Na-Ca} were activated by application of 5 mM caffeine at –80 mV (modified from [11]).

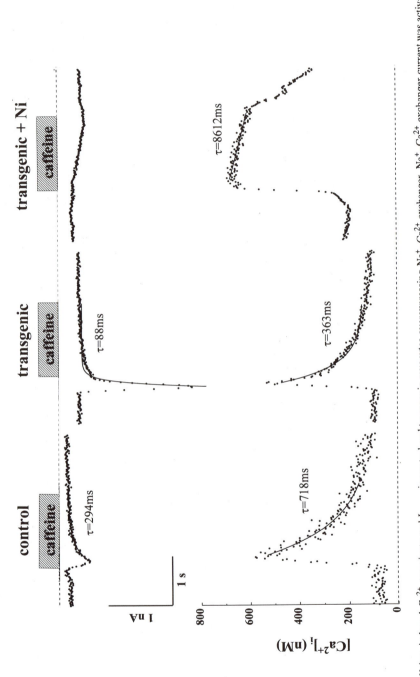

Figure 1. Caffeine-induced Ca^{2+}-transients and I_{Na-Ca} in control and transgenic myocytes overexpressing Na^+–Ca^{2+} exchanger. Na^+–Ca^{2+} exchanger current was activated by Ca^{2+} release from the SR triggered by rapid application of 5 mM caffeine at a holding potential of –90 mV. **A)** $I_{Na/Ca}$ (upper tracing) and Ca_i^{2+}-transients (lower tracing) recorded from a control myocyte. The timing of caffeine application is indicated by the shaded bar. **B)** Similar recordings from transgenic myocyte in the absence and **C)** presence of 5 mM $NiCl_2$. [Fura–2] = 0.2 mM (modified from Adachi-Akahane *et al.* [11]).

the exchanger current and strongly suppressed the rate of decay of Ca^{2+} transients, suggesting that the exchanger contributes significantly to the reduction of myoplasmic Ca^{2+}. Interestingly, when Ni^{2+} was used to block the efflux of Ca^{2+} via the exchanger the magnitude of Ca^{2+} transients was also significantly larger in transgenic vs. control myocytes. One likely explanation for larger Ca$_i^{2+}$–transients in transgenic myocytes treated with Ni^{2+}is that the activity of Ca^{2+}–ATPase may have been also enhanced in these myocytes. Such a compensatory mechanism may arise in order to maintain or overcome the larger efflux of Ca^{2+} from the myoplasm that must necessarily result from the overexpression of the exchanger.

Figure 2 compares the ability of Ca^{2+} influx via the Ca^{2+} channel and the exchanger in triggering Ca^{2+} release in transgenic myocytes at two selected voltages, 0 mV (where I_{Ca} is maximum) and +50 mV (where I_{Ca} is small but the exchanger operates in the Ca^{2+} influx–mode). Figure 2 shows a large Ca^{2+}–transients activated by I_{Ca} which is completely blocked in the presence of 100 μM Cd^{2+}. Figure 2, on the other hand, shows a much smaller Ca^{2+} release during the pulse (most likely due to the residual I_{Ca} at +50 mV) but a larger Ca^{2+} transient generated in response to I_{Ca} "tail" currents upon repolarization. Note that the Ca^{2+} channel tail–current, which triggers large Ca$_i^{2+}$–transients, also activates a large exchanger current. All parameters, I_{Ca} , I_{Na-Ca} , and Ca$_i$ –transients are strongly suppressed by 100 μM Cd^{2+}, suggesting that Ca^{2+} channel tail–current which triggers the release of Ca^{2+} also activates I_{Na-Ca}.

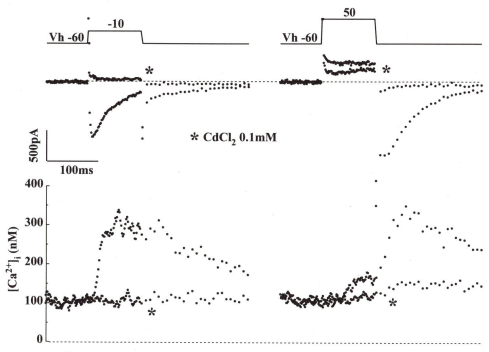

Figure 2. Cd^{2+} blocks Ca^{2+} release by blocking I_{Ca} at –10 and +50 mV in transgenic myocytes overexpressing Na$^+$–Ca^{2+} exchanger. Membrane currents and Ca^{2+}–transients activated by depolarizing pulses in transgenic myocytes dialyzed with 0.2 mM Fura–2 were recorded at 10 s intervals before and following addition of 0.1 mM Cd^{2+}. [Fura–2] = 0.2 mM (from Adachi–Akahane *et al.* [11]).

Thus, Ca^{2+} influx via the exchanger, irrespective of the level of its functional expression in various species or in transgenic mice, does not seem to have the same accessibility to the ryanodine receptor as the L–type Ca^{2+} channel.

FUNCTIONAL CONSEQUENCES OF THE OVEREXPRESSION OF CALSEQUESTRIN

Calsequestrin is the primary Ca^{2+}–binding protein of the SR, the structure of which has been identified and the gene cloned [12]. Cardiac calsequestrin binds 35 – 40 mol of Ca^{2+} per molecule with moderate affinity of $K_D =$ ˜1 mM [13]. Recently, it has been pos–sible to develop transgenic mice which overexpress cardiac calsequestrin (a gift from Larry Jones of Krannert Institute, Indiana). Such mice, though living into adulthood, show cardiac hypertrophy and ventricular fibrosis. The level of calsequestrin expression in transgenic mouse heart was 18–fold higher than that in control mouse heart as judged by the western blot analysis (Larry Jones, personal communication). Isolated myocytes from calsequestrin–overexpressing hearts release nearly five–fold or higher concentration of Ca^{2+} as compared to their non–transgenic littermates. Figure 3 compares the time course and magnitude of caffeine–induced Ca^{2+} release and its accompanying exchanger–mediated Ca^{2+} efflux in control and calsequestrin–overexpressing mice. The large caffeine–induced rise in $[Ca^{2+}]_i$ in 100 µM Fura–2 dialyzed transgenic myocytes often saturated the dye and irreversibly damaged the cell. In fact, in the vast majority of myocytes, caffeine–induced Ca^{2+} release was the final experimental step. Nevertheless, prior to loss of giga–seal and increase in leak current, large and rapidly activating exchanger currents were often recorded. Figure 3 sug–gests $I_{Na–Ca}$ density is in the range of 6–7 pA/pF. The currents generated by the exchanger are significantly larger than even those measured in transgenic mice overexpressing the

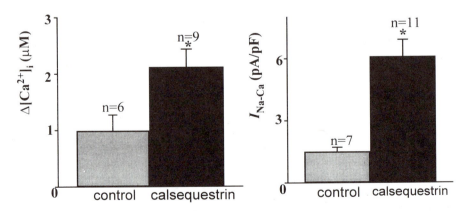

Figure 3. Caffeine–induced Ca_i^{2+}–transients and $I_{Na/Ca}$ in control and transgenic myocytes overexpressing calsequestrin. $Na^+–Ca^{2+}$ exchanger current was activated by Ca^{2+} release from the SR triggered by rapid application of 5 mM caffeine at a holding potential of –90 mV. Ca_i^{2+}–transients (upper panel) and $I_{Na/Ca}$ (lower panel) recorded from representative control and calsequestrin–overexpressing myocytes. [Fura–2] = 0.1 mM.

exchanger (≈ 5 pA/pF, see Table 2). The large magnitude of $I_{\text{Na-Ca}}$ in calsequestrin–overexpressing myocytes appears to be secondary to the large Ca^{2+} release, rather than compensatory overexpression of the exchanger. Consistent with this idea, exchanger–induced Ca^{2+} release was undetected at physiological potentials and was not significantly larger than those of control myocytes at positive potentials (> 80 mV).

Comparing the various electrophysiological parameters of calsequestrin–overexpressing myocytes to control myocytes (Table 3) suggests significantly larger membrane capacitance (sarcolemmal surface area), similar Ca^{2+} channel current densities, but significantly smaller I_{Ca}–induced Ca^{2+} release especially when compared to the over-powering and dye–saturating caffeine–induced Ca^{2+} release. Since the density of I_{Ca} is within the normal range in these transgenic myocytes and caffeine easily triggers large Ca^{2+} release from the ryanodine receptor, the data suggests possible defects in the mechanisms of Ca^{2+} channel–signaling of Ca^{2+} release. It should be noted that even though the Ca^{2+} channel gating of the ryanodine receptor is defective, the exchanger does not appear to replace the Ca^{2+}–signaling function of the Ca^{2+} channel. It is likely that the failure of I_{Ca}–induced Ca^{2+} release mechanism may eventually lead to cardiac hypertrophy and failure.

Table 3. Properties of cardiac calsequestrin–overexpressing transgenic mice

	Control		Calsequestrin (+)	
Heart Mass	170.7 ± 6.7	(n=6)	284.5 ± 13.4	(n=13)
Capacitance	151.1 ± 6.0 pF	(n=23)	239.9 ± 12.4 pF	(n=54)
I_{Ca} (HP–60; 2 mM Fura)	7.1 ± 3.2 pA/pF	(n=4)	7.3 ± 2.0 pA/pF	(n=6)
$\Delta[Ca^{2+}]_i$ (HP–60; 2 mM Fura)	110.5 ± 23.5 nM	(n=4)	17.6 ± 7.6 nM	(n=6)
Caffeine–induced $I_{\text{Na/Ca}}$ (0.1 mM Fura)	1.4 ± 0.2 pA/pF	(p=7)	6.1 ± 0.8 pA/pF	(n=11)
(2 mM Fura)	0.6 ± 0.4 pA/pF	(n=6)	8.9 ± 1.7 pA/pF	(n=14)
Caffeine–induced $\Delta[Ca^{2+}]_i$ (0.1 mM Fura)	993.0 ± 278.2 nM	(n=6)	2121.4 ± 313.6 nM	(n=9)
(2 mM Fura)	237.3 ± 70.2 nM	(n=5)	882.6 ± 249.1 nM	(n=14)
$[\Delta[Ca^{2+}]_i]_{\text{Ca}}/[\Delta[Ca^{2+}]_i]_{\text{caffeine}}$ (2 mM Fura)	0.47		0.02	

Control and transgenic ventricular myocytes were dialyzed with 0.1 or 2.0 mM Fura–2 as indicated. I_{Ca} was activated at 0 mV from a holding potential of –60 mV. Caffeine (5 mM)–induced Ca_i–transients and $I_{\text{Na-Ca}}$ were activated at –90 mV. Heart mass was measured in mg.

CONCLUSION

Ca^{2+}–signaling in mammalian cardiac myocytes appears to be mediated via influx of Ca^{2+} through the DHP receptor, which in turn activates the ryanodine receptor allowing release of Ca^{2+} from the SR. There appears to be a preferential access of Ca^{2+} entering via the DHP receptor to the ryanodine receptor, compared to that flowing in via the Na^+–Ca^{2+} exchanger protein. Our data clearly show that varying the degree of the expression of the exchanger by almost five–fold in various species and transgenic mice does not qualitatively alter the primacy of the Ca^{2+} channel in initiating and controlling Ca^{2+} release. In transgenic models, even though large inward currents can be observed following the release of Ca^{2+} triggered either by I_{Ca} or by caffeine, the exchanger fails to cause significant Ca^{2+} release in the physiological range of membrane potentials. It should be noted that even when I_{Ca}–induced Ca^{2+} release is defective in calsequestrin–overexpressing mice, we could not observe significant activation of ryanodine–receptor by Ca^{2+} influx via the exchanger.

Thus, neither when the exchanger is overexpressed in transgenic myocytes nor when the I_{Ca}-gating of Ca^{2+} release is compromised in calsequestrin–overexpressing myocytes, did we find critical data to support a physiological role for the exchanger in signaling of Ca^{2+} release. On the other hand, the overexpressed exchanger appears to modify ionic currents responsible for determining the duration of action potential.

Acknowledgments

This work was supported by NIH grant RO1–16152. We thank Dr. Larry Jones and his collaborators at Indiana University for generously supplying us with the calsequestrin transgenic mice. The Na^+–Ca^{2+} exchanger overexpressing mice were a generous gift of Dr. Ken Philipson of UCLA Medical Center.

DISCUSSION

Dr. H. Ter Keurs: The calsequestrin mice are unhappy, probably because they have heart failure, and have lost a large number of cells already in their normal lifetime before they meet you. If they have heart failure, what is the contribution of modification of protein expression in the failing cardiac cells to what you have measured and express simply as calsequestrin overexpression?

Dr. M. Morad: The amount of overexpression of calsequestrin measured by Dr. Larry Jones of Indiana University, is about 18–fold above control (Western blot analysis). If every calsequestrin molecule binds 40–50 calciums we may have about 1000–fold increase in the calcium content of the SR. We don't as yet know what other protein changes have occurred. I agree with you that these mice have lost a lot of cells, but the cells we are looking at are the surviving cells. These cells look like sacks, are hypertrophied, and the striations are not as clear as those seen in normal mice myocytes. If you measure the membrane capacity of each cell, it is about 50–75% larger than the membrane capacity of normal mouse myocytes.

Dr. H. Ter Keurs: Did you look for FK binding proteins involved in this feedback?

Dr. M. Morad: No.

Dr. N. Alpert: Is it possible that instead of having a problem in your DHP or ryanodine receptor, it is because of the increase in calsequestrin that you do not have any calcium available for release and the muscle is not being activated? That would be comparable to observations in heart failure where there is a decrease in SERCA–II proteins and phospholamban, etc. , so that the amount of calcium in the sarcoplasmic reticulum is low enough to result in inadequate activation.

Dr. M. Morad: This is clearly not the case. If anything, the SR is full of Ca^{2+}. Calsequestrin is supposedly a buffering molecule. Overexpression, I would have thought, would simply result in an increase in the number of calsequestrin molecules without significant change in its binding kinetics. Therefore, one might have guessed that nothing in particular should have happened in these mice. What we found, to our surprise, was that even though caffeine–induced Ca^{2+} release was extremely large, Ca^{2+} current–induced release was small. This finding suggests that the Ca^{2+} content of the SR or its release via the ryanodine receptors is not compromised. Thus we have concluded that the signaling of Ca^{2+} release via the Ca^{2+} channel is defective.

Dr. H. Strauss: This is a wonderful story teaching us about heart failure and hypertrophy. I have two questions. First, with regard to the mechanism of hypertrophy or adaptive changes in your overexpressed calsequestrin model. The pathways may be different in this species than in others because of the importance of the IP$_3$ pathway in intracellular calcium release in this species, in contrast to other mammalian species such as man and dogs. Second, with regard to the mice with overexpressed Na$^+$–Ca^{2+} exchanger, I wonder if you have any data about the distribution of the protein in mice. Does it couple to the Ca^{2+} channel and are the distributions around the Ca^{2+} channel similar in the overexpressed mouse? If the domains are not fully reconstituted then you might not be able to draw some of the conclusions that you otherwise would.

Dr. M. Morad: Let me take your second question first. In the Na$^+$–Ca^{2+} exchanger expressing mouse, the immunofluorescence shows that the molecule is all over the place; located in the same place, more or less, as the calcium channel. So why was it that we were not able to bring enough calcium to trigger Ca^{2+} release especially when we could show that the exchanger current had reached the nano–ampere range (about the same range as I$_{Ca}$)? An interesting hint came from experiments where we blocked the exchanger current with Ni^{2+}. To our surprise, in the presence of Ni^{2+} we found that calcium release from the SR via the ryanodine receptor went up by 30–40% suggesting that the overexpressed exchanger molecules were close enough to he DHP–Ryanodine receptor micro–domain, as to be able to extrude some of the released calcium, thus diminishing the magnitude of the release. We believe, therefore, that the overexpressed exchanger is close enough to the micro–domain created by the Ca^{2+} channel/Ryanodine receptor to pump out the Ca^{2+} but is not close enough to trigger the release of Ca^{2+} from the Ryanodine receptor. Why can't we bring in enough Ca^{2+} on the exchanger to trigger Ca^{2+} release effectively remains a mystery. With respect to your first question, you are absolutely right that the human heart–failure model may be quite different on the molecular level. However, this model has taught us some of the intricacies in Ca^{2+} signaling steps. At the least, we have learned that calsequestrin may have, in addition to its Ca^{2+} binding properties, a regulatory role in signaling of Ca^{2+} release.

REFERENCES

1. Sham JSK, Cleemann L, Morad M. Gating of cardiac release channels by Na$^+$ current and Na$^+$–Ca^{2+} exchange. *Science* 1992;255:850–853.
2. Sham JSK, Cleemann L, Morad M. Functional coupling of Ca^{2+} channels and ryanodine receptors in cardiac myocytes. *Proc Natl Acad Sci USA* 1995;92:121–125.
3. Adachi–Akahane S, Cleemann L, Morad M. Cross–signaling between L–type Ca^{2+} channels and ryanodine receptors in rat ventricular myocytes. *J Gen Physiol* 1996;108:435–454.
4. Bridge JHB, Smolley JR, Spitzer KW. The relationship between charge movements associated with I_{Ca} and I_{Na-Ca} in cardiac myocytes. *Science* 1990;248:376–378.
5. Lipp P, Pott L, Callewaert G, Carmeliet E. Simultaneous recording of Indo–1 fluorescence and Na$^+$/Ca^{2+} exchange current reveals two components of Ca^{2+} release from sarcoplasmic reticulum of cardiac atrial myocytes. *FEBS Lett* 1990;275:181–184.
6. Levi AJ, Spitzer KW, Kohmoto O, Bridge JHB. Depolarization–induced Ca^{2+} entry via Na–Ca exchange triggers SR release in guinea pig cardiac myocytes. *Am J Physiol* 1994;266:H1422–H1433.
7. Wassertrom JA, Vites AM. The role of Na$^+$–Ca^{2+} exchange in activation of excitation–contraction coupling in rat ventricular myocytes. *J Physiol* 1996;493:529–542.
8. Lederer WJ, Cheng H, He S, Valdivia C, Kofuji P, Schulze DH, Cannel MB. Na/Ca exchanger: Role in excitation–contraction coupling in heart muscle and physiological insights from the gene structure. *Heart Vessels Suppl* 1995;9:161–162.
9. Wier WG. Local calcium transients in voltage–clamped cardiac cells: Evoked calcium sparks. In: Morad M, Ebashi S, Trautwein W, Kurachi, Y, eds. *Molecular Physiology and Pharmacology of Cardiac Ion Channels and Transporters*, Dordretch, Netherlands: Kluwer Academic Publishers, 1996; 381–388.
10. Sham JSK, Hatem SN, Morad M. Species differences in the activity of the Na$^+$–Ca^{2+} exchanger in mammalian cardiac myocytes. *J Physiol* 1995;488:623–631.
11. Adachi–Akahane S, Lu L, Li Z, Frank JS, Philipson KD, Morad M. Calcium signaling in transgenic mice overexpressing cardiac Na$^+$–Ca^{2+} exchanger. *J Gen Physiol* 1997; in press.

12.   Scott BT, Simmerman HKB, Collins JH, Nadal–Ginard B, Jones LR. Complete amino acid sequence
        of canine cardiac calsequestrin deduced by cDNA cloning. *J Biol Chem* 1988;263:8958–8964.
13.   Mitchell RD, Simmerman HKB, Jones LR. Ca^{2+} binding effects on protein conformation and protein
        interactions of canine cardiac calsequestrin. *J Biol Chem* 1988;263:1376–1381.

CHAPTER 2

Diastolic Viscoelastic Properties of Rat Cardiac Muscle; Involvement of Ca^{2+}

Bruno D.M.Y. Stuyvers, Masahito Miura, and Henk E.D.J. ter Keurs[1]

ABSTRACT

Diastolic cardiac sarcomere stiffness, sarcomere length changes, and calcium concentration $[Ca^{2+}]_i$ were investigated in 18 trabeculae, dissected from the right ventricle of rat heart. $[Ca^{2+}]_i$ declined following a mono–exponential diastolic time course with a time constant of 210–350 ms. During diastole, ($[Ca^{2+}]_o = 1$ mM), sarcomere length (SL) increases (amplitude: 5–65 nm; time constant: 600 ms). Eighty percent of muscles showed discrete spontaneous motion of sarcomeres near the end of diastole; this phenomenon occurred earlier at higher $[Ca^{2+}]_o$. The stiffness modulus of the sarcomere (MOD) increased by 30% during diastole (n=158; p<0.05), while the phase difference, Φ, between force and SL decreased by 13% (n=158; p<0.05). The increase of MOD and the decrease of Φ reversed when spontaneous activation occurred. These results show that the mechanical diastolic properties of the cardiac sarcomere are time dependent. The time dependence of the diastolic properties can be faithfully reproduced by a simple linear four element viscoelastic model. The diastolic changes of MOD and of Φ could be reproduced by assuming an exponential change of the elastic and viscous coefficients of the model over time with a time constant similar to the time constant of change of $[Ca^{2+}]_i$. We suggest that the simplest combination of structural counterparts of the model in the sarcomere consists of titin bound to both actin and myosin in the myofibril, while the sarcomere is in parallel with another purely elastic element. We propose that the Ca^{2+}–dependence of diastolic stiffness might be the result of an inverse relation between $[Ca^{2+}]_i$ and the affinity of titin for actin.

---

[1]The University of Calgary, Health Sciences Centre, 3300 Hospital Drive, N.W., Calgary AB, Canada

Analytical and Quantitative Cardiology
Edited by Sideman and Beyar, Plenum Press, New York, 1997

INTRODUCTION

The present study was undertaken to investigate the diastolic viscoelastic properties of intact unstimulated cardiac muscle, in particular because the viscous force–velocity relation appeared to depend on the extra cellular Ca^{2+} concentration ($[Ca^{2+}]_o$) [1] suggesting an inverse Ca^{2+}–dependence of viscosity. From investigations of intracellular free Ca^{2+}–concentration ($[Ca^{2+}]_i$) in cardiac trabeculae injected with Fura-2 [2] it is obvious that relaxation of the Ca^{2+}–transient is not complete at the end of the twitch and $[Ca^{2+}]_i$ decreases continuously during diastole separating two beats. Recently, the large endo–sarcomeric protein titin [3] has been identified as the major generator of elastic force at SL<2.1 µm [4] whereas the collagen network surrounding myocytes appeared predominant at SL >2.1 mm [4, 5]. The mechanisms by which titin–based elasticity is generated in intact myocardium are still unclear. We show that stiffness of intact rat cardiac trabeculae increases during diastole together with an increase of SL and a decline of $[Ca^{2+}]_i$ in submicromolar range. The results could be reproduced with a mechanical model of the sarcomere which incorporates Ca^{2+}–dependent alterations of elastic and viscous properties.

METHODS

Lewis Brown Norway rats (250–350 g) of either sex were anesthetized with ether and the hearts were rapidly removed. The aorta was cannulated and the heart perfused with either a modified Krebs–Henseleit solution or a HEPES buffer solution. The standard Krebs–Henseleit solution (K–H solution) was composed of (mM) 112 NaCl, 1.2 $MgCl_2$, 5 KCl, 2.4 Na_2SO_4, 2 NaH_2PO_4, 1 $CaCl_2$, 10 Glucose, 19 $NaHCO_3$, and equilibrated with 95% O_2 and 5% CO_2; pH 7.4 (adjusted with KOH 1M). The standard HEPES buffer solution was composed of (mM) 120 NaCl, 1.2 $MgCl_2$, 5 KCl, 2.8 Na–Acetate, 10 Glucose and 10 HEPES, oxygenated with 100% O_2; pH 7.4 (adjusted with NaOH 1M) at 25.3 ± 0.6°C. Eighteen right ventricular trabeculae (length, 2.36 ± 0.25 mm; width, 349 ± 43 mm; thickness, 102 ± 32 mm) were dissected and mounted in an experimental chamber as described previously [1]. The preparations were stimulated at 0.5 Hz with 5 ms pulses 50% above threshold.

Force, Muscle Length, SL Measurements

The methods used to measure Force (F), Muscle Length (ML) and SL of trabeculae have been described earlier [1, 6, 7]. Muscle length was determined from the displacement of a motor arm controlled by a dual servo–amplifier (model 300s, Cambridge Technology, Watertown, MA, USA). Force was measured by a silicon strain gauge (model X17625, SenSoNor, Horten, Norway). The resolution was 0.63 µN. SL was measured by laser diffraction techniques as previously described [6–8]. The combination of two detectors—a CCD array and a lateral effect photodiode—permitted precise positioning of the preparation with respect to the laser beam, lowering the error due the Bragg angle phenomenon [9]. The resulting resolution of the SL measurement was 2–3 nm. A 0.8 ms delay on the SL signal collected by the CCD array was systematically corrected digitally. SL signals and force were monitored on a digital oscilloscope (Data Precision Model 6000, Danvers, MA, USA) and on a chart recorder (Gould Model 2800S, Cleveland, OH, USA) and recorded via an A–D converter (sampling rate 9 kHz) installed in an IBM PC–AT.

Stiffness Measurements

The time course of diastolic stiffness was determined by imposing 30 ms bursts of sinusoidal perturbations of muscle length at 500 Hz (Fig. 1A) during the period between two contractions. Sine waves were provided by a sweep/function generator (model 3030 BK Precision, Chicago, IL, USA) synchronized with the stimulator. A mean stiffness modulus (MOD) was calculated from the average of 13 individual ratios dF/dSL obtained from a burst of 30 ms (dF: maximal amplitude of force oscillations; dSL: maximal corresponding SL oscillations; see Fig. 1B). A mean phase shift (Φ) was evaluated from the delays, peak–to–peak, between Force and SL oscillations (Fig. 1B). Stiffness was expressed in units of Stress (mN.mm^{-2}) per unit of sarcomere strain (mm).

Experimental Protocol

After the stabilization period, 500 Hz length perturbations were imposed at 10% of the diastole. The SL and force signals were monitored on the digital oscilloscope and duration of diastole was carefully measured according to the criteria mentioned above. The amplitude of SL oscillations was adjusted to the predetermined amplitude by setting the output voltage of the function generator. The same burst was imposed consecutively at 10, 30, 50, 70 and 90% during resting periods of 5 consecutive cycles, i.e., at 652 ± 15 ms, 948 ± 13 ms, 1250 ± 9 ms, 1548 ± 6 ms, and 1850 ± 2 ms (n=18) from stimulation in standard conditions (25°C, pH 7.4, [Ca^{2+}]$_o$ =1 mM). In order to perform our measurements in the linear range, we have used SL perturbations smaller than 30 nm to obtain the viscoelastic response of the sarcomere.

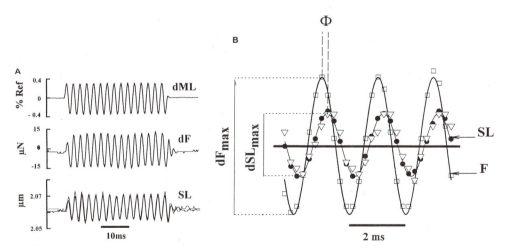

Figure 1. Response of trabeculae to 500 Hz muscle length perturbations. **A)** Records of SL and force, F, during 0.8% amplitude muscle length perturbations. SL was recorded from both photodiode array (continuous line) and lateral photodetector (broken line). Note that the photodiode array and lateral photodetector signals remain superposed during 500 Hz oscillations. **B)** Shows, from oscillations of Panel A represented on a slower time base, the method used for calculation of stiffness. The stiffness modulus (MOD) and phase shift (Φ) between F and SL signals were calculated from a burst of oscillations lasting 30 ms. MOD was determined from the averaged ratio of maximal amplitudes of force oscillations (dF) over maximal corresponding amplitudes of SL oscillations (dSL). Φ was measured in degrees (DEG) from the time delay between dSL and dF peak–to–peak.

$[Ca^{2+}]_i$ Measurement from Fura–2 Fluorescence

The free acid form of Fura–2 was microinjected iontophoretically into trabeculae, [2]. Excitation ultra–violet light from a 150 W Xenon (Xe) arc lamp (model 6255, Oriel Corp., Stratford, CT) was filtered using bandpass filters (Melles Griot, Irvine, CA) centered at 340, 360, or 380 nm. The band width of all bandpass filters was 10 nm and the bandpass filters were switched manually. The filtered light was projected onto the trabeculae via a 10X UV–Fluor objective lens (Nikon, Canada) in the inverted microscope using a dichroic mirror (400 DPLC, Omega Opticals, VT). The epifluorescence of Fura–2 from trabeculae was collected by the objective and projected onto a photomultiplier tube (PMT–R2693 with a C1053–01 socket, Hamamatsu) through a 500 nm bandpass filter (Melles Griot, Irvine, CA). The signal from the photomultiplier tube was fed into the computer via an A/D converter (2801A Data–Translation) and into a chart recorder (Gould, model 2800S, Cleveland, Ohio, USA). $[Ca^{2+}]_i$ was given by the following equation (after subtraction of the autofluorescence of the muscle):

$$[Ca^{2+}]_i = K'd \, (R-Rmin) \, / \, (Rmax-R) \tag{1}$$

where K'd is the apparent dissociation constant, R is the ratio of the fluorescence at 340 nm excitation to that at 380 nm excitation (340/380), Rmin is R at zero $[Ca^{2+}]_i$ and Rmax is R at a saturating $[Ca^{2+}]_i$. The values for K'd, Rmin, and Rmax were determined by *in vitro* calibrations [2]. Rmin and Rmax were 0.129 and 3.71, respectively, and K'd was 4.57 μM.

RESULTS

Diastolic $[Ca^{2+}]_i$

Diastolic $[Ca^{2+}]_i$ varied linearly in the 0.2–2 mM range of $[Ca^{2+}]_o$ indicating that an increase of $[Ca^{2+}]_o$ from 1 to 2 mM in our experiments induced a rise of $[Ca^{2+}]_i$ from 143.5 ± 35 to 256.5 ± 89 nM (n=7; p<0.05). Note that 5 of the 8 trabeculae studied showed a small degree of spontaneous activity of the sarcomeres at $[Ca^{2+}]_o$ =1–2 mM. This spontaneous activity appeared to consist, on the video monitor at high magnification of the microscope, of contractile waves which started in single cells and usually propagated within the cell of origin.

As illustrated in Fig. 2, $[Ca^{2+}]_i$ decreased continuously during diastole. The amplitude of the diastolic decline was approximately 120 nM. The $[Ca^{2+}]_i$ decay was complete approximately 200 ms before the end of diastolic interval, i.e., at 90% of total duration. The time constant of the decay during diastole ranged from 210–325 ms. At higher $[Ca^{2+}]_o$ (above 2 mM depending of the muscles), a similar exponential shape relation was found, but an increase of $[Ca^{2+}]_i$ occurred at the end of diastole, while spontaneous sarcomere activity was seen.

Diastolic SL Changes

Figure 3 shows the typical SL changes following a twitch. Complete relaxation of twitch force was accompanied by a sarcomere shortening transient followed by an exponential lengthening (time constant ~ 600 ms; amplitude 4–65 nm). A similar SL increase still occurred when the distance between the two attachments to the muscle was reduced

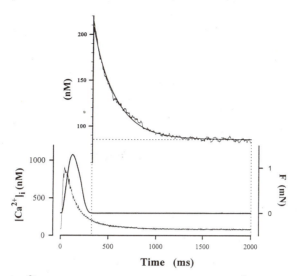

Figure 2. Assessment of $[Ca^{2+}]_i$ during diastolic interval. Assessment of $[Ca^{2+}]_i$ through Fura 2 fluorescence measurements simultaneously with the force shows an exponential decline of $[Ca^{2+}]_i$ during diastole (see smooth line in the insert; amplitude = 123 nM; $[Ca^{2+}]_i = 738.e^{(-t/224)}+86$; r=0.98). The diastolic decline of $[Ca^{2+}]_i$ is amplified in the insert.

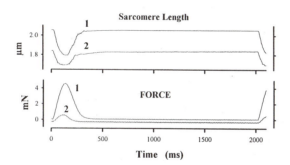

Figure 3. Sarcomere lengthening in the central segment of a trabeculae during the diastolic period at two SLs Keeping muscle at slack length (**1:** 2.05 µm) caused buckling of the trabeculae during diastole. In this configuration, the muscle shortened and developed small amount of force as the sarcomere reached the maximum of active shortening. Diastolic sarcomere lengthening still occurred in muscles below slack length (**2:** 1.83µm) ruling out that sarcomere lengthening is due to contracture of the damaged ends of the trabeculae.

below slack length of the muscle; lengthening was, then, accompanied by increased buckling of the muscle. Hence, this lengthening must have resulted from a true SL increase rather than from a stretch due to a slow shortening of the ends of the trabeculae. During the SL increase, no force change larger than 0.3 $^0/_{00}$ twitch force was detected.

Diastolic Time Course of Viscoelastic Properties

The time courses of MOD and F during diastole were complex (Fig. 4). In standard conditions ($[Ca^{2+}]_o$=1 mM), a 30% increase of MOD occurred in the initial 450 ms of diastole (10%: 9.3±0.6 vs 50%: 12.2±0.5 mN·mm^{-2}·mm^{-1}, n=158; p<0.05, 18 muscles).

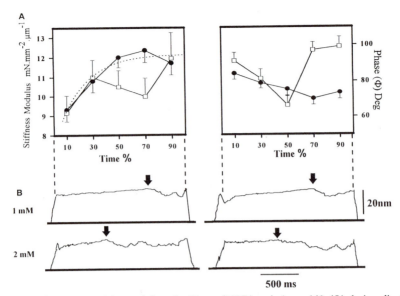

Figure 4. A) The time course of the modulus of stiffness (MOD) and phase shift (Φ) during diastole in the presence of 1 mM (circles) and 2 mM (squares) of $[Ca^{2+}]_o$. The results are expressed as mean±sem; n=173, 18 muscles. The difference between results obtained at 1 mM and 2 mM $[Ca^{2+}]_o$ was considered as significant when student test provided p<0.05. The time scale is expressed in % of diastolic interval. **B)** shows the time courses of SL of a muscle representative of Panel **A**, showing slight spontaneous motions of the sarcomeres (arrowhead) at 1 mM (upper trace) and 2 mM $[Ca^{2+}]_o$ (lower trace) during two consecutive diastoles. In order to compare timings of stiffness and sarcomere length, time scales of **A** and **B** were made identical. In both cases, an inversion in courses of MOD and Φ occurred simultaneously with spontaneous activity of the sarcomeres. Spontaneous activity was absent in only 3 out of 18 trabeculae.

Then, MOD slightly decreased at the end of diastole to 11.6 ± 0.65 mN·mm^{-2}·mm^{-1}. Φ between F and SL oscillations significantly decreased with time during diastole (from $84 \pm 3°$ to $73 \pm 4°$; n=18, p<0.05). At $[Ca^{2+}]_o = 1$ mM, 15 of 18 trabeculae studied showed discrete sarcomere spontaneous activity, restricted to a brief period at the end of diastole (Fig. 6B, top trace). When $[Ca^{2+}]_i$ was increased by approximately 120 nM, by increasing $[Ca^{2+}]_o$ from 1 to 2 mM, the spontaneous sarcomere activity (Fig. 4B: lower trace) and the decrease of the modulus (Fig. 4A) were detected earlier into diastole (from 30%).

Viscoelastic Response to Linear Stretches

We used small linear stretches during diastole in four trabeculae in order to assess stiffness (k_p) of steady elasticity and the viscous force (Fv) developed were calculated as described previously [1]. The viscous coefficient (η) was derived from the ratio of viscous force over the velocity (v) of SL increase (Fv/v with v ~ 25–70 µm.s^{-1}). The stiffness coefficient k_p was calculated by dividing the static elastic force by the corresponding SL variation (see Fig. 5A). In the presence of $[Ca^{2+}]_o = 1$ mM and at the beginning of diastolic interval (10–30%), k_p and η were 15–60 mN·mm^{-2}·mm^{-1} and 155–350 mN·ms·mm^{-2}·mm^{-1} respectively. As shown in Fig. 5B, both η and k_p increased significantly during diastole. A significant decrease of η was seen when spontaneous activity occurred, whereas the rise of k_p appeared almost unchanged. The maximal values of k_p and η reached at 90% if no spontaneous activity would have occurred, were determined by extrapolation using smooth exponential variations of the diastolic time courses of k_p and η represented in

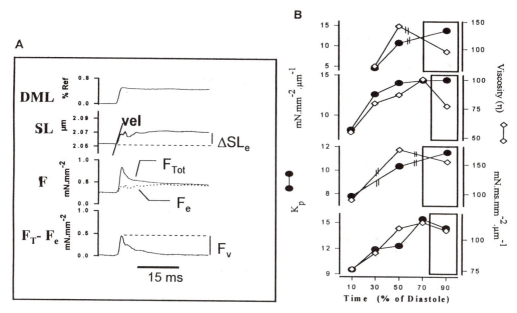

Figure 5. Time course of diastolic viscoelastic properties of cardiac trabeculae investigated from linear stretches. **A)** Static elasticity (k_p) and viscosity (η) were evaluated from the ratios dF/dSL and Fv/v, respectively in four trabeculae according to the method of De Tombe and Ter Keurs [1]. dF: maximal static elastic force [A:F_e trace (dotted line)]; ΔSL_e: sarcomere length variations at steady state; Fv: maximal viscous force calculated from the total force (solid line) minus elastic force predicted from a model of linear elastic element (dotted line) in parallel with the sarcomere. **B)** Time courses of k_p and η determined in four trabeculae at different times of diastolic interval. The time scale is expressed in % of diastolic period. The occurrence of spontaneous motions of the sarcomeres, as described in Fig. 4, is indicated individually as a rectangular area overlying the curves. Note the variability from muscle to muscle in the quantitative determination of k_p and η.

Fig. 5B. Thus, the total amplitude of the variations during diastole, was estimated to be 63–75% for k_p and 76–175% for η, assuming that there was no spontaneous sarcomere activity.

Modeling the Diastolic Viscoelasticity

In order to understand how the results from both techniques of stiffness measurement used in the current study were linked, we modeled the viscoelastic behavior of the sarcomere (Fig. 6). In the models that we have evaluated we have ignored the mass of the trabeculae because of the low frequencies at which the behavior of the sarcomeres was tested. Two four element models reproduced the experimental data accurately. The model that we have selected for reasons that are outlined below is depicted in Fig. 6; it consists of a Voigt model in branch A [with a viscous element VE(A) in parallel with the spring (PE(A)) and in series with the spring (SE(A))] in parallel with spring (PE(B)) in branch B. This arrangement implies that, with sarcomere stretch, PE(A) and PE(B) are extended and SE(A) is compressed. The model was subjected to the following constraints: given the experimental values for η and k_{SA}, the sum of the values of k_{PB} and k_{SA} had to be small (3–4 mN·mm^{-2}·μm^{-1}) in order to allow for a value of Φ of 40–45° as had been observed in the experiments (in the absence of spontaneous activity of the (sarcomeres).

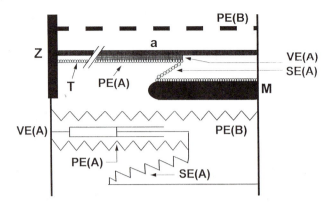

Figure 6. Components of the mechanical model and a proposed structural basis. The viscoelastic response of the sarcomere to 500 Hz ML oscillations can be predicted from a mechanical model based on the arrangement of two branches in parallel. One damper (VE(A), viscous coefficient η) in parallel with a spring (PE(A), stiffness coefficient k_{PA}), both in series with another spring (SE(A), stiffness coefficient k_{SA}) working in an opposite direction composed branch A. Branch B involved one spring (PE(B), stiffness coefficient k_{PB}). The arrangement of titan (T) in the half sarcomere may be the ultrastructural counterpart for the mechanical model. a: actin; M: myosin; z: z–line.

This constraint meant that either k_{PB} had to be slightly smaller than k_{SA}, or k_{PB} was slightly larger than k_{series}. Given the value for k_p, the former condition required that k_{PA} was about twice as large as k_{SA}; the latter condition required a small positive value for k_{PA}. Both models reproduced the experimental SL changes in response to a sinusoidal force at the beginning of diastole faithfully.

　　　　Above the mechanical model in Fig. 6, we have depicted a working hypothesis with assumed equivalence between structures of the sarcomere and the components of the model. This hypothesis is based on the affinity of titin's filament 4 for actin. In this model, it is speculated that an elastic titin filament binds to the thin filament far enough into A–Band region to cause titin to reverse its orientation between actin and myosin. In this conforma–tion, the free part of titin filament strained between actin and myosin filaments would be the equivalent of SE(A) with a negative elasticity k_{SA}, while the actin associated segment would be equivalent to PE(A) with an elasticity k_{PA}. The viscosity η would be located in the interaction between titin and actin. A bond of 'sliding' type might be regulated by the affinity of titin for actin. An inverse Ca–dependence of this affinity would explain the Ca–dependent time course of stiffness during diastole. According to this hypothesis, the lower level of stiffness measured few milliseconds after the end of the twitch relaxation is interpreted by a dissociated state between titin and actin in the A–Band region induced by the rise in $[Ca^{2+}]_i$ during the twitch and/or the increase of mechanical strain generated by cross–bridges during active process of contraction. Inversely, the continuous increase of stiffness evidenced during diastole would reflect the kinetics of reattachment of titin on actin driven by the decrease of $[Ca^{2+}]_i$. The elasticity equivalent to the element k_{PB} is provided by a structure in parallel with the sarcomere that might correspond to intermediate filament network.

　　　　The characteristics of the model in Fig. 7 calculated at 10% of diastole were: 1) η of VE(A) (200 mN·ms·mm^{-2}·mm^{-1}) was derived directly from linear stretches. 2) the stiffness coefficient of SE(A) (k_{SA}) was 50 mN·mm^{-2}·mm^{-1}, consistent with the value calculated by De Tombe and ter Keurs [1]. When a sinusoidal driving force, F=Fo.cos(ω.t) (Fo: initial force; ω: angular frequency), with an amplitude similar to experimental force

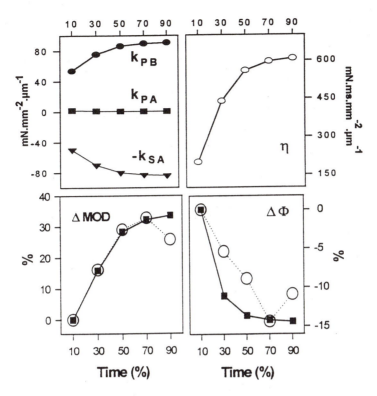

Figure 7. Modeled diastolic viscoelastic behavior of intact cardiac trabeculae. The displacement was determined by the mechanical impedance of the device shown in Fig. 6 and the driving force F=Fo.cos ω.t (Fo: initial force; ω: angular frequency, ω = 2 πf with f = 500 Hz). When k_{PA}= 2, k_{SA}= −50, k_{PB}=54 mN·mm^{-2}·mm^{-1} and η=200 mN·ms·mm^{-2}·mm^{-1}, the modulus of the device was 11.54 mN·mm^{-2}·mm^{-1} and X lags F by Φ = 43°. These values fitted well with results obtained at 10% of diastolic interval in trabeculae without spontaneous activity (see Fig. 4). Both elasticities (k's) and viscosity (η) of the device were modified according to a model of variation based on the diastolic mono exponential decay of [Ca^{2+}]$_i$ described in Fig. 2: | k_{SA} | and k_{PB} were increased and k_{PA} was decreased by a percentage % = −328.e$^{(-t/365)}$+70.5 and η was increased by %= −984. e$^{(-t/310)}$+208. These modifications predicted an increase of the modulus (ΔMOD: black squares): and a reduction of the phase difference (ΔΦ: black squares) with time that were closely correlated with the courses of MOD and Φ (white circles) determined experimentally (correlation coefficient 0.96 and 0.89, respectively).

oscillations (10 − 20 μN) was injected into the model, the calculated MOD was 11.69 mN·mm^{-2}·mm^{-1} and the Φ between force and displacement was 43°. In order to allow for a value of Φ of 40–45°, as observed in the experiments, the sum of the values of k_{PB} and k_{SA} had to be small (3–4 mN·mm^{-2}·μm^{-1}). These values are similar to MOD and Φ ob-tained experimentally from trabeculae without spontaneous activity at 10%. These results were only obtained under the condition that the sum k_{PB}+k_{SA} was small and positive. This led to the conclusion that k_{PB} and k_{SA} must be oriented in opposite directions. This resulted in the model depicted in Fig. 6 (bottom part) in which only k_{SA} had a reverse orientation. The experimental results were reproduced accurately in the latter model, when k_{PB} = 54 mN·mm^{-2}·mm^{-1} and k_{SA}= 50 mN·mm^{-2}·mm^{-1} (in the calculations k_{SA} appeared with a negative sign), respectively. The value of k_{PA} (2 mN·mm^{-2}·mm^{-1}) was deduced from the fact that static elastic coefficient, k_p (k_p: 17–56 mN·mm^{-2}·mm^{-1}), determined from linear stretches, reflects the parallel arrangement of k_{PB} together with k_{PA} and k_{SA} in series. k_{PA} appeared to be small compared to k_{PB}. Actually, modification of the values of MOD and Φ induced by large changes (50%) of k_{PA} were less than 0.1%, while the same variation of k_{PB} induced a variation of the modulus > 400% and of the phase shift > 80%.

Time Dependence of Diastolic Stiffness

The values of k_{PA}, k_{SA}, k_{PB} and η were subsequently changed exponentially according to the decline of $[Ca^{2+}]_i$. The corresponding variations of MOD and Φ were calculated from the model for t (in ms) equivalent to 30, 50, 70 and 90% of diastole in response to a sinusoidal driving force. As illustrated in Fig. 7, the time course of both modulus and Φ was reproduced when the values of k_{PB}, and k_{SA} at 10% of diastole were exponentially increased by 68% and η was increased by 204% over time (cf. Fig. 7). These values are close to the maximal variations of k_p (48–75%) and η (76–175%) estimated from the experiments (see above). In both cases, the time constants (340 and 310 ms respectively) were similar to the time constant of diastolic decay of $[Ca^{2+}]_i$ (210–325 ms). Assuming that PE(A) and SE(A) belong to the same spring, k_{PA} was decreased by 68% with the same exponential time course (cf. Fig. 7), even though variation of k_{PA} in the calculations of MOD and Φ was irrelevant compared to the effect of variations of k_{PB}, k_{SA} and η. As seen in Fig. 7, this procedure reproduced the diastolic time course of MOD (r=0.96) except for the decrease represented by the last data point. In the same conditions, the model also provided a maximal decrease of Φ ($-15°$) similar to the experimentally observed decrease of Φ (r=0.89; Fig. 7). A slight discrepancy appeared, however, between experimental and predicted time courses of Φ. The differences between the data provided by the model and the experimental results are probably related to spontaneous activity.

DISCUSSION

In the present study, we have investigated the sarcomere stiffness during diastolic interval of a stimulated cardiac trabeculae. We show that viscoelastic properties vary with time. An increase of stiffness occurred simultaneous with a SL increase and a decrease of $[Ca^{2+}]_i$. The occurrence of discrete sarcomere spontaneous activity reversed the time course of diastolic stiffness.

Diastolic SL Lengthening

This is the first time that the observation of a slow SL increase following the twitch is reported. Evidently the external force measured during diastolic interval results from a balance of forces in the sarcomere. So it is possible that one structure causes stretch of the sarcomere which is opposed by an elastic element in parallel with the sarcomere. The observation that the external force is virtually constant, in spite of the lengthening of the sarcomere, indicates that the forces generated by these two opposing elastic elements balance during diastole.

Time Dependence of Diastolic Stiffness

Our results (Figs. 4 and 5) clearly show variation of stiffness during diastole. On average, an increase of 32% of the modulus and a decrease of 18% of the Φ were detected between 10 and 70% of diastole at $[Ca^{2+}]_o$ =1 mM. At the end of diastole, the respective courses of MOD and Φ reversed, while spontaneous motion of sarcomeres occurred (see discussion below). k_p during diastole was similar to the MOD, i.e., 20 mN·mm^{-2}·mm^{-1} and η was approximately 200 mN·ms·mm^{-2}·mm^{-1}, similar to the previously reported values [1]. In the absence of spontaneous sarcomere activity, k_p and η increased significantly during diastole, explaining the increase of the lumped stiffness reflected by MOD. Figure 5 shows that the time course of η appeared to reverse when trabeculae exhibited the spontaneous motion of the sarcomeres, suggesting that influence of spontaneous activity on the modulus of stiffness is exerted predominantly through the viscous element and the phase shift determined during 500 Hz oscillations appears inversely related to the viscosity.

Crossbridge Activity and Diastolic Properties

Skinned rat cardiac cells bathed in a $[Ca^{2+}]=100$ nM usually start to show recurrent spontaneous Ca^{2+} release from the sarcoplasmic reticulum [10–12]. Figure 2 shows that under our experimental conditions, $[Ca^{2+}]_i$ in the intact trabeculae was 130 nM at $[Ca^{2+}]_o$ =1 mM, so that it is reasonable to expect spontaneous activity in the form of random spontaneous activity of small groups of sarcomeres. It is probable that the spontaneous activity observed here is similar to spontaneous activity in single cells seen as Ca^{2+} waves accompanied by propagating contractions of the sarcomeres. It has been shown that at the threshold of spontaneous activity the frequency at which these waves occur is around 0.1 Hz and the waves, which last about 200–300 msec, propagate at a velocity of 50 µm/s. It follows that the 1–2% of all sarcomeres would randomly be involved in spontaneous activity. These sarcomeres would shorten along their force–length relationship by <~0.4 µm and stretch the cells in series with them by ~4 nm and cause both a small force increase (~0.1% of twitch force) and an increase of k_p of 1%. So, it is unlikely that spontaneous activity is responsible for the decrease of MOD and the change of Φ observed in this study. Weakly attached crossbridges do not provide an explanation for the observed properties of the muscle either, because the viscosity due to weakly attached crossbridges would be two orders of magnitude lower than the observed viscosity [13]. Uniform crossbridge activation by 1% is even less likely as a candidate to explain the changes in MOD and Φ given the high instantaneous stiffness of the active cardiac sarcomere [14] similar to that of the sarcomere in skeletal muscle [15], because it would be accompanied by a force equal to 1% of twitch force and a hundred fold increase of muscle stiffness above the diastolic level. On the other hand, Ca^{2+} dependent attachment of crossbridges was probably responsible for the secondary rise of MOD seen between 70 and 90% of diastole when trabeculae is bathed with $[Ca^{2+}]_o= 2$ mM (Fig. 4).

Ca^{2+} Dependence of Diastolic Stiffness

The mechanical model reproduced the diastolic changes of MOD and Φ (at $[Ca^{2+}]_o= 1$ mM) accurately when the elastic and viscous terms in the model were modified using an exponential time course based on the diastolic $[Ca^{2+}]_i$ decay curve (Fig. 7), suggesting that an inverse relation exists between $[Ca^{2+}]_i$ and stiffness. The slight discrepancy between the predicted and the experimental results probably resulted from the fact that spontaneous activity observed in the experiments was not included in the model calculations. The exact course of stiffness during diastole is reproduced, in the model shown in Fig. 6, when the magnitude of the modification applied on viscous coefficient is threefold larger compared to the simultaneous modifications of elastic coefficients. This suggests that the effect of a variation of $[Ca^{2+}]_i$ on viscosity is at substantially larger than on elasticity; which may explain that, while η showed a decrease during spontaneous sarcomere activity, k_p remained constant or declined only slightly (Fig. 5). Figure 4 shows that MOD was sensitive to spontaneous activity due an increase of $[Ca^{2+}]_i$, suggesting that viscosity dominated dynamic stiffness.

Structural Origin of Diastolic Viscoelastic Properties

The simplest model that explains the behavior of the viscoelastic properties of the sarcomere is a four element model, as discussed above. The properties of the sarcomere could be mimicked by two alternative versions of a four element model: one in which the parallel elastic elements had the usual positive stiffness coefficients, while the element in series with the viscous term appeared to have a negative orientation, hence acting like a compressive spring. Such a compressive spring may result either from a simple linear structure which is oriented in such a way that stretch of the sarcomere causes relaxation of this structure or from an elastic mesh which is strained when the sarcomeres shorten and is released when the sarcomeres are stretched. There is substantial evidence supporting a simple parsimonious mechanical equivalent for the model depicted in Fig. 6. It has been recently reported that titin and collagen are the main contributors to passive tension over the working range of the sarcomeres (1.9–2.2 mm) in the heart, with titin being dominant at SL<2.1 mm and collagen dominating at SL>2.1 mm [5]. It is known that titin forms filaments in the sarcomere that span from the Z–line to the M–line. The association of titin with the thick filament is so stiff that it does not participate in length changes. On the other hand, it has been demonstrated recently that, in vitro, titin binds to F–Actin [16]. In the intact sarcomere, this property allows for binding to thin filament in I–Band region up to I/A junction and, considering that the molecule is intrinsically elastic, even into the A–Band region. If the latter is the case the arrangement leads to a structure depicted in Fig. 6. The mechanical features of the structure proposed in Fig. 6 are consistent with the properties of the model shown in Fig. 7. We propose, first, that the extensible segment of titin bound to actin equals the spring PE(A). Second, the free segment of titin with its reverse orientation between actin and myosin provides the spring SE(A) with its negative elasticity indicating that sarcomere stretch tends to release this spring, while a restoring elastic force is generated during sarcomere shortening. Third, we propose that the viscous behavior is conferred upon the sarcomere by association of titin with actin responding to force exerted by the segment of titin between actin and myosin. Figure 6 shows PE(A) and SE(A) as parts of the same molecule (titin); however, calculations of k_{PA} (2 mN·mm^{-2}·µm^{-1}) from k_p show that the stiffness of the segment of titin associated with actin is 25 times smaller than the stiffness of the free part extending between actin and myosin (kSA: 50 mN·mm^{-2}·µm^{-1}). This may be explained by recent observations [17] that the structure of titin, particularly in the vicinity of I/A junction, is more complex than the structure expected from a regular repetition of the Ig–FN3 domains to which the intrinsic elasticity of titin has been ascribed [18]. Labeit and Kolmerer [17] have shown that the PEVK domain of titin is probably much more compliant than Ig–FN3 domains and is localized in the I–Band near the I/A junction, which would make the molecule much more compliant in the region where titin is associated with actin. In addition, the fact that the actin-associated–part is longer than the actin–myosin segment of titin enhances this difference.

Although the nature of the association between titin and actin has not been established yet, sliding of titin along actin during a variation of strain provides a plausible explanation for viscosity of the sarcomere. For example, a force exerted along the long axis of the sarcomere on the titin–actin bonds could induce a detachment of titin from actin, followed by re–attachment of the molecule at an adjacent site. If the rate at which the latter process takes place, i.e., the rate at which displacement occurs, is force dependent one would envisage the equivalent of a viscous behavior. In this case, it is clear that the magnitude of the viscous resistance is determined by the affinity of titin for actin. It is of interest that in the model depicted in Fig. 6, an exact prediction of the experimental data required that the elasticity of the element corresponding to PE(B) varies in synchrony with the other elements of the model during diastolic interval. We speculate that PE(B) is caused by one of the cytoskeletal structures of the cell [19]). This structural model provides a possible mechanism for the Ca^{2+}–dependent time course of stiffness during diastole (Fig. 6).

CONCLUSIONS

We propose that the inverse relationship between stiffness and $[Ca^{2+}]_i$ is caused by an inverse Ca^{2+}–dependence of the affinity of titin for actin. In this way, the strength of the bond between titin and actin decreases when $[Ca^{2+}]_i$ increases, leading to the progressive dissociation of titin from the thin filament. A decrease of the affinity of titin for actin would facilitate the sliding of titin along actin, thus reducing the viscous resistance generated by the bond. After the twitch, titin would reattach progressively to the thin filament as Ca^{2+} is extruded from the cytosol and the stress exerted by the crossbridges has disappeared. The exponential lengthening of the sarcomere would result from the increase of the restoring force generated by the progressive reattachment of titin to actin into A–Band which causes myosin to be pulled toward the center of the sarcomere by means of the titin segment with the reverse orientation between actin and myosin.

The observation that SL increases after the twitch indicates that a restoring force is set up in the muscle during diastole. The simultaneous observation that SL increased without a noticeable (<0.3 $^0/_{00}$ twitch force) change in force suggested this restoring force is balanced by an elastic element in parallel with the sarcomere. This observation is adequately explained by the presence of PE(B).

DISCUSSION

Dr. R. Beyar: Do you also foresee that titin may have a similar role? I cannot see how the titin can be accounted for such a large lengthening of the sarcomere. Is it also a multiple step process, the same as contraction, or maybe its a much longer molecule that can allow for a larger step?

Dr. H. ter Keurs: Titin is composed of a large number of titin monomers. The titin monomers have a physical dimension in the same order of magnitude as the g–Actin monomers, 5 nm in each. So one could expect that titin monomer binds to actin, and that binding can take place for a substantial length and easily explain the 30 nm or stretch that we see in the experimental work. At the moment we are testing that hypothesis more directly by skinning cardiac muscle and applying the three relevant dimers that one can construct on the titin monomers. Titin is produced in the form of titin–1 and titin–2 which form stable titin 1–2 (Ti I–II) in solution. Using the dimers as a receptor blocking agent, that means that we expose the skinned fiber to the dimers and anticipate that titin filaments will come off completely so that we can obtain proof that titin is involved in this process because the prediction is that it should expect a low elastic modulus and a low viscous modulus. But a direct answer to your question is, yes, in terms of length, titin is the largest molecule we have in our system and it is easily able to make that stretch even 50 nm.

Dr. N. Westerhof: Do the blood vessels contribute to this phenomenon? We used the papillary muscle that we perfused and during coronary perfusion we saw a small but very consistent change in the diastolic properties of the muscle [*Allaart CP, Sipkema P, Westerhof N. Effect of perfusion* *pressure on diastolic stress–strain relations of isolated rat papillary muscle. Am J Physiol 1995;268:H945–H954*]. I wonder whether part of the viscoelasticity is inherent with the vasculature.

Dr. H. ter Keurs: That is an interesting thought. First of all, when we perfuse trabeculae, we also find a very clear change in its elastic properties. When you perfuse these muscles, always with a K–H solution, you inflate the tiny blood vessels in these muscles quite substantially. So you prestrain that elastic term to a very substantial amount. Firstly, if you do not perfuse it, that elastic term is released and relaxed to a large extent. I think that would reduce the role of the blood vessels. Secondly, in a muscle in which, as one of the examples shows, the muscle is held completely slack, you would have a hard time explaining stretch of the sarcomeres on the basis of lengthening of the blood vessels. So that part definitely does not fit. I can not completely rule out the role of the blood vessels.

Dr. N. Westerhof: Pre–stretching of filled blood vessels could explain the negative elasticity too.

Dr. H. ter Keurs: The perfused blood vessels prestretched in these experiments were without perfusion.

Dr. N. Westerhof: But they might be prestretched; even vessels like the aorta are prestretched in the body. If you take it out it shortens considerably. It is a negative type of elasticity.

Dr. H. ter Keurs: That is a possible thought.

Dr. A. McCulloch: Your interpretation of your model suggests that there is a calcium dependent critical buckling length for titin that changes during diastole. Have you thought of a way that you might be able to experimentally assay this critical buckling length or perhaps its a critical buckling sarcomere length.

Dr. H. ter Keurs: What you ask for is probably this element. If you stretch the sarcomere from 2.0 μm and therefore pull the myosin, you will find discontinuity in the elastic behavior when the severed titin element turns straight and then is stretched. It is interesting to note, I did not put it in the slides, but if you look very carefully at the force sarcomere length relation of the sarcomeres in these muscles, you find above slack length the initial rise in elastic force which plateaus at approx. 2–2. 1 μm, then declines slightly and is then followed by further increase of elastic force. Its no proof, but it is consistent with the idea that there is buckling of the element that you discussed here.

Dr. Y. Lanir: What you have presented is very challenging and interesting. Can you comment on the relevance of your data that was taken at 500 Hz to the physiological domain?

Dr. H. ter Keurs: Thank you for this question. We have also done the experiments at slightly lower frequencies and similar modules and phase shift behavior came out. At 500 Hz, we chose 500 Hz for a very simple, practical reason. Note that the length oscillations of the sarcomeres are always, in these experiments, less than 30 nm. That means we are working at about 1–2% sarcomere length; that creates a technical problem. We have chosen 500 Hz and a burst of around 30 ms in order to be able to extract the data accurately. The remainder of your criticism, I accept.

Secondly, a short burst allows you to look at the behavior of the modulus and the phase shift over time during diastole, so that we can get a time course of the behavior of the system. I am not quite aware of the physics of water to answer the question whether at 500 Hz the behavior of water would be time dependent so I will leave that in the middle, but I don't think so personally.

Dr. H. ter Keurs: We are testing this system in skinned fibers. We find that at low calcium levels, the behavior of viscoelasticity is indeed dependent on the actual calcium level around a filament. We are also constructing complete transfer function starting at a very low frequency perturbation, but you can only do that in a very limited manner in the period of long diastole because you cannot evaluate the response to 1 Hz standard and 1 Hz sinus and you have only 1. 5 sec to sample this. Yes, in principle your critique is acceptable, but I do not think that it will change the conclusion completely.

Dr. M. Morad: Does *in vitro* titin as a protein show different aggregation with respect to calcium? Isn't that the simplest experiment?

Dr. H. ter Keurs: That would be the simplest experiment and it has not been shown to be the case. The answer is no. Calcium by itself does not influence titin. Granzier [*personal communication*] has studied that.

Dr. M. Morad: So how do you make titin calcium sensitive?

Dr. H. ter Keurs: By making the affinity of titin for actin or vice versa calcium dependent.

Dr. M. Morad: But that can certainly be done *in vitro* as well.

REFERENCES

1. De Tombe PP, ter Keurs HEDJ. An internal viscous element limits unloaded velocity of sarcomere shortening in rat myocardium. *J Physiol* 1992;454:619–642.
2. Backx PH, ter Keurs HEDJ. Fluorescent properties of rat cardiac trabeculae microinjected with fura-2 salt. *Am J Physiol* 1993;264:H1098–H1110.
3. Wang K, McClure J, Tu A. Titin: Major myofibrillar components of striated muscle. *Proc Nat Acad Sci USA* 1979;76:3698–3702.
4. Brady AJ. Length dependence of passive stiffness in single cardiac myocytes. *Am J Physiol* 1991;260:h1062–h1071.
5. Granzier HLM, Irving TC. Passive tension in cardiac muscle: contribution of collagen, titin, microtubules, and intermediate filaments. *Biophysical J* 1995;68:1027–1044. (Abstract)
6. ter Keurs HEDJ, Rijnsburger WH, van Heuningen R, Nagelsmit MJ. Tension development and sarcomere length in rat cardiac trabeculae. Evidence of length–dependent activation. *Circ Res* 1980;46:703–714.
7. Daniels MCG, Noble MIM, ter Keurs HEDJ, Wohlfart B. Velocity of sarcomere shortening in rat cardiac muscle: relationship to force, sarcomere length, calcium, and time. *J Physiol* 1984;355:367–381.
8. van Heuningen R, Rijnsburger WH, ter Keurs HEDJ. Sarcomere length control in striated muscle. *Am J Physiol* 1982;242:H411–H420.
9. Goldman YE. Measurement of sarcomere shortening in skinned fibers from frog muscle by white light diffraction. *Biophysical J* 1987;52:57–68.
10. Chiesi M, HO MM, Inesi G, Somlyo AV, Somlyo AP. Primary role of sarcoplasmic reticulum in phasic contractile activation of cardiac myocytes with shunted myolemma. *J Cell Biol* 1981;91:728–742.
11. Fabiato A, FAbiato F. Contractions induced by a calcium–triggered release of calcium from the sarcoplasmic reticulum of single skinned cardiac cells. *J Physiol* 1975;249:469–495.
12. Fabiato A. Myoplasmic free calcium concentration reached during the twitch of an intact isolated cardiac cell and during calcium–induced release of calcium from the sarcoplasmic reticulum of a skinned cardiac cell from the adult rat or rabbit ventricle. *J Gen Physiol* 1981;78: 457–497.
13. Schoenberg M, Brenner B, Chalovich JM, Greene LE, Eisenberg, E. Cross–bridge attachment in relaxed muscle. *Advances in Exp & Med & Biol* 1984;170:269–284.
14. Backx PH, ter Keurs HEDJ. Restoring forces in rat cardiac trabeculae. *Circulation* 1988;78:II–68.

15.   Ford LE, Huxley AF, Simmons RM. Tension response to sudden length change in stimulated frog muscle fibers near slack length. *J Physiol* 1977;269:441–515.

16.   Jin JP. Cloned rat cardiac titin class I and class II motifs. Expression, purification, characterization, and interaction with F–Actin. *J Biological Chem* 1995;270:1–9.

17.   Labeit S, Kolmerer B. Titins: giant proteins in charge of muscle ultrastructure and elasticity. *Science* 1995;270:293–296.

18.   Erickson HP. Reversible unfolding of fibronectin type III and immunoglobulin domains provides the structural basis for stretch and elasticity of titin and fibronectin. *Proc Nat Acad Sci USA* 1994;91:10114–10118.

19.   Price MG. Molecular analysis of intermediate filament cytoskeleton – a putative load bearing structure. *Am J Physiol* 1984;246:H566–H572.

CHAPTER 3

The Beta Subunit, Kvβ1.2, Acts as a Rapid Open Channel Blocker of NH$_2$–Terminal Deleted Kv1.4 α–Subunits

Randall L. Rasmusson,[1] Shimin Wang,[2] Robert C. Castellino,[3]
Michael J. Morales,[4] and Harold C. Strauss[2]

ABSTRACT

A recently discovered class of ancillary subunits has been shown to modify the inactivation properties of α–subunits belonging to the Kv1 family of potassium channels. One of these subunits, Kvβ1.2, modifies intrinsic α–subunit C–type inactivation. N–type inactivation and open channel block have been proposed to increase the rate of development of C–type inactivation. We demonstrate here that Kvβ1.2 has kinetic properties which are consistent with rapid open channel block.

INTRODUCTION

Inactivation of voltage sensitive ion channels has been a subject of active investigation since Hodgkin and Huxley's elegant voltage–clamp analysis of sodium channel inactivation [1]. However, recent molecular biological studies on potassium channels have significantly advanced our understanding of inactivation of voltage–sensitive ion channels [2–12]. In the heart, studies of inactivation of native potassium channels have focused on the calcium independent potassium selective voltage–sensitive transient outward current [13, 14]. Inactivation time course of the transient outward K$^+$ current is voltage insensitive

---

[1]The Department of Biomedical Engineering, Room 136, School of Engineering, Box 90281, Duke University, Durham, NC 27708, USA and the Departments of [2]Medicine, [3]Cell Biology and [4]Pharmacology, Duke University Medical Center, Box 3845 Durham, NC 27710, USA

Analytical and Quantitative Cardiology
Edited by Sideman and Beyar, Plenum Press, New York, 1997

and reasonably well described by a monoexponential function [13, 14]. Elucidation of the molecular basis of this gating transition is based on recent advances in our understanding of inactivation of *Shaker* B channels and the identification of the appropriate pore forming α subunit responsible for the current [2, 3, 15].

The time course of inactivation is extremely variable and at least two types appear to have been identified. The first and best understood is N–type inactivation [5, 6]. It is usually rapid and appears to be mediated by a ball and chain type mechanism [5, 6, 16]. In essence the terminal ~30 residues in the NH_2 terminus bind to the inner vestibule region of the open channel to occlude ion permeation [5, 6]. Although there appears to be little sequence homology between the NH_2–terminal residues of *Shaker* B channels and other inactivating voltage–sensitive mammalian K^+ channels, such as Kv1.4, and Kv3.3 clones, the rapid component of inactivation appears to be N–type and mediated by the same molecular mechanism [17–20].

In addition to the N–type mechanism, another type has been identified in *Shaker* K^+ channels. This mechanism was initially identified as being responsible for inactivation in two alternatively spliced variants of NH_2 terminal deleted *Shaker* K^+ channels lacking N–type inactivation. Subsequent experiments have suggested that this type of inactivation is variable in time course and appears to be mediated by an occlusion of the external mouth of the pore [6, 7]. Although the criteria defining C–type inactivation are less stringent than those for N–type, five criteria have emerged. First, the inactivation process while accelerat– ed by N type is not mediated by the NH_2–terminus [6]. Second, elevation of extracellular $[K^+]$ slows the inactivation process [9]. Third, competition with external TEA^+ block in those channels which possess an extracellular binding site for TEA^+[8]. Fourth, sensitivity to mutations of an amino acid in a critical region of the P loop near the extracellular mouth of the pore region [9, 10]. Fifth, the recovery from inactivation is inversely related to the time course of inactivation [12]. The latter effect is seen whether inactivation is modulated by changes in extracellular $[K^+]$ or by mutations in a critical region of the P loop [12]. These properties strongly suggest that in contrast to N–type inactivation, C–type inactivation results from occlusion of the extracellular mouth of the pore.

It is now recognized that voltage–gated K^+ channels consist of complexes of pore forming membrane bound α subunits and cytoplasmic β subunits [22, 24]. The primary phenotypic effect of coexpression of α and β subunits is an increase in the inactivation rate of the expressed current. In the case of the Kvβ1.1 subunit a classical N–type inactivation mechanism was demonstrated [24]. However, in the case of Kvβ1.2, which differs only in its NH_2 terminus, the enhancement of inactivation rate has been demonstrated to be dependent on several factors linked to C–type inactivation [22].

We demonstrate here that Kvβ1.2 induces kinetic behavior consistent with rapid open channel block [22, 23]. Coupling between β subunit NH_2 terminal mediated open channel block and C–type inactivation can account for the increase rate of C–type inactivation.

METHODS

Cloning of Kvβ1.2 (formerly referred to as Kvβ3) from ferret ventricle was described previously [21]. Isolation of the Kv1.4 α subunit, FK1, and construction of the N–terminal deletion mutant of Kv1.4, FK1Δ2–146, were described previously [20]. Defolliculated *Xenopus laevis* oocytes (stage V–VI) were injected with 50 nL cRNA solution prepared as described [21, 22], containing up to 50 ng cRNA, with and without Kvβ1.2, at a ratio of 1:4 (α:Kvβ1.2) for studies using Kv1.4 and 1:16 for studies using the NH_2–terminal deletion mutant of Kv1.4. These injection ratios of α:Kvβ1.2 are saturating in inactivation rate [12]. Voltage–clamp experiments were performed at room temperature, within 3–6 days of injection, using a two–electrode "bath clamp" amplifier (OC–725A, Warner Instruments Corp.) or a cut–open oocyte clamp amplifier (CA–1a, Dagan Corp.) [12] as described previously [21–23]. Oocytes were perfused with extracellular ND–96 (in mM: 96 NaCl, 2 KCl, 1 MgCl$_2$, 1.8 CaCl$_2$, 5 HEPES–NaOH, pH 7.4) for two–electrode voltage clamp measurements. Activation was measured in extracellular ND–96 and high [K$^+$] intracellular solution (in mM: 98 KCl, 1.8 MgCl$_2$, 1 EGTA, 5 HEPES–NaOH, pH 7.4), using the cut–open oocyte clamp. Deactivation was also measured using the cut–open oocyte clamp, but with symmetric high [K$^+$] solutions. Data were not leakage or capacitive subtracted unless otherwise noted. Data acquired using the two–electrode voltage clamp was filtered at 2 kHz and at 5 kHz using the cut–open oocyte clamp. Simulations were carried out in Basic using an Euler algorithm. Results were tested for numerical accuracy by demonstrating insensitivity to stepsize [13].

RESULTS

FK1, a Kv1.4 channel, has been previously reported to display bi–exponential inactivation, with a large fast N–type component. Removal of the amino terminus from FK1 (FK1Δ2–146) greatly reduces inactivation rate (Fig. 1A) as described previously [14, 20]. This fast N–type component is insensitive to a shift from 2 to 98 mM [K$^+$]$_o$ [12] (Fig. 1B). However, a slow component of inactivation remains after NH$_2$–terminal deletion, as can be seen on an expanded time scale for the NH$_2$–terminal deletion mutant (Fig. 1C). This slowly developing C–type inactivation is strongly inhibited by increasing [K$^+$]$_o$ from 2 to 98 mM as shown previously [12] and in Fig. 1C.

Kvβ1.1 was the first ancillary voltage gated K$^+$ channel subunit that was demonstrated to increase the rate of inactivation of Kv1 α subunits. This was demonstrated to occur through a N–type mechanism [24]. As shown in Fig. 2A, Kvβ1.1 results in a very rapid and complete inactivation of an NH$_2$–terminal deletion mutant of Kv1.4 (FK1Δ2–146). Subsequently, we demonstrated that Kvβ1.2 can accelerate inactivation of Kvα1.4 and *Shaker* B that lack N–type inactivation due to removal of their NH$_2$–terminal "ball" domains [4, 20, 21]. We have reproduced this result for an NH$_2$–terminal deleted mutant

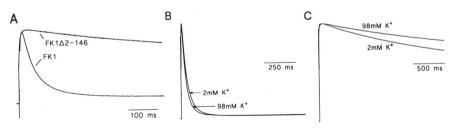

Figure 1. NH$_2$–terminal deletion unmasks C–type inactivation in FK1. **A)** Removal of the NH$_2$–terminus removes fast inactivation (from [20] with permission of the American Physiological Society). **B)** FK1 current traces recorded at +50 mV in the presence of control (2 mM [K$^+$]$_o$) and high (98 mM [K$^+$]$_o$) show no change in the rate of fast inactivation. Currents recorded during a pulse from −90 to +50 mV (stimulation rate = 0.03 Hz) and normalized for comparison (peak conductance and E$_{rev}$ changed with elevated [K$^+$]$_o$). **C)** FK1Δ2–146 current traces recorded at +50 mV in the presence of 2 mM [K$^+$]$_o$ and 98 mM [K$^+$]$_o$ show a marked decrease in the rate of development of inactivation. Currents recorded during a pulse from −90 to +50 mV (rate 0.03 Hz) and normalized for comparison (adapted from [12] with permission of the Physiological Society, UK).

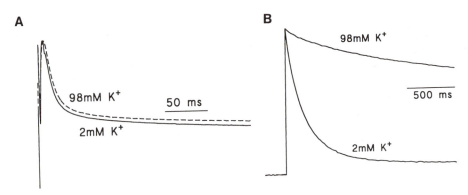

Figure 2. Different sensitivities of β–subunit mediated inactivation to $[K^+]_o$. **A)** overxpression of Kvβ1.1 with Kv1.4 shows a rapid $[K^+]_o$ insensitive inactivation. Data shown for a step from –90 to +50 mV in 2 and 98 mM $[K^+]_o$. **B)** FK1Δ2–146 current traces recorded at +50 mV in the presence of 2 mM $[K^+]_o$ and 98 mM $[K^+]_o$ show a marked decrease in the rate of development of inactivation. Currents were normalized for comparison (currents in Panel B were adapted from [22]).

of Kv1.4 (FK1Δ2–146) in Fig. 2B. However, the enhancement is much slower than would be predicted for the wild–type N–type inactivating channels and is much less complete than that demonstrated for Kvβ1.1 [24]. This type of inactivation also demonstrated a strong sensitivity to increasing $[K^+]_o$ from 2 to 98 mM ([12] and Fig. 2B). These properties sug–gested that Kvβ1.2 might be increasing the rate of C–type inactivation through an intracellular domain [12].

One potential explanation for the increased rate of C–type inactivation was that the N–terminal domain of Kvβ1.2 might be acting like an ordinary fast N–type inactivation "ball" but that it might not have a high affinity for the open channel. In such a model, the NH_2–terminal "ball" domain of Kvβ1.2 binds rapidly to the intracellular vestibule, orienting the channel into a conformation favorable for C–type inactivation. Unbinding before the C–type inactivated conformation occurs frequently due to the relatively low affinity of Kvβ1.2 compared with other NH_2–terminal inactivation domains. The result is an acceleration of net C–type inactivation due to a mechanism which is similar to that proposed for α subunit "ball" domains [4, 5]. This rapid block model of acceleration of C–type inactivation makes two important kinetic predictions for macroscopic currents: 1) If activation is sufficiently fast relative to binding of the NH_2–terminal domain then a transient component of current should be observable; and 2) The deactivation tails should be slowed in the presence of Kvβ1.2.

A simple computer model can demonstrate the expected results. In the N–terminal deletion mutant in the presence of 98 mM $[K^+]_o$ we can neglect C–type inactivation and model the NH_2–terminal binding as:

$$C \underset{\alpha_v}{\overset{\beta_v}{\rightleftharpoons}} O \underset{k_{on}}{\overset{k_{off}}{\rightleftharpoons}} N \tag{1}$$

where C is a resting closed state, O is the open and conducting state and N is the β–subunit NH_2–terminal bound state. α_v and β_v are voltage dependent first order activation rate constants and k_{on} and k_{off} are the on and off rates for binding of the NH_2–terminal respectively. k_{on} and k_{off} are voltage insensitive rate constants, consistent with the general

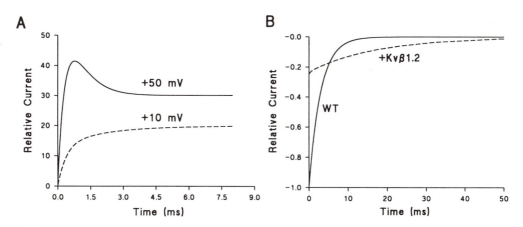

Figure 3. Model simulations predict that rapid block or low affinity N–type inactivation causes a potential dependent transient and slowing of deactivation tails. **A)** Slow activation at potentials near the threshold potential do not show transient behavior (dotted line) ($\alpha_v = 0.4808$ ms^{-1}, $\beta_v = 0.004808$ ms^{-1}, $V_m = 10$ mV). Faster activation at more positive potentials shows a transient behavior ($\alpha_v = 1.443$ ms^{-1} $\beta_v = 0.0001443$ ms^{-1}, $V_m = 50$ mV). **B)** Deactivation is slowed by open channel block. Simulations show the absence (solid lines) and presence (dashed lines) of β–subunit. Current amplitudes are not to the same scale as in Panel A. Simulations following a negative step ($\alpha_v = 0.00025$ ms^{-1}, β_v $0.25 = $ ms^{-1}, $V_m = -90$ mV) from equilibrium values calculated in the previous simulation at +50 mV (initial conditions C = 0.000001, O = 0.25 and N = 0.749999). A significant slowing of deactivation is predicted. For all simulations at positive potentials, $E_{rev} = -70$ mV. For all simulations $k_{on} = 2.0$ ms^{-1} and $k_{off} = 0.6667$ ms^{-1}, initial conditions started with 100% probability of the C state except as noted.

voltage insensitivity of N–type inactivation. As shown in Fig. 3A, at relatively negative potentials where activation is very slow relative to NH$_2$–terminal binding, no transient component is observed. However, at more positive potentials, where activation is faster, a transient component is present. Following activation of the channel, deactivation of the current is delayed due to the need to exit the inactivated state before channel opening and subsequent deactivation. This leads to a slowing of the deactivation tail (shown in Fig. 3B).

This predicted behavior cannot be clearly resolved using the two–electrode voltage clamp technique due to its limited bandwidth. In order to resolve changes in rapid activation and deactivation we used the cut–open oocyte clamp technique [23]. Figure 4A shows a superposition of FK1Δ2–146 currents in the presence and absence of Kvβ1.2 for a range of potentials from −10 mV to +50 mV. The two currents were normalized at 2 ms of activation and the FK1Δ2–146+Kvβ1.2 currents (dashed lines) were re–normalized in amplitude to allow a comparison of a range of typical FK1Δ2–146 currents (solid lines). As shown in Fig. 4A, a clear transient was observed upon depolarization in the presence of Kvβ1.2 that was not present for the α–subunit alone. The rate of deactivation of FK1Δ2–146 was altered by Kvβ1.2. Time constants of deactivation were obtained by pulsing first to a depolarized potential of +50 mV (HP=−90 mV) for 10 ms and then to a range of potentials, from −30 mV to −150 mV. The deactivation tails of FK1Δ2–146 (Fig. 4B and empty circles in Fig. 4D) were significantly slowed (P<0.05 at all potentials, n=5) when FK1Δ2–146 was expressed with Kvβ1.2 (Fig. 4C and filled circles in Fig. 4D).

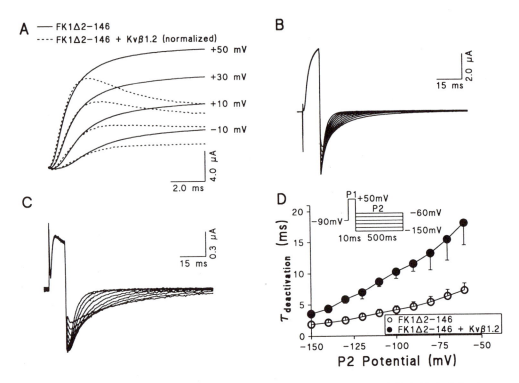

Figure 4. A) Currents recorded from FK1Δ2–146 (solid lines) and FK1Δ2–146+Kvβ1.2 (dashed lines) were superimposed for comparison. FK1Δ2–146+Kvβ1.2 currents were averaged and normalized at 2 ms of activation to match the activation phase of FK1Δ2–146 current. This analysis suggested that Kvβ1.2 induced a small, fast inactivating component which overlaps with activation. **B)** Deactivation tail currents of FK1Δ2–146 measured in high [K^+] solution. **C)** Deactivation tail currents of FK1Δ2–146+Kvβ1.2 measured in high [K^+] solution. **D)** Kvβ1.2 slows the time course of deactivation of FK1Δ2–146 (P<0.05 at all potentials, n = 5). All currents were recorded using the cut–open oocyte clamp. The data in panels A–D were capacitance and leakage resistance compensated (adapted from [23] with permission of the American Physiological Society).

DISCUSSION

We propose that the NH_2 terminus of Kvβ1.2 acts as a relatively low affinity inactivation ball that intermittently occludes the channel pore. The main evidence for this is a rapid transient component which occurs at positive potentials. The absence of complete inactivation suggests that the affinity of Kvβ1.2 NH_2–terminal domain for the α subunit is lower than the Kvβ1.1 NH_2–terminal domain. This rapid low affinity of the NH_2–terminal domain for the α subunit is further manifested by the slowing of the deactivation tails. Such a proposed mechanism makes an important prediction at the single channel level. Coexpression of the Kvβ1.2 with the α subunit should result in a shortened open duration or burst duration and significant numbers of reopening events. In fact, a recent single channel study by Wang *et al.* [25] confirms these predictions.

N–type inactivation in Shaker and Kv1.4 channels has been demonstrated to increase the rate of development of C–type inactivation. Two potential explanations have been proposed to explain the increased rate of C–type inactivation observed in the presence of NH_2–terminal inactivation domains. The first proposes that the increase in rate may be caused by a reduced K^+ occupancy of the pore due to occlusion of the cytoplasmic side of the pore region. The second proposed mechanism is that the NH_2–terminal domain either immobilizes the channel or induces a conformational change that enhances C–type inactivation. The two mechanisms are not mutually exclusive. Due to variability in permeation and kinetic behavior, some channels may be more sensitive to immobilization, while in others permeation may be more strongly influenced. Binding of the NH_2–terminal domain of Kvβ1.2 may enhance C–type inactivation through either or both of these two mechanisms.

Acknowledgments

This work was supported by NIH grants HL–19216, 52874 and 54314.

DISCUSSION

Dr. O. Binah: Is I_{Kr} expression modified during any disease states?

Dr. H. Strauss: Not that I know of, but people are obviously going to look at this question.

Dr. M. Morad: As I was looking at the current records, it appeared that maximum *HERG* density current was about 20 pico–ampere. For an average cell of about 200 pico–farad, you have about 0. 1–1. 0 pico–farad of I_{Kr}. The inward rectifier (I_{K1}) at the range voltages (–20 to –10 mV) which inactivates is about 10 pico–ampere per pico farad. At the range of –20 mV, the inward rectifier is more or less at the low point. At that point, the rectifier is carrying about 10 pA/pF. I have measured it in a guinea pig ventricle at about 10 pA/pF vs 1 pA/pF and I am amazed at the difference between the two. I am amazed at the level of problem that *HERG* channel causes clinically, since it has such a spotty expression in the heart. How do you explain this? How do you fit all of this together?

Dr. H. Strauss: The question of current density is somewhat complicated because most of these studies were done in the atrium where the cell capacitance is smaller. But the current is still small raising concern about its overall contribution to repolarization. An additional concern is the regional distribution of protein. Presumably, the impedance of the membrane is so high, that one would argue that it does not take very much current to initiate repolarization. Clearly there are two pieces of data that suggest that this channel is an important contributor to repolarization. Mutations in *HERG* in the human heart prolong repolarization, clearly implicating it in repolarization. The other is the data obtained with selective I_{Kr} blockers, E–4031 and dofetilide, when administered to patients or to animals cause QT interval prolongation, at doses that are thought to be comparable to those producing selective blockade of the I_{Kr} channel.

All I can say is that there are still some unanswered questions, such as does this α subunit comprise the entire channel or are there associated β subunits. In addition, a truncated form of the α subunit has been identified. We may or may not have detected that alternate splice variant with our fluorescent in–situ hybridization and immunofluorescent techniques and we certainly do not know its pharmacologic profile. In addition, the distribution of the channel and the magnitude of the current and the relative contribution to cardiac repolarization also remain unresolved.

Dr. D. Noble: If one goes just 20 mV more positive, then I_{Kr} would be very tiny. Isn't that going to be part of the answer?

Dr. H. Strauss: The maximum steady–state I_{Kr} is +10 mV.

Dr. D. Noble: But at, say, +20 mV it will dominate nevertheless?

Dr. H. Strauss: No. It is a simulation of an action potential clamp that showed relative current amplitude.

Dr. M. Morad: If you look at *HERG* expressed on 0 side, at +20 the current is 0.

Dr. D. Noble: But it gets bigger after activation?

Dr. H. Strauss: If you look at the studies where inward rectifier current expression was decreased, as has been shown in myocytes obtained from patients with heart failure and in analyses of the current contributions to repolarization, these data suggest that the inward rectifier current really makes its major contribution in the last 30 mV of repolarization. Are the densities of the currents in the human myocyte different than in the quinea pig myocyte. Even the KvLQT1 story is more complicated as we do not see evidence for minK and KvLQT1 transcripts in all cells of the ferret heart. This leaves unanswered the question concerning the relationship of those two currents to repolarization in the heart.

Dr. Y. Rudy: You have shown that during action potential clamp I_{Kr} exerts its maximal effect during phase–3 repolarization. At that time I_{K1} is greater than I_{Kr} and dominates the repolarization process. This tends to minimize the role of I_{Kr}. On the other hand, we know that I_{Kr} block has a major effect on action potential duration and slows repolarization starting from the plateau phase. So something does not quite fit.

Dr. H. Strauss: The issues are probably more complicated than we have heretofore discussed. Professor Noble's paper in the *Journal of Physiology* [26] suggests that calcium and magnesium modulate the gating kinetics of the I_{Kr} channel. To implement our studies on I_{Kr} in myocytes, ion substitution as well as appropriate voltage clamp protocols needed to be used to ensure adequate voltage clamp control and isolation of I_{Kr} from overlapping currents.

Sodium and calcium were removed to minimize contamination from overlapping currents. As a result of these ionic substitutions, we may have the gating modified somewhat. Hence, the protocol that we used may have led us to derive values for gating kinetics that do not accurately reflect their values under physiological conditions. Work is under way now to look at the potential effects of ion substitution on gating properties of I_{Kr}.

REFERENCES

1. Hodgkin AL, Huxley AF. The dual effect of membrane potential on sodium conductance in the giant axon of *Loligo*. *J Physiol (Lond)* 1952;116:497–506.
2. Pongs O. Molecular biology of voltage–dependent potassium channels. *Physiol Rev*.1992;72:S69–S88.
3. Jan LY, Jan YN. Potassium channels and their evolving gates. *Nature* 1994;371:119–122.
4. Hoshi T, Zagotta WN, Aldrich RW. Biophysical and molecular mechanisms of *Shaker* potassium channel inactivation. *Science* 1990;250:533–538.
5. Zagotta WN, Hoshi T, Aldrich RW. Restoration of inactivation in mutants of *Shaker* potassium channels by a peptide derived from ShB. *Science* 1990;250:568–571.
6. Hoshi T, Zagotta WN, Aldrich RW. Two types of inactivation in *Shaker* K^+ channels: Effects of alterations in the carboxy–terminal region. *Neuron* 1991;7:547–556.
7. Busch AE, Hurst RA, North RA, Adelman JP, Kavanaugh MP. Current inactivation involves a histidine residue in the pore of the rat lymphocyte channel RGK5. *Biochem Biophys Res Comm* 1991;179:1384–1390.
8. Choi K, Aldrich RW, Yellen G. Tetraethylammonium blockade distinguishes two inactivation

mechanisms in voltage–gated K$^+$ channels. *Proc Natl Acad Sci (USA)* 1991;88:5092–5095.

9. Lopez–Barneo l, Hoshi T, Heinemann SH, Aldrich RW. Effects of external cations and mutations in the pore region on C–type inactivation of *Shaker* potassium channels. *Receptors and Channels* 1993;1:61–71.

10. DeBiasi M, Hartmann HA, Drewe JA, Tagliatella M, Brown AM, Kirsch GE. Inactivation determined by a single site in K$^+$ pores. *Pflügers Archiv* 1993;422:354–363.

11. Gomez–Lagunas F, Armstrong CM. The relation between ion permeation and recovery from inactivation of *Shaker* B K$^+$ channels. *Biophys J* 1994;67:1806–1815.

12. Rasmusson RL, Morales MJ, Castellino RC, Zhang Y, Campbell DL, Strauss HC. C–type inactivation controls recovery in a fast inactivating cardiac K$^+$ channel (Kv1.4) expressed in *Xenopus* oocytes. *J Physiol (Lond)* 1995;489:709–721.

13. Campbell DL, Rasmusson RL, Qu Y, Strauss HC. The calcium–independent transient outward potassium current in isolated ferret right ventricular myocytes. *J Gen Physiol* 1993;101:571–601.

14. Campbell DL, Rasmusson RL, Comer MB, Strauss HC. The cardiac calcium–independent transient outward potassium current: Kinetics, molecular properties, and role in ventricular repolarization. In: Zipes DP, Jalife J, eds. *Cardiac Electrophysiology. From Cell to Bedside 1994*;83–96.

15. Brahmajothi MV, Morales MJ, Liu S, Rasmusson RL, Campbell DL, Strauss HC. In situ hybridization reveals extensive diversity of K$^+$ channel mRNA in isolated ferret cardiac myocytes. *Circ Res* 1996;78:1083–1089.

16. Armstrong CM. Interaction of the tetraethylammonium ion derivatives with the potassium channels of giant axons. *J Gen Physiol* 1971;58:413–437.

17. Ruppersberg JP, Frank R, Pongs O, Stocker M. Cloned neuronal I$_{K(A)}$ channels reopen on recovery from inactivation. *Nature* 1991;353:603–604.

18. Ruppersberg JP, Stocker M, Pongs O, Heinemann SH, Frank R, Koenen M. Regulation of fast inactivation of cloned mammalian I$_{K(A)}$ channels by cysteine oxidation. *Nature* 1991;#52:711–714.

19. Tseng–Crank J, Yao J–A, Berman MF, Tseng G–N. Functional role of the NH$_2$–terminal cytoplasmic domain of a mammalian A–type K channel. *J Gen Physiol* 1993;102:1057–1083.

20. Comer MB, Campbell DL, Rasmusson RL, Lamson DR, Morales MJ, Zhang Y, Strauss HC. Cloning and characterization of an I$_{to}$–like channel from ferret ventricle. *Am J Physiol* 1994;267:H1383–H1395.

21. Morales MJ, Castellino RC, Crews AL, Rasmusson RL, Strauss HC. A novel β subunit increases rate of inactivation of specific voltage–gated potassium channel α subunits. *J Biol Chem* 1995;270:6272–6277.

22. Morales MJ, Wee JO, Wang S, Strauss HC, Rasmusson RL. The N–terminal domain of a K$^+$ channel β–subunit increases the rate of C–type inactivation from the cytoplasmic side of the channel. *Proc Natl Acad Sci (USA)* 1996;93:15119–15123.

23. Castellino RC, Morales MJ, Strauss HC, Rasmusson RL. Time– and voltage–dependent modulation of a Kv1.4 channel by a β subunit (Kvβ3) cloned from ferret ventricle. *Am J Physiol* 1995;269:H385–H391.

24. Rettig J, Heinemann SH, Wunder F, Lorra C, Parcej DN, Dolly JO, Pongs O. Inactivation properties of voltage–gated K$^+$ channels altered by presence of beta–subunit. *Nature* 1994;369:289–294.

25. Wang Z, Kiehn J, Yang Q, Brown AM, Wible BA. Comparison of binding and block produced by alternatively spliced Kvβ subunits. *J Biol Chem* 1996;271:28311–28317.

26. Ho WK, Earm YE, Lee SK, Brown HF, Noble D. Voltage– and time–dependent block of delayed rectifier K$^+$ current in rabbit sino–atrial node cells by external Ca^{2+} and Mg^{2+}. *J Physiol* 1996;494:727–742.

CHAPTER 4

Signal Transduction in Ischemic Preconditioning

James M. Downey and Michael V. Cohen[1]

ABSTRACT

Ischemic preconditioning is a phenomenon in which exposure of the heart to a brief period of ischemia causes it to quickly adapt itself to become resistant to infarction from a subsequent ischemic insult. The mechanism is not fully understood but, at least in the rabbit, it is known to be triggered by occupation of adenosine receptors, opioid receptors, bradykinin receptors and the generation of free radicals during the preconditioning ischemia. All of these are thought to converge on and activate protein kinase C (PKC), which in turn activates a tyrosine kinase. This kinase cascade eventually terminates on some unknown effector, possibly a potassium channel or a cytoskeletal protein, which makes the cells resistant to infarction. If this process can be understood, it should be possible to devise a method for conferring this protection to patients with acute myocardial infarction.

INTRODUCTION

The concept of ischemic preconditioning was first described by Murry and his colleagues in 1986 [1]. In that study they found that the amount of infarction resulting from a 45 min occlusion of a dog's coronary artery could be greatly reduced if the heart were first exposed to four cycles of combined 5 min coronary occlusion and 5 min reperfusion. This sublethal ischemic insult, by some unknown mechanism, caused the heart to very quickly adapt to become resistant to infarction from a more prolonged ischemic insult, and this phenomenon was labeled "ischemic preconditioning". The observation was a turning point for the cardioprotection community. Ever since the classic study by Maroko *et al*. in

---

[1]Departments of Physiology and Medicine, University of South Alabama, College of Medicine, Mobile, AL 36688, USA

1971 [2] it had been proposed that it should be possible to devise a treatment that would limit necrosis in the patient with acute myocardial infarction. Attempts to identify such an intervention, however, were met with continuing frustration. While free radical scavengers, β–blockers, and calcium antagonists had all been considered, by the mid 1980s it was clear that none of these would result in meaningful limitation of infarct size in laboratory animals [3–5]. Until the study by Murry *et al*. it was not known whether tissue salvage in the normothermic beating heart was even theoretically possible. However, if the mechanism of this ischemic preconditioning can be elucidated, it should be possible to devise a clinically useful intervention based on it.

Early on it was shown that the protection was not the result of increased collateral flow [1], altered anti–oxidant status [6], presence of stunning [7], or production of a protective protein [8]. The preconditioning phenomenon has been found to exist in every species examined so far, including pig [9, 10], rabbit [11], rat [12–14] and human [15–18]. Thus, the heart's preconditioning mechanism appears to be a highly conserved one. Li *et al*. [19] showed that four cycles of preconditioning were not required in the dog, and that similar protection could be derived from a single 5 min occlusion, suggesting a very sharp threshold for entering the preconditioned state. The protection is relatively short–lived, and lasts only about one hour after the preconditioning ischemia in anesthetized animals [7, 11, 20].

PRECONDITIONING THE HEART

Is Protection Receptor–Mediated?

An important breakthrough in determining the ischemic preconditioning mechanism occurred when Liu *et al*. [21] discovered that adenosine acts as a trigger for protection in the rabbit heart. Adenosine has long been recognized to be a metabolite of ATP degradation that is produced by ischemic cells and, therefore, was considered to be a possible candidate for initiation of this process. Liu tested whether an adenosine receptor blocking agent could modify infarction in preconditioned hearts. Figure 1 shows the results of that study. Note that (upper panel) preconditioning (PC) with a single cycle of 5 min ischemia/10 min reperfusion reduced infarct size in the rabbit experiencing a 30 min regional ischemic insult from approximately 35% of the ischemic region (control) to less than 10% (PC). The non–specific adenosine antagonist 8–(p–sulfophenyl)theophylline (SPT) was administered to two groups of hearts prior to the 30 min coronary occlusion. SPT had no effect on infarct size in non–PC hearts but aborted the protective effect of ischemic preconditioning. These data suggest that adenosine indeed plays a role in ischemic preconditioning, an impression confirmed by the lower panel of Fig. 1 which shows data from isolated blood–perfused rabbit hearts. Again, 5 min of preconditioning ischemia conferred protection against a 45 min period of regional ischemia as shown by the two left–hand groups. In the third group, a transient 5 min exposure to intracoronary adenosine was as protective as transient ischemia. In the latter hearts a 10 min washout period was allowed before the ischemic insult, indicating that adenosine receptor stimulation had triggered a transition to the preconditioned state that persisted even after the adenosine was withdrawn. The last group shows that an intracoronary infusion of the A_1–selective adenosine agonist r–phenylisopropyl adenosine (PIA) could duplicate the protection indicating that it was the A_1 adenosine receptor that was responsible. There has been widespread confirmation of adenosine's role in rabbit [22], pig [10, 23, 24], dog [25] and human [16, 18, 26]. Oddly enough, adenosine appears not to play a role in the rat heart [13, 14].

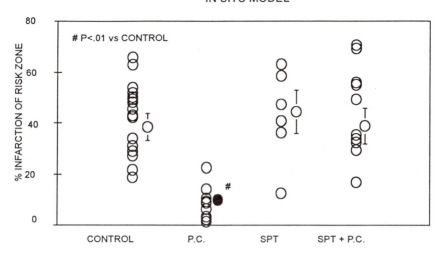

Figure 1. Infarct size (normalized as % of the ischemic region at risk) that results from a 30 min (**top** panel) or 45 min (**bottom** panel) period of regional ischemia in rabbit hearts. Infarction was determined by triphenyltetrazolium staining. Open circles on the left of each pane are data from individual hearts and symbols on the right represent group means and SEM. The top panel is data from *in situ* hearts while the bottom panel shows data from blood–perfused isolated hearts which allowed intracoronary infusion of drugs. Adapted from [21].

The Protein Kinase C (PKC) Hypothesis of Preconditioning

When adenosine binds to A_1 receptors in the cell membrane it causes activation of inhibitory G–proteins which among other things are known to activate membrane phospho–

lipases C [27] and D [28]. The latter degrade membrane phospholipids with ultimate production of diacylglycerol, a co–factor which binds to and stimulates several isoforms of PKC. PKC is of immense importance to the cell and is responsible for many critical cell functions. Early in our studies with preconditioning we wondered whether PKC might be involved in the protection. Ytrehus and colleagues [29] addressed this question by treating ischemically preconditioned rabbit hearts with the PKC antagonist staurosporine. Figure 2 reveals that staurosporine had no effect on non–preconditioned hearts but completely aborted protection in preconditioned hearts. The right–hand panel shows that a 5 min infusion of either oleoyl acetyl glycerol (OAG), a water soluble diacylglycerol, or the phorbol ester, phorbol 12–myristate 13–acetate (PMA), both direct activators of PKC, were as protective as ischemic preconditioning. Staurosporine has been criticized as being a potent but not a very specific inhibitor of PKC. We found, however, that two other PKC antagonists, polymyxin B [29] and chelerythrine [30] also blocked the protective effect of brief ischemia. Polymyxin B has no known inhibitory action against protein kinase A and chelerythrine is extremely selective. Based on this evidence we concluded that PKC is part of the activation pathway required for protection.

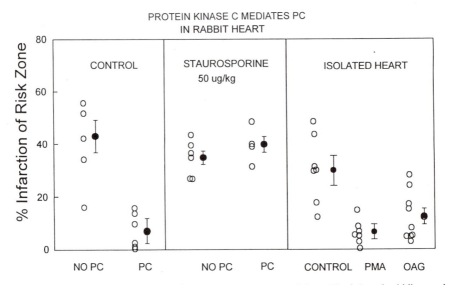

Figure 2. Infarct sizes as in Fig. 1 are plotted for seven treatment conditions. The left and middle panels are data from *in situ* hearts while the right panel contains data from Krebs–perfused isolated hearts. All hearts underwent 30 min regional ischemia followed by 2–hr (isolated hearts) or 3–hr (*in situ* hearts) reperfusion. Note that the PKC blocker staurosporine blocks protection and that either the direct PKC activator phorbol 12–myristate 13–acetate (PMA) or the water–soluble diacylglycerol, 1–oleoyl–2–acetyl–sn–glycerol (OAG), could mimic the protection of preconditioning. Adapted from [29].

All PKC–Coupled Receptors can Trigger Protection

It is well known that there are many PKC–coupled receptors on the myocyte. These include receptors for bradykinin, opioids, angiotensin II, endothelin, and norepinephrine. Even free radicals can activate PKC. It was reasoned that if activation of PKC were a key step in preconditioning, then an agonist to any of these receptors, and not just adenosine, should be capable of initiating protection. This led us to a methodical evaluation of each of these agonists in our isolated heart model.

Goto *et al*. [31] demonstrated that a transient infusion of bradykinin could indeed protect the heart in a fashion similar to that seen with ischemic preconditioning. They also found that the PKC antagonist polymyxin B could block this protection confirming that protection was dependent upon PKC activation. Tsuchida *et al*. [32] found that phenylephrine, an α_1–adrenergic agonist, could also mimic ischemic preconditioning, and that PKC blockade with polymyxin B could again abort phenylephrine's protective effect. And in similar fashion we demonstrated that activation of each of the PKC–coupled receptors including the endothelin receptor [33], the angiotensin II receptor [34] and most recently the opioid receptor [35] could trigger the preconditioning effect. Furthermore a PKC inhibitor blocked protection from each of these. These observations strongly support the PKC hypothesis of preconditioning.

Free Radicals can also Precondition the Heart

Our most recent investigation deals with free radicals. Free radicals are known to stimulate phospholipase D [36] as well as PKC directly [37]. Figure 3 reveals that a 5 min exposure to a free radical generating system consisting of hypoxanthine and xanthine oxidase provides mild protection of the isolated ischemic rabbit heart. While the infarcts were significantly smaller than those in the control hearts, they were not as small as those typically seen with ischemic preconditioning. One possibility is that too few radicals were produced to fully precondition the hearts. Since free radicals are known to be injurious to the heart, another more interesting explanation is that some direct injury from the generator was being masked by the preconditioning process. Figure 3 reveals that when preconditioning's protection was blocked by a PKC inhibitor, infarct size was much larger than that in the non–preconditioned heart, confirming the latter hypothesis. We studied only one concentration of enzyme and substrate for our generating system and it is likely that a less robust generator might have protected with less concurrent injury.

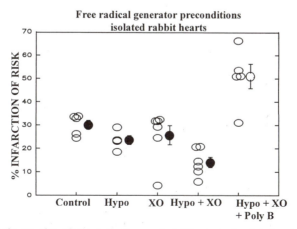

Figure 3. Free radicals can also trigger protection against 30 min regional ischemia in the rabbit heart. Infusion of either hypoxanthine (HYPO) or xanthine oxidase (XO) alone had no effect on infarction but the combination of the two was protective. When PKC was blocked with polymyxin B (Poly B) the protection was converted to an injury with larger than normal infarcts. Adapted from [38].

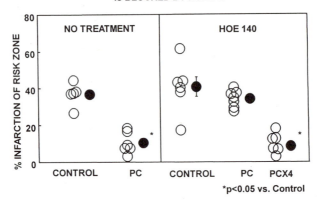

Figure 4. Bradykinin receptors are also involved in preconditioning in the *in situ* rabbit heart. HOE 140, a bradykinin receptor antagonist, blocks protection from a single 5 min ischemic preconditioning cycle (PC) but not from four cycles of ischemia (PCx4). All hearts experienced 30 min regional ischemia and 3–hr reperfusion. Adapted from [31].

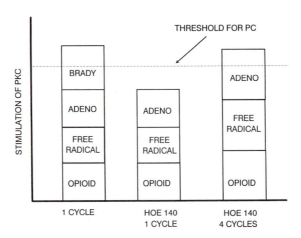

Figure 5. A possible explanation for why both adenosine and bradykinin receptor antagonists can block protection from a single cycle of preconditioning ischemia. There are four identified sources of PKC stimulation in the *in situ* ischemic rabbit heart. All four are required to reach the threshold for protection from a single preconditioning cycle. Removal of one component results in a subthreshold stimulation of PKC from a single cycle of preconditioning. Amplifying the ischemic stimulus with multiple cycles of ischemia increases the remaining components such that protection is restored.

DISCUSSION

Multiple Receptors Participate in Ischemic Preconditioning

It was demonstrated above that there are many receptors on the myocardial cells capable of triggering the preconditioned state. It is known that agonists to most of these receptors are released in the ischemic myocardium. The question must be asked then whether any of these plays a physiologic role in preconditioning's protection? Figure 4 shows what happens when HOE 140, a bradykinin receptor blocker, is given to an *in situ* rabbit heart [31]. When the heart was preconditioned with a single 5 min occlusion, protection was blocked indicating that endogenous bradykinin does contribute to the protection. However, when we preconditioned with four 5 min cycles of ischemia protection persisted despite the bradykinin blockade. At first these observations would seem to be at odds with our earlier finding that adenosine blockade prevented preconditioning's protective effect. Figure 5 attempts to explain that behavior on the basis of parallel receptor pathways. Assume that both adenosine and bradykinin's stimulation are additive in their activation of PKC. If the preconditioning stimulus is near threshold, which is the case for a single 5 min ischemic period [11], then loss of either the adenosine or the bradykinin component will block protection. If, however, the stimulus is amplified by multiple preconditioning cycles so that adenosine receptors are exposed to adenosine for a longer time, then those receptors can precondition on their own even in the absence of a bradykinin component.

Through experiments like these we have found that opioids [35] and even free radicals [38] in addition to adenosine and bradykinin contribute to endogenous preconditioning in the rabbit following brief ischemia. Norepinephrine [32], angiotensin II [34], and endothelin [33] are also produced by the ischemic heart, but are apparently released in quantities which are too small to have a measurable physiological impact since blockade of those receptors has no effect on protection from a single 5 min preconditioning ischemic period. The proportions and, therefore, importance of these agonists could be much different in species other than the rabbit. For example, protection in the rat seems to be very dependent upon opioids [39], with little apparent adenosine effect [14]. In crystalloid-perfused isolated rabbit hearts, opioids [35] and bradykinin [31] seem to be much less important, leaving only adenosine and free radicals as triggers of preconditioning. Furthermore, we were able to show a role for endogenous norepinephrine in isolated rabbit hearts preconditioned with 10 min of hypoxia rather than ischemia [40]. In those hearts a combination of adenosine and α_1 receptor blockers was needed to block protection.

What is Preconditioning's Memory?

One of the peculiar features of preconditioning is that a transient stimulation of receptors puts the heart in a protected state that persists even after the agonists are washed away. So it must be asked what is different about the preconditioned heart? One might hypothesize that during the first ischemia PKC phosphorylated some protein, and protection would last as long as that protein remained phosphorylated. Timing studies, however, do not support that view. In recent experiments we have administered the PKC antagonist staurosporine to isolated hearts, either at the time of the preconditioning ischemia or during the long ischemia. PKC is unique in that its activation is associated with a physical trans-location from the cytosol to a membrane or cytoskeletal location where it comes in contact with its substrate. Staurosporine blocks the ATP-binding site and therefore the ability of PKC to phosphorylate its substrate but not of PKC's ability to translocate. Also, the blockade can be reversed by washing out the staurosporine. Giving staurosporine only during the preconditioning ischemia did not block the protection. If staurosporine were present during the subsequent 30 min ischemia, however, protection was completely blocked [41]. Therefore, phosphorylation by PKC appears to be required only during the long ischemia. The activation of PKC during the long ischemia appears to be dependent on receptor occupancy. While adenosine clearly serves as a trigger to protection (see Fig. 1), we have also found that the myocardial cell's receptors must be reoccupied during the long ischemia making adenosine a mediator as well [42]. Furthermore, we have found that even if adenosine receptors were blocked during the long ischemia, protection could be restored by having an α_1 agonist present at that time [32], suggesting that occupancy of any PKC–coupled receptor was sufficient and again implying that PKC was the target.

We have tried to explain this behavior by the translocation hypothesis [43, 44]. We initially proposed that the delay associated with translocation causes PKC to be activated too late in ischemia to be protective. Preconditioning would cause the PKC to translocate to the membrane where it would be poised to begin phosphorylation as soon as receptors were reoccupied during the subsequent occlusion. This membrane or cytoskeletal location prior to the long ischemia would then be the feature that distinguished preconditioned from naive cells. Most investigators, however, have been unable to document the presence of a sustained translocation in preconditioned hearts [45] (see [46] for a review).

While the translocation model may not be correct, the heart clearly behaves as if preconditioning caused an up–regulation of the coupling between the membrane receptors and preconditioning's end–effector. Adenosine is released in quantity in the non-preconditioned heart [47, 48], but yet occupation of the adenosine receptors causes no measurable protection [21]. PKC inhibitors have no effect in non–preconditioned hearts, indicating that either no PKC stimulation occurred or if stimulation was evident the end-effector was not activated. Only with a second stimulation does PKC appear to "wake up" and protect the heart. Elucidation of preconditioning's memory remains one of the major goals in this field.

What is the End–Effector of this Protection?

The end–effector of this pathway is currently unknown, but there is much speculation that it may be an ATP–sensitive potassium (K_{ATP}) channel. Blockers of the channel prevent protection from ischemic preconditioning [49] or adenosine [50] in dogs and exposure to channel activators mimics the protection of ischemic preconditioning [49]. Controversy arises from the observations that the K_{ATP} blocker glibenclamide either does not modify protection in rats [14, 51] or only does so if an inordinate preincubation time is used [52]. Furthermore, glibenclamide blocks preconditioning's protection in rabbit heart, but only if the animal had been anesthetized with a ketamine–xylazine mixture [53, 54].

Armstrong et al. [55] propose that preconditioning acts to delay the appearance of osmotic fragility which accompanies deep ischemia. This would most likely be related to modification of some cytoskeletal protein. Murry et al. [56] have reported that ATP utiliza-tion is reduced in the preconditioned dog heart suggesting an energy–sparing effect. Such an effect was observed by Yellon et al. [17] in human hearts ischemically preconditioned during cardiac surgery. Kolocassides et al. [57], however, found that ATP was actually depleted sooner during ischemia in preconditioned rat hearts. A similar effect was seen in preconditioned rabbit cardiomyocytes [55]. Kitakaze and colleagues propose that activation of PKC acts to increase 5'-nucleotidase activity in the heart which results in increased adenosine production during the second ischemia [58]. They postulated that elevated adenosine then protects the heart by some unidentified mechanism. Unfortunately, most investigators have found adenosine production to be decreased rather than increased during ischemia in the preconditioned heart [47, 48]. Thus, at the time of this writing there seems to be little consensus as to what the end–effector might be.

Criticism of the PKC Hypothesis

The PKC hypothesis has not been universally accepted. In a recent review Brooks and Hearse [46] have pointed out some of the weaknesses of the current evidence. To date direct measurement of PKC's translocation has failed to show any clear differences between preconditioned and non–preconditioned hearts. This means that the evidence must rest on two observations: 1) PKC–selective inhibitors block protection and 2) all methods of activating PKC tested to date result in protection mimicking that of ischemic preconditioning. Table 1 shows that in most of the studies in rat [59–64], rabbit [29–32, 34, 44, 65, 66], and human [18, 67] myocardium PKC inhibitors block protection and PKC activators mimic it. However, Table 2 reveals that there have been some discrepant results. Most of the negative small animal studies [68–72] did not use infarction as the end–point. Because PKC activators and antagonists have direct effects on contractility it is not surprising that these studies may yield discrepant results. The dog studies have been both positive [73] and negative [74], while the pig studies are all negative [75–77]. The study by Vahlhaus et al. [77] is of particular note. In that study sufficient staurosporine was infused into the coronary perfusate to ensure PKC inhibition, and yet protection from preconditioning was not aborted. Thus it would appear that a true species difference exists, at least in the pig. While the evidence obtained with PKC inhibitors has been criticized on the grounds that the antagonists are not totally specific [46], it must be noted that all of the PKC inhibitors that have been tested so far have blocked preconditioning's anti–infarct effect in rats and rabbits (see Table 1). Because the only thing that this diverse group of compounds has in common is inhibition of PKC, the data with inhibitors can not be so easily dismissed.

Table 1. Studies supporting PKC hypothesis

Investigator	Animal	PKC	
		Antagonist	Activator
Ytrehus et al. [29]	Rabbit	Staurosporine	PMA
		Polymyxin B	OAG
Liu et al. [30]	Rabbit	Chelerythrine	
Liu et al. [44]	Rabbit	Staurosporine	
Goto et al. [65]	Rabbit	Staurosporine	
Tsuchida et al. [32]	Rabbit	Polymyxin B	
Liu et al. [34]	Rabbit	Polymyxin B	
Goto et al. [31]	Rabbit	Polymyxin B	
Armstrong et al. [66]	Rabbit	Calphostin C	
Speechly–Dick et al. [59]	Rat	Chelerythrine	DOG
Li and Kloner [60]	Rat	Calphostin C	
Mitchell et al. [61]	Rat	Staurosporine	SAG
		Chelerythrine	
Hu and Nattel [62]	Rat	H–7	PMA
Cave and Apstein [63]	Rat	Polymyxin B	
Brew et al. [64]	Rat	Chelerythrine	
Kitakaze et al. [73]	Dog	Polymyxin B	
		GF109203X	
Ikonomidis et al. [18]	Man	Chelerythrine	PMA
		Calphostin C	
Speechly–Dick et al. [67]	Man	Chelerythrine	DOG

Table 2. Studies not supporting PKC hypothesis

Investigator	Animal	PKC	
		Antagonist	Activator
Tsuchida et al. [68]	Rat	Polymyxin B	
Kolocassides and Galiñanes [69]	Rat	Chelerythrine	
Mitchell et al. [70]	Rat		PdBu
Moolman et al. [71]	Rat	Bisindolylmaleimide Chelerythrine	
Galiñanes et al. [72]	Rat		DOG
Przyklenk et al. [74]	Dog	H–7 Polymyxin B	
Vogt et al. [75, 76]	Pig	Bisindolylmaleimide Staurosporine	PMA
Vahlhaus et al. [77]	Pig	Staurosporine	

It should be pointed out that our tools for working with PKC are extremely limited. Ideally we would like to monitor kinase activity directly in the cell so that we could know when it is turned on and when it is turned off. Unfortunately, identification of a suitable endogenous PKC substrate has not been forthcoming. There are assays for PKC in tissue homogenates, but regrettably they give no indication of the enzyme's activation state *in situ*. As a result we have had to rely on translocation studies which are difficult to interpret.

What Lies Beyond PKC?

We are now attempting to probe the signal transduction pathway beyond PKC. In a recent experiment we found that at least one tyrosine kinase is also involved in preconditioning [78]. Fifty µM genistein, a potent antagonist of tyrosine kinase, blocks protection from ischemic preconditioning when given to isolated hearts during the long ischemia, but, like PKC antagonists, had no effect when present only at the time of the preconditioning ischemia. Because genistein can also inhibit PKC at high concentrations, we tested another tyrosine kinase blocker, lavendustin A, which has no known anti–PKC activity. Lavendustin A also blocked the protection of ischemic preconditioning. It aborted protection at a dose which blocks cytosolic tyrosine kinases (500 nM), but not at a lower dose (100 nM) which is selective for most of the receptor tyrosine kinases. To determine which of the kinases, PKC or tyrosine kinase, was upstream, preconditioning was triggered with the phorbol ester PMA, a direct activator of PKC. While PMA mimicked preconditioning's protection, this protection could be blocked by either genistein or high–dose lavendustin A. These results would suggest that the critical tyrosine kinase is downstream of PKC.

The involvement of a tyrosine kinase step downstream of PKC may explain why the pig does not seem to require PKC for its protection. In some species there may be alternate pathways around PKC that feed directly into the tyrosine kinase step. We have no idea which tyrosine kinase might be involved at this point since there are many tyrosine kinases in the cell. Each will have to be examined. It is likely that there are more than just two kinases in the pathway and we suggest that PKC may just be the first step in a kinase cascade which is dependent on many kinases in series. This scheme is reminiscent of other signal transduction pathways such as those involving MAP kinases.

CONCLUDING REMARKS

PKC appears to be an integral part of preconditioning's signal transduction pathway, at least in small laboratory animals and in human myocardium. PKC's activation invites cellular protection, while its blockade results in an inability of otherwise protective stimuli to salvage ischemic myocardium. Perhaps in other species like the pig nature may have found a way to bypass PKC and to directly activate downstream tyrosine kinases. We have come to appreciate that this preconditioning pathway is highly redundant, and no single route need be followed each time. Future investigations will undoubtedly resolve many of the existing questions and controversies, and will uncover the elusive end–effector so that a targeted approach to attenuation of myocardial infarction in the clinical setting will be possible.

DISCUSSION

Dr. H. ter Keurs: The final path in a protective mechanism must be something that keeps the cell membrane intact for a longer period of time. The cell membrane is composed of a lipid bilayer supported by a cytoskeleton that provides mechanical support and, probably, glycoproteins also play a role in this. If you are able to protect a cell through intracellular mechanisms which involve PKC and a number of protein kinases, how do they act to change what holds the cell membrane together?

Dr. J. Downey: We do not know much about the end–effector at this point. The actual end–effector in all of this has been a subject of debate for some time and there are some who say that it is a preservation of high energy phosphates; that the cell becomes more efficient and loses ATP more slowly during ischemia. Others say that it is the opening of a potassium channel. If anybody can think of why opening a K_{ATP} channel would be so protective, we would sure like to know because nobody can figure out why that would be so.

We find that one of the things that happens with ischemia is that the cell becomes very osmotically fragile and we think this is due to modification of the cytoskeleton during ischemia. Preconditioning will delay the appearance of this cytoskeletal change. The cytoskeletal effect is my favorite candidate for the end–effector. There is very little hard data on any of these factors, so we do not know which one of these, or any of these, is the actual protective mechanism. Part of the reason for that is because, believe it or not, we do not know why ischemia kills cells. We do not know exactly what it is about ischemia that is giving the lethal insult to the heart. But whatever it is, preconditioning obviously interferes with that process.

Dr. H. ter Keurs: If it is the cytoskeleton that is affected, you would be able to test at least part of that assumption by making the cytoskeleton more vulnerable by, for example, depolymerizing actin using cytochalasin or taxol.

Dr. J. Downey: Right. Obviously, as we get a better handle on these signal transduction pathways, we should be able to devise experiments to actually test that hypothesis.

Dr. J. Bassingthwaighte: My question is about the energetics. What is the evidence for and against the premise that there might be some reduction in the requirement for ATP?

Dr. J. Downey: The evidence for down regulation is in the first studies that Jennings and Reimer made in dogs [*Circulation 74:1124, 1986*], showing that ATP is being depleted somewhat more slowly in preconditioned hearts during simulated ischemia. More recent studies in rats, by David Hearse [*Am J Physiol 269:H1415, 1995*] show that the ATP is actually depleted more quickly in preconditioned hearts. During ischemia, preconditioned hearts go into contracture about 5 min sooner than those that are not preconditioned. ATP at that time is in fact down and that is why they go into contracture. But for some reason, they recover from the contracture beautifully whereas a non–preconditioned heart will not. That is the same in rabbits; they go into early contracture but yet they will recover completely. Thus the ATP–sparing hypothesis fits for dogs but it does not fit for rabbits or rats.

Dr. A. Pinson: What is the role of heat stress proteins in preconditioning?

Dr. J. Downey: There are actually two phases of protection. We have data that the protection lasts for about an hour and then it wanes. But if you follow those hearts, about 24 hrs later, the protection will come back. That is the "second window" of protection and it is thought to be related to expression of some protective protein such as a heat shock protein, although that has never actually been proven. The early phase does not seem to be related to any gene expression. We have preconditioned these hearts in the presence of cycloheximide or actinomycin D and neither one of these will block the protection.

Dr. A. Pinson: Heat shock or stress proteins are preserving the cells and this may be one of the mechanisms of protection.

Dr. J. Downey: Yes, heat shock proteins seem to be protective. Transgenic mice, for instance, that overexpress HSP–70, seem to be very resistant to infarction [*J Clin Invest 95:1446, 1995*]. What is interesting is that the second window of protection is also associated with an increased HSP–70 level in the heart. Interestingly, if you give animals adenosine, you can also get a clear second window of protection, but HSP–70 is not increased in those animals [*Derek Yellon, personal communication*] so there must be another factor involved, perhaps expression of some other protective protein. HSP–70 itself seems to be protective, but it is not necessarily what is causing the second window.

Dr. A. Pinson: But adenosine works through PKC.

Dr. J. Downey: Yes, it does. And of course PKC activation is a good way to get expression of many genes so it is not surprising that adenosine will trigger a second window type of protection.

Dr. H. Strauss: You have ascribed a great deal of the protective effect to the activation of two receptors, the adenosine and the bradykinin receptors. These A_1 and A_2 adenasine receptors desensitize fairly quickly. I am surprised that you have a model system where you have multiple increments or multiple conditioning phases prior to the actual event. Do you think that the impact of the adenosine and bradykinin receptors are maximal in the early phase whereas other receptors, or other components of the system participate in the later phases of the conditioning process? For example, if you give an adenosine or bradykinin receptor blocker after the initial exposure, do you see the same kind of protective effect as if you give it prior to the whole series of conditioning phases? Also, did the blood flow change as a result of this conditioning phase or is this effect solely mediated at the myocardial cell level.

Dr. J. Downey: Let me answer your second question first. This protection does not seem to be associated with any change in blood flow. If you look at collateral flow for example in non–preconditioned dog hearts vs preconditioned hearts, it is exactly the same. More importantly, in animals like the rabbit there are no collaterals so the ischemia in rabbits and pigs is always very deep and again we see no effect of preconditioning on the amount of residual perfusion. At reperfusion after the long ischemia, blood flow is of course better in the preconditioned hearts, but that is probably because there is less necrosis.

Now, to the first question, desensitization. As far as we can tell with these models, the bradykinin, opioid, and adenosine receptors are on a pretty equal footing. We cannot see any real difference in those. As far as downregulation, we have tried multiple preconditioning protocols where we precondition the heart, let it wear off and see if we can recondition. The repreconditioning is found in those experiments, but we have not looked to see if the same receptors are participating. If we give a constant infusion of an adenosine agonist we can maintain the protection for at least 6 hr before we lose it due to desensitization of the adenosine receptors. That would indicate that the time course of desensitization is probably much longer than what would be seen in a 5 min period of preconditioning ischemia. But desensitization is a real problem when it comes to therapy. Desensitization is the main reason we do not use adenosine agonists clinically to protect the heart. The only way we could use them in the setting of an acute MI would be prophylactic treatment of high-risk patients but, unfortunately, they would develop tolerance to these drugs very quickly.

Dr. O. Binah: First, is there an equivalent tissue culture model for preconditioning? Second, there has been a lot of talk about the role of apoptosis in ischemia. Can you comment on this?

Dr. J. Downey: The answer to the first question is, yes. We have an isolated adult myocyte model from rabbits. We simulate ischemia in it and can show a clear delay of cell death if we precondition the cells by a brief exposure to simulated ischemia, then let them recover and simulate the ischemia again. Adenosine or any of the other agonists work equally well in the cell model. In that model, the change seems to be primarily in the cytoskeleton by the way. We use fresh adult myocytes that are not beating and, interestingly, even K_{ATP} openers are protective in that model. That again is part of the enigma as to how opening the potassium channel protects. It is clearly not through reduction of action potential duration.

    Apoptosis is a big question. The main data on that is from Engler [*Proc Nat Acad Sci 92:5965, 1995*] who has shown that ICE-protease inhibitors seem to prolong survival in these cell systems and mimic preconditioning. The only problem that I have with apoptosis being an important component of ischemic cell death is that cardiac myocytes can live for quite a while without a nucleus and as far as we can tell the ischemic death in ischemia/reperfusion is really complete within a couple of hours after reperfusion. So the time course seems a little fast for dying by apoptosis, but anything is possible.

Dr. J. E. Saffitz: You have indicated that PKC plays a central role in mediating preconditioning. And yet, during the actual preconditioning event, phosphorylation does not seem to play a role. So what else does PKC do?

Dr. J. Downey: That is a real problem since the trigger to the preconditioned state seems to be activation of PKC itself. As far as we know, PKC can only phosphorylate something or translocate. PKC is relatively slow to turn on in the myocyte and we are sure that the problem in the non-preconditioned heart is that by the time PKC gets activated it is too late to be protective. In the preconditioned heart the prior activation seems to mobilize it to protect early in the subsequent ischemic period. Chuck Ganote [*Paper in review*] did a very fascinating study with calphostin-C, a PKC inhibitor which has to be light-activated. He preconditioned his cells in the dark, started the ischemia, and then at different times in his experiment would turn the light on. What he found was that, basically, you have to phosphorylate something in the first 10 min of ischemia, or protection does not occur. We are not sure where the delay is. It might be in one of the phospholipases upstream of PKC; these also have very slow turn-on kinetics, especially phospholipase-D which is pretty important in this process. The other possibility is that the delay is in the translocation of PKC, a slow step required in PKC's activation. Other than that we are at a loss why PKC would turn on more quickly in preconditioned hearts.

REFERENCES

1.   Murry CE, Jennings RB, Reimer KA. Preconditioning with ischemia: a delay of lethal cell injury in ischemic myocardium. *Circulation* 1986;74:1124–1136.

2.   Maroko PR, Kjekshus JK, Sobel BE, Watanabe T, Covell JW, Ross J Jr, Braunwald E. Factors influencing infarct size following experimental coronary artery occlusions. *Circulation* 1971;43:67–82.

3.   Hearse DJ, Yellon DM, Downey JM. Can beta blockers limit myocardial infarct size? *Eur Heart J* 1986;7:925–930.

4.   Reimer KA, Murry CE, Richard VJ. The role of neutrophils and free radicals in the ischemic–reperfused heart: why the confusion and controversy? *J Mol Cell Cardiol* 1989;21:1225–1239.

5.   Kloner RA, Braunwald E. Effects of calcium antagonists on infarcting myocardium. *Am J Cardiol* 1987;59:84B–94B.

6.   Turrens JF, Thornton J, Barnard ML, Snyder S, Liu G, Downey JM. Protection from reperfusion injury by preconditioning hearts does not involve increased antioxidant defenses. *Am J Physiol* 1992;262:H585–H589.

7.   Murry CE, Richard VJ, Jennings RB, Reimer KA. Myocardial protection is lost before contractile function recovers from ischemic preconditioning. *Am J Physiol* 1991;260:H796–H804.

8.   Thornton J, Striplin S, Liu GS, Swafford A, Stanley AWH, Van Winkle DM, Downey JM. Inhibition of protein synthesis does not block myocardial protection afforded by preconditioning. *Am J Physiol* 1990;259:H1822–H1825.

9.   Schott RJ, Rohmann S, Braun ER, Schaper W. Ischemic preconditioning reduces infarct size in swine myocardium. *Circ Res* 1990;66:1133–1142.

10.   Van Winkle DM, Chien GL, Wolff RA, Soifer BE, Kuzume K, Davis RF. Cardioprotection provided by adenosine receptor activation is abolished by blockade of the K_{ATP} channel. *Am J Physiol* 1994;266:H829–H839.

11.   Van Winkle DM, Thornton JD, Downey DM, Downey JM. The natural history of preconditioning: cardioprotection depends on duration of transient ischemia and time to subsequent ischemia. *Coron Artery Dis* 1991;2:613–619.

12.   Yellon DM, Alkhulaifi AM, Browne EE, Pugsley WB. Ischaemic preconditioning limits infarct size in the rat heart. *Cardiovasc Res* 1992;26:983–987.

13.   Li Y, Kloner RA. The cardioprotective effects of ischemic "preconditioning" are not mediated by adenosine receptors in rat hearts. *Circulation* 1993;87:1642–1648.

14.   Liu Y, Downey JM. Ischemic preconditioning protects against infarction in rat heart. *Am J Physiol* 1992;263:H1107–H1112.

15.   Deutsch E, Berger M, Kussmaul WG, Hirshfeld JW Jr, Herrmann HC, Laskey WK. Adaptation to ischemia during percutaneous transluminal coronary angioplasty: clinical, hemodynamic, and metabolic features. *Circulation* 1990;82:2044–2051.

16.   Walker DM, Walker JM, Pugsley WB, Pattison CW, Yellon DM. Preconditioning in isolated superfused human muscle. *J Mol Cell Cardiol* 1995;27:1349–1357.

17.   Yellon DM, Alkhulaifi AM, Pugsley WB. Preconditioning the human myocardium. *Lancet* 1993;342:276–277.

18.   Ikonomidis JS, Shirai T, Weisel RD, Derylo B, Rao V, Whiteside CI, Mickle DAG, Li R–K. "Ischemic" or adenosine preconditioning of human ventricular cardiomyocytes is protein kinase C dependent. *Circulation* 1995;92 (Suppl I):I–12. Abstract.

19.   Li GC, Vasquez JA, Gallagher KP, Lucchesi BR. Myocardial protection with preconditioning. *Circulation* 1990;82:609–619.

20.   Miura T, Adachi T, Ogawa T, Iwamoto T, Tsuchida A, Iimura O. Myocardial infarct size–limiting effect of ischemic preconditioning: its natural decay and the effect of repetitive preconditioning. *Cardiovasc Pathol* 1992;1:147–154.

21.   Liu GS, Thornton J, Van Winkle DM, Stanley AWH, Olsson RA, Downey JM. Protection against infarction afforded by preconditioning is mediated by A_1 adenosine receptors in rabbit heart. *Circulation* 1991;84:350–356.

22.   Tsuchida A, Miura T, Miki T, Shimamoto K, Iimura O. Role of adenosine receptor activation in myocardial infarct size limitation by ischaemic preconditioning. *Cardiovasc Res* 1992;26:456–461.

23.   Schulz R, Rose J, Post H, Heusch G. Involvement of endogenous adenosine in ischaemic preconditioning in swine. *Pflügers Arch* 1995;430:273–282.

24.   Schwarz ER, Mohri M, Sack S, Arras M. The role of adenosine and its A1–receptor in ischemic preconditioning. *Circulation* 1991;84(Suppl II):II–191. Abstract.

25.   Auchampach JA, Gross GJ. Adenosine A_1 receptors, K_{ATP} channels and ischemic preconditioning in dogs. *Am J Physiol* 1993;264:H1327–H1336.

26. Kerensky RA, Kutcher MA, Braden GA, Applegate RJ, Solis GA, Little WC. The effects of intracoronary adenosine on preconditioning during coronary angioplasty. *Clin Cardiol* 1995;18:91–96.

27. Kohl C, Linck B, Schmitz W, Scholz H, Scholz J, Tóth M. Effects of carbachol and (–)-N^6–phenyl-isopropyladenosine on myocardial inositol phosphate content and force of contraction. *Br J Pharmacol* 1990;101:829–834.

28. Cohen MV, Liu Y, Liu GS, Wang P, Weinbrenner C, Cordis GA, Das DK, Downey JM. Phospholipase D plays a role in ischemic preconditioning in rabbit heart. *Circulation* 1996;94:1713–1718.

29. Ytrehus K, Liu Y, Downey JM. Preconditioning protects ischemic rabbit heart by protein kinase C activation. *Am J Physiol* 1994;266:H1145–H1152.

30. Liu Y, Cohen MV, Downey JM. Chelerythrine, a highly selective protein kinase C inhibitor, blocks the antiinfarct effect of ischemic preconditioning in rabbit hearts. *Cardiovasc Drugs Ther* 1994;8:881–882.

31. Goto M, Liu Y, Yang X–M, Ardell JL, Cohen MV, Downey JM. Role of bradykinin in protection of ischemic preconditioning in rabbit hearts. *Circ Res* 1995;77:611–621.

32. Tsuchida A, Liu Y, Liu GS, Cohen MV, Downey JM. α_1–Adrenergic agonists precondition rabbit ischemic myocardium independent of adenosine by direct activation of protein kinase C. *Circ Res* 1994;75:576–585.

33. Wang P, Gallagher KP, Downey JM, Cohen MV. Pretreatment with endothelin–1 mimics ischemic preconditioning against infarction in isolated rabbit heart. *J Mol Cell Cardiol* 1996;28:579–588.

34. Liu Y, Tsuchida A, Cohen MV, Downey JM. Pretreatment with angiotensin II activates protein kinase C and limits myocardial infarction in isolated rabbit hearts. *J Mol Cell Cardiol* 1995;27:883–892.

35. Miki T, Sato H, Cohen MV, Downey JM. Opioid receptor contributes to ischemic preconditioning through protein kinase C activation in rabbits. *Circulation* 1996;94 (Suppl I):I–392–I–393. Abstract.

36. Natarajan V, Taher MM, Roehm B, Parinandi NL, Schmid HHO, Kiss Z, Garcia JGN. Activation of endothelial cell phospholipase D by hydrogen peroxide and fatty acid hydroperoxide. *J Biol Chem* 1993;268:930–937.

37. Gopalakrishna R, Anderson WB. Ca^{2+}– and phospholipid–independent activation of protein kinase C by selective oxidative modification of the regulatory domain. *Proc Natl Acad Sci* 1989;86:6758–6762.

38. Baines CP, Goto M, Downey JM. Oxygen radicals released during ischemic preconditioning contribute to cardioprotection in the rabbit myocardium. *J Mol Cell Cardiol* 1997;29:207–216.

39. Schultz JEJ, Rose E, Yao Z, Gross GJ. Evidence for involvement of opioid receptors in ischemic preconditioning in rat hearts. *Am J Physiol* 1995;268:H2157–H2161.

40. Cohen MV, Walsh RS, Goto M, Downey JM. Hypoxia preconditions rabbit myocardium via adenosine and catecholamine release. *J Mol Cell Cardiol* 1995;27:1527–1534.

41. Yang X–M, Sato H, Downey JM, Cohen MV. Protection of ischemic preconditioning is dependent upon a critical timing sequence of protein kinase C activation. *J Mol Cell Cardiol* 1997; in press.

42. Thornton JD, Thornton CS, Downey JM. Effect of adenosine receptor blockade: preventing protective preconditioning depends on time of initiation. *Am J Physiol* 1993;265:H504–H508.

43. Cohen MV, Downey JM. Ischaemic preconditioning: can the protection be bottled? *Lancet* 1993;342:6.

44. Liu Y, Ytrehus K, Downey JM. Evidence that translocation of protein kinase C is a key event during ischemic preconditioning of rabbit myocardium. *J Mol Cell Cardiol* 1994;26:661–668.

45. Armstrong SC, Hoover DB, DeLacey MH, Ganote CE. Translocation of PKC, protein phosphatase inhibition and preconditioning of rabbit cardiomyocytes. *J Mol Cell Cardiol* 1996;28:1479–1492.

46. Brooks G, Hearse DJ. Role of protein kinase C in ischemic preconditioning: player or spectator? *Circ Res* 1996;79:627–630.

47. Van Wylen DGL. Effect of ischemic preconditioning on interstitial purine metabolite and lactate accumulation during myocardial ischemia. *Circulation* 1994;89:2283–2289.

48. Goto M, Cohen MV, Van Wylen DGL, Downey JM. Attenuated purine production during subsequent ischemia in preconditioned rabbit myocardium is unrelated to the mechanism of protection. *J Mol Cell Cardiol* 1996;28:447–454.

49. Gross GJ, Auchampach JA. Blockade of ATP–sensitive potassium channels prevents myocardial preconditioning in dogs. *Circ Res* 1992;70:223–233.

50. Auchampach JA, Gross GJ. Adenosine A$_1$ receptors, K$_{ATP}$ channels, and ischemic preconditioning in dogs. *Am J Physiol* 1993;264:H1327–H1336.

51. Grover GJ, Dzwonczyk S, Sleph PG. ATP–sensitive K$^+$ channel activation does not mediate preconditioning in isolated rat hearts. *Circulation* 1992;86 (Suppl I):I–341. Abstract.

52. Schultz JEJ, Hsu AK, Gross GJ. Morphine mimics the cardioprotective effect of ischemic preconditioning via a glibenclamide–sensitive mechanism in the rat heart. *Circ Res* 1996;78:1100–1104.

53. Thornton JD, Thornton CS, Sterling DL, Downey JM. Blockade of ATP–sensitive potassium channels increases infarct size but does not prevent preconditioning in rabbit hearts. *Circ Res* 1993;72:44–49.

54. Walsh RS, Tsuchida A, Daly JJF, Thornton JD, Cohen MV, Downey JM. Ketamine–xylazine anaesthesia permits a K$_{ATP}$ channel antagonist to attenuate preconditioning in rabbit myocardium. *Cardiovasc Res* 1994;28:1337–1341.

55. Armstrong S, Ganote CE. Preconditioning of isolated rabbit cardiomyocytes: effects of glycolytic blockade, phorbol esters, and ischaemia. *Cardiovasc Res* 1994;28:1700–1706.

56. Murry CE, Richard VJ, Reimer KA, Jennings RB. Ischemic preconditioning slows energy metabolism and delays ultrastructural damage during a sustained ischemic episode. *Circ Res* 1990;66:913–931.

57. Kolocassides KG, Galiñanes M, Hearse DJ. Preconditioning accelerates contracture and ATP depletion in blood–perfused rat hearts. *Am J Physiol* 1995;269:H1415–H1420.

58. Kitakaze M, Hori M, Morioka T, Minamino T, Takashima S, Sato H, Shinozaki Y, Chujo M, Mori H, Inoue M, Kamada T. Alpha$_1$–adrenoceptor activation mediates the infarct size–limiting effect of ischemic preconditioning through augmentation of 5'-nucleotidase activity. *J Clin Invest* 1994;93:2197–2205.

59. Speechly–Dick ME, Mocanu MM, Yellon DM. Protein kinase C: its role in ischemic preconditioning in the rat. *Circ Res* 1994;75:586–590.

60. Li Y, Kloner RA. Does protein kinase C play a role in ischemic preconditioning in rat hearts? *Am J Physiol* 1995;268:H426–H431.

61. Mitchell MB, Meng X, Ao L, Brown JM, Harken AH, Banerjee A. Preconditioning of isolated rat heart is mediated by protein kinase C. *Circ Res* 1995;76:73–81.

62. Hu K, Nattel S. Mechanisms of ischemic preconditioning in rat hearts: involvement of α_{1B}–adrenoceptors, pertussis toxin–sensitive G proteins, and protein kinase C. *Circulation* 1995;92:2259–2265.

63. Cave AC, Apstein CS. Polymyxin B, a protein kinase C inhibitor, abolishes preconditioning–induced protection against contractile dysfunction in the isolated blood perfused rat heart. *J Mol Cell Cardiol* 1996;28:977–987.

64. Brew EC, Mitchell MB, Rehring TF, Gamboni–Robertson F, McIntyre RC Jr, Harken AH, Banerjee A. Role of bradykinin in cardiac functional protection after global ischemia–reperfusion in rat heart. *Am J Physiol* 1995;269:H1370–H1378.

65. Goto M, Miura T, Sakamoto J, Iimura O. Infarct size limitation by adenosine A$_1$ receptor agonist was blocked by staurosporine. *J Mol Cell Cardiol* 1994;26:CLII. Abstract.

66. Armstrong S, Downey JM, Ganote CE. Preconditioning of isolated rabbit cardiomyocytes: induction by metabolic stress and blockade by the adenosine antagonist SPT and calphostin C, a protein kinase C inhibitor. *Cardiovasc Res* 1994;28:72–77.

67. Speechly–Dick ME, Grover GJ, Yellon DM. Does ischemic preconditioning in the human involve protein kinase C and the ATP–dependent K$^+$ channel? Studies of contractile function after simulated ischemia in an atrial in vitro model. *Circ Res* 1995;77:1030–1035.

68. Tsuchida A, Miura T, Miki T, Sakamoto J, Iimura O. Role of $\alpha 1$–adrenergic receptor and protein kinase C in infarct size limitation by ischemic preconditioning in rat heart. *Circulation* 1994;90 (Suppl I):I–647. Abstract.

69. Kolocassides KG, Galiñanes M. The specific protein kinase C inhibitor chelerythrine fails to inhibit ischemic preconditioning in the rat heart. *Circulation* 1994;90 (Suppl I):I–208. Abstract.

70. Mitchell MB, Brew EC, Harken AH, Banerjee A. Does protein kinase C mediate functional preconditioning? *J Mol Cell Cardiol* 1993;25(Suppl III):S.64. Abstract.

71. Moolman JA, Genade S, Tromp E, Lochner A. No evidence for mediation of ischemic preconditioning by alpha$_1$–adrenergic signal transduction pathway or protein kinase C in the isolated rat heart. *Cardiovasc Drugs Ther* 1996;10:125–136.

72. Galiñanes M, McGill C, Brooks G, Hearse DJ. Can the protein kinase C activator diacylglycerol precondition the rat heart? *J Mol Cell Cardiol* 1996;28:A73. Abstract.

73. Kitakaze M, Node K, Minamino T, Komamura K, Funaya H, Shinozaki Y, Chujo M, Mori H, Inoue M, Hori M, Kamada T. Role of activation of protein kinase C in the infarct size–limiting effect of ischemic preconditioning through activation of ecto–5'–nucleotidase. *Circulation* 1996;93:781–791.

74. Przyklenk K, Sussman MA, Simkhovich BZ, Kloner RA. Does ischemic preconditioning trigger translocation of protein kinase C in the canine model? *Circulation* 1995;92:1546–1557.

75. Vogt A, Barancik M, Weihrauch D, Arras M, Podzuweit T, Schaper W. Protein kinase C inhibitors reduce infarct size in pig hearts in vivo. *Circulation* 1994;90 (Suppl I):I–647. Abstract.

76. Vogt A, Barancik M, Weihrauch D, Arras M, Podzuweit T, Schaper W. Activation of protein kinase C fails to protect ischemic porcine myocardium from infarction in vivo. *J Mol Cell Cardiol* 1994;26:CXVIII. Abstract.

77. Vahlhaus C, Schulz R, Post H, Onallah R, Heusch G. No prevention of ischemic preconditioning by the protein kinase C inhibitor staurosporine in swine. *Circ Res* 1996;79:407–414.

78. Baines CP, Cohen MV, Downey JM. Protein tyrosine kinase inhibitor, genistein, blocks preconditioning in isolated rabbit hearts. *Circulation* 1996;94 (Suppl I):I–661. Abstract.

CHAPTER 5

CA^{2+} SPARKS WITHIN 200 NM OF THE SARCOLEMMA OF RAT VENTRICULAR CELLS: EVIDENCE FROM TOTAL INTERNAL REFLECTION FLUORESCENCE MICROSCOPY

Lars Cleemann,[1,2] Giancarlo DiMassa,[1] and Martin Morad[1,2]

ABSTRACT

Total internal reflection fluorescence microscopy (TIRFM) was used to measure local calcium releases in resting cardiac myocytes stained with fluo–3AM. The measured fluorescence originated from regions where cells were close to, and develop adhesions to, a totally reflecting glass surface. The excitation of the fluorescent Ca^{2+} indicator dye by the exponentially attenuated evanescent wave penetrated approximately 200 nm into the fluid phase. In rat ventricular cells, Ca^{2+} waves and Ca^{2+} sparks were observed within the adhesions. Ca^{2+} sparks recorded with TIRFM compared favorably to sparks recorded under similar conditions with confocal microscopy. Computer simulation supported this assessment. It is concluded that TIRFM can provide an economical, flexible tool for detailed measurement of Ca^{2+}–transients in the subsarcolemmal space of live cells.

INTRODUCTION

Mammalian ventricular cardiomyocytes contract when Ca^{2+} is released from the sarcoplasmic reticulum (SR) in response to sarcolemmal Ca^{2+} influx. This calcium–induced calcium–release (CIRC) [1] is believed to involve diadic junctions where L–type Ca^{2+} channels (DHP–receptors) in the transverse tubules (t–tubules) are found in juxtaposition to Ca^{2+} release channels (ryanodine receptors) in the terminal cisternae of the SR. Both Ca^{2+} channels have been cloned, expressed in model systems and examined at the single

---

[1]The Department of Pharmacology Georgetown University Medical Center, Washington, DC, 20007, and [2]Mount Desert Island Biological Laboratory, Salsbury Cove, ME, 04672, USA

Analytical and Quantitative Cardiology
Edited by Sideman and Beyar, Plenum Press, New York, 1997

channel level [2–4]. The cellular distributions of these channels have been determined with fluorescent antibodies and electron microscopy. The sarcolemma of each diadic junction contains approximately twelve DHP receptors opposite to, but physically separated from, approximately 100 ryanodine receptors in the SR membrane [5, 6]. Recent studies emphasize the "local control" of the Ca^{2+} release process and the putative role of Ca^{2+} "micro–domains." These "micro–domains" have been visualized with confocal microscopy as highly localized, sporadic "Ca^{2+} sparks" in resting cells [7, 8]. The larger Ca^{2+} releases elicited by voltage–clamp activation of Ca^{2+} current (I_{Ca}) show "inhomogeneities," which may represent closely spaced or fused "Ca^{2+} sparks" [8–10]. Finally, the Ca^{2+} release process remains intact when the diffusion distance is limited to less than 0.05 μm by dialysis with millimolar concentrations of fast Ca^{2+} buffers [11].

The detailed interaction between DHP and ryanodine receptors, however, still remains poorly understood. It is unsure whether a) a Ca^{2+} spark is produced by a single or a cluster of ryanodine receptors [12], b) the unitary releases elicited by I_{Ca} have the same properties as the spontaneous Ca^{2+} sparks [13], c) local releases are regenerative [14] and d) release depends on unitary or ensemble current of DHP receptors [15]. The uncertainties are linked to the technical difficulties involved in accurate measurement of local Ca^{2+} releases. While confocal measurements with fluorescent Ca^{2+}–indicator dyes have uncovered new details, the limitations of the technique should be recognized. The majority of confocal Ca^{2+} measurements have been found in the line–scan mode (600–1000 Hz line frequency) which can miss the exact centers of release sites and obscure their two–dimensional organization. The typical point–spread function of a confocal instrument gives a poorer resolution in depth ($\Delta z \cong 1$ μm) than in the lateral direction ($\Delta x \cong \Delta y \cong 0.4$ μm). The acquisition of two and three–dimensional Ca^{2+} distribution is relatively slow unless the conventional scanning mirrors are replaced by faster devices [16]. It appears that the current resolution of Ca^{2+} releases must be improved by an order of magnitude in order to detect the Ca^{2+} transfer produced by single channel openings of ryanodine and DHP–receptors (Table 1).

We explore herein whether TIRFM can be used to detect local Ca^{2+} releases with improved resolution. TIRFM has been used to study focal and near–adhesions of cells to glass surfaces which reflect a beam of light coming from the other side [17, 18]. When the critical angle of incidence is exceeded, there is, ideally, no net energy flux out of the glass. Yet, an electromagnetic field is created near the surface. The magnetic field is strongly

Table 1. Ca^{2+} Release and detection systems in a rat ventricular cell (all numbers are approximate)

Region	Dimensions	Time	Ca^{2+} Ions
Whole Cell (10^6 Ry, 10^5 DHP)	10μm·20μm·100μm	20 ms	1,000,000,000
Sarcomeric Unit	1μm·1μm·2μm	20 ms	100,000
t–SR junction (100 Ry, 10 DHP)	0.4μm·0.4μm·0.05μm		(?) 100,000
Ca^{2+}–spark		10–20 ms	50,000
Confocal microscope (resolution)	0.4μm·0.4μm·1μm	4–30 ms	(?) >20,000
TIRFM–microscope (resolution)	0.4μm·0.4μm·0.2μm	1 ms(?)	(?) >5,000
Ryanodine receptor (2 pA)		3 ms	20,000
Calcium channel (0.3 pA)		1 ms	1,000

attenuated as the distance to the interface is increased to a fraction of a wavelength. This evanescent illumination can be seen as defining a single focal plane with a depth of resolution ($\cong$ 200 nm) which compares favorably to that of confocal microscopes ($\cong$ 1000 nm). We hypothesize that evanescent illumination might be used for fluorescence excitation of intracellular Ca^{2+}–indicator dyes in live cells adhering to glass. It might be possible to observe Ca^{2+} sparks with improved resolution using an inexpensive CCD camera. This possibility was explored using rat ventricular cells (which contain highly developed SR) and shark ventricular cells which (because of their lack of SR) are activated directly by sarcolemmal Ca^{2+} influx.

METHODS

Rat ventricular cells were prepared by enzymatic dissociation [19]. Batches of cells were transferred to a perfusion chamber in which a glass prism serves as the bottom of the chamber and is mounted on the stage of an upright microscope (Olympus BX50WI) equipped with a long distance (2 mm) water immersion objective (LUMPlanFl, 60x, N.A. 0.9). The cells were allowed to settle on the prism and were incubated 30 to 60 min at room temperature with Tyrode solutions containing 20 μM fluo–3AM. A focused, attenuated laser beam (λ = 488 nm, argon ion, Omnichrome) was directed through the side of the prism hitting the glass/fluid interface at the center of the microscope's field of vision from below (Fig. 1). Total reflection was achieved by adjusting the angle of incidence, θ, with a mirror mounted on a translation stage. The microscope was equipped with lamps (incandescent and Hg–arc) and filters (488 nm interference excitation filter, barrier filter: > 510 nm) for bright field and epi–fluorescence microscopy. Images were detected with an intensified CCD camera (Attoflour) and acquired as individual frames by an IBM compatible computer or were stored on video tape (sVHS/NTSC, 30 frames/sec) for later analysis on a Silicon Graphics computer (Indy, Unix). The pixel size was 0.3 μm.

The electromagnetic field in the fluid phase may be determined directly from Fresnel's formulas [20]. With total internal reflection, there is no average flow of energy from the glass phase into the fluid phase, yet the steady state condition requires the presence of an exponentially attenuated "evanescent" wave:

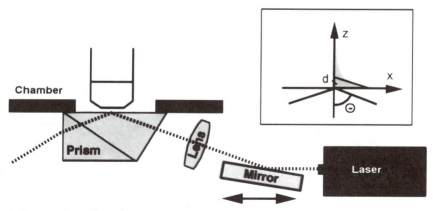

Figure 1. The experimental setup. The optics for TIRFM was mounted on an upright microscope. The beam of blue light from an argon ion laser is shown in a dotted line. The inset defines the angle of incidence (θ), the depth of penetration (d) and vertical (z) and horizontal (x) coordinates.

$$E_{water} = E_{0,\ water} \cdot exp(-z/d + i(bx - \omega t)) \tag{1}$$

where $E_{0,\ water}$ is a constant vector, d is the space constant of attenuation, z is the vertical distance from the interface and $(bx - \omega t)$ gives the phase angle with time, t, and horizontal position, x. The space constant depends on the angle of incidence, θ:

$$d = \lambda \ / \ \left(2\Pi \cdot n_{glass} \cdot \sqrt{\sin^2\theta - (n_{water}/n_{glass})^2} \right) \tag{2}$$

There is no attenuation at the critical angle ($\theta_c = 61°$; $\sin(\theta_c) = n_{water}/n_{glass}$; $n_{water} = 1.38$; $n_{glass} = 1.58$). At larger angles the space constant falls rapidly to a fraction of the wave length: 184 nm at 66°, 134 nm at 71° and 101 nm at 90°. During experiments the critical angle was first found by observation, and the angle of incidence was increased by 5° to 10° to lower the space constant below 200 nm while considering that the refractive index of tissue is slightly larger than that of water or the Tyrode solution.

RESULTS

The images produced with TIRFM have a multitude of signals with rapidly changing fluorescence intensity. The fluorescence of microscopic organisms flashed as they moved rapidly in and out of the focal plane as defined by particles resting on the bottom of the chamber. Spontaneously contracting cardiomyocytes produced flashes where their freely moving ends hit the glass surface. Streaks of fluorescent and excitation light, in the general direction of the laser beam, were found to penetrate into the fluid phase at air bubbles, imperfection in the glass surface and, to a lesser degree, at all points of cellular contact. The background illumination resulting from this violation of the total internal reflection condition was minimized by focusing the attenuated laser beam to a small elliptical spot (100 μm x 200 μm) within the field of vision.

Figure 2 compares images obtained from a shark ventricular myocyte using bright field illumination (panel A), epi–fluorescence illumination (panel B) and evanescent illumination (panel C). The bright field image shows the outline and striation pattern of the cell and is used to assess viability and provide a framework for the interpretation the fluorescent images. Epi–illumination produces bright uniform fluorescence within the entire outline of the cell. In contrast, the TIRFM images show only small patches of fluorescence which initially had diffuse outlines and changed position during contractions. These fluorescent patches are generally oriented in the longitudinal direction of the cell and often include

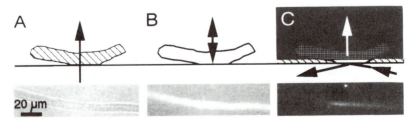

Figure 2. A) Shark ventricular myocyte images with bright field illumination, **B)** epi–fluorescence illumination, and **C)** evanescent illumination. The diagrams show the directions of the light beams. The cell was incubated with 20 μM fluo–3AM for 30 min.

corners and ends. This pattern may simply reflect areas where the cell is resting on the glass surface.

Within 30 to 90 min the cells often developed well–defined areas of intense fluorescence which had sharp outlines, roughly reproduced the sarcomere pattern and remained stable during normal contractions. These patches probably represent areas of strong adhesion because they seem to resist the permanent contraction which terminates most experiments after 5–30 min (Fig. 3). This type of adhesion was seen in ventricular myocytes from both rat and shark and could contain domains where Ca^{2+} signals can be observed without complications from motion artifacts.

Within areas of adhesion, rat ventricular myocytes showed Ca^{2+} waves and Ca^{2+} sparks similar to those seen with confocal microscopy. At a recording frequency of 30 Hz, individual Ca^{2+}–sparks in rat myocytes typically lasted for only one or two frames. No Ca^{2+}–sparks in shark myocytes were found using TIRFM. The Ca^{2+} sparks in rat myocytes were particularly prominent when Ca^{2+}–overloaded states started to develop. Shark cardiomyoctes, when subjected to Ca^{2+}–overloaded states, showed a slow continuous rise in the fluorescence signals without the occurrence of sparks.

The occurrence of Ca^{2+} sparks was evaluated using either confocal microscopy or TIRF microscopy (Fig. 4). It often appeared that the Ca^{+2} sparks recorded with TIRFM were more distinct than those recorded with confocal microscopy. This may be due to the superior resolution in the vertical direction as defined by evanescent fluorescence excitation (Eq. (2)).

It should also be noted that the conditions compared in Fig. 4 (staining with Fluo–3 AM, 30 frames per second) may not be ideal for recording Ca^{2+} sparks at the highest possible resolution. Dialysis of the indicator dye through a patch pipette may give higher and more reproducible dye concentrations and the frame rate can in both cases be increased. Thus we have used an acousto–optically steered confocal microscope, to measure Ca^{2+} sparks at frame rates of 120 and 240 Hz [16]. TIRFM, however, may lend itself to even higher frame rates since the readout from a CCD camera is limited neither by a mechanical scanner nor the spread of an acoustic wave.

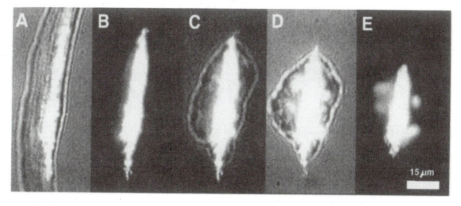

Figure 3. Stability of cellular adhesion. Frames A to E were recorded over a period of 2 min from the rat ventricular cell which slowly underwent irreversible contraction. Frames B and E were recorded exclusively in the TIRFM–mode while the other frames included some bright field illumination to show the contours of the cell. Notice that the area of stable adhesion appears to resist contraction and is only slowly pealed away as the as the length of the cell is reduced to a fraction of its resting value.

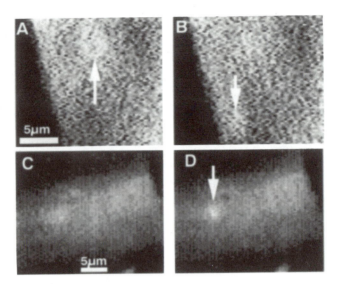

Figure 4. Comparison of Ca^{2+} sparks (arrows) in rat ventricular myocytes measured (A, B) – with confocal and TIRFM (C, D). In both cases the panels show two consecutive frames which were recorded at 30 Hz in cells incubated with fluo–3 AM.

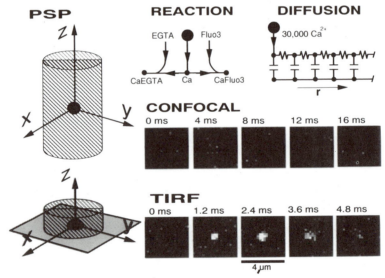

Figure 5. Simulation of measurements of Ca^{2+} sparks with confocal and TIRF microscopy. The detection of Ca^{2+} was followed from the release at point source (black dot) to the representation in a sequence of frames. Ca^{2+} was assumed to bind to both fluorescent (fluo–3) and non–fluorescent (EGTA) Ca^{2+} buffers and the diffusion of all compounds involved (Ca^{2+}, CaEGTA, EGTA, Cafluo–3 and fluo–3) were simulated by step-wise integration assuming spherical or hemispherical symmetry. The calculated Ca^{2+} distributions were convoluted by point spread functions (PSF) which were approximated by truncated cylinders 0.4 µm in diameter. The length of the cylinder was 1 µm for confocal microscopy and 0.2 µm for TIRF microscopy. Compton noise was superimposed on the calculated fluorescence signals based on the assumption that signal-to–noise ratio for the resting Ca^{2+} activity was the same for confocal and TIRF microscopy. The duration of the simulated release was 2 ms. The frame rate for the confocal simulation was 240 Hz in order to match measurements performed with a NORAN instrument. The frame rate for TIRFM was set to 800 Hz match the characteristics of readily available, inexpensive CCD cameras.

The detection of Ca^{2+} sparks with confocal and TIRF microscopy was simulated to evaluate the capacity to measure small and brief releases (Fig. 5). The simulation suggested that TIRFM may give better resolution because a) it has better definition in the vertical direction, b) Ca^{2+} released right under the membrane may spread in a solid angle of 2Π rather than 4Π and c) a higher frame rate may serve to detect Ca^{2+} immediately after it has been released and before it diffuses away. The higher resolution may reduce the detection limit, perhaps by a factor of 3–5, thereby making it possible to detect, perhaps, the Ca^{2+} transported by the opening of a single Ca^{2+} release channel (Table 1).

CONCLUSIONS

The results show that TIRFM can be successfully applied to live cardiomyocytes and can measure brief local Ca^{2+} transients of the type labeled as "sparks" in confocal microscopy. The presence of such signals in ventricular myocytes from rat, but not in those from sharks, support the notion that these transients depend on the presence of functional internal Ca^{2+} stores. We estimate the vertical resolution of the technique to be approximately 200 nm, which is significantly better than that achieved with confocal microscopy.

TIRFM is less expensive than confocal microscopy, is likely to give less bleaching and toxicity since only the "focal plane" is illuminated, has a frame rate determined by the readout of the camera and not the scan–rate of the illumination/detection beam and, finally, has superior depth resolution, albeit, only in a single superficial layer.

Acknowledgment

Supported by NIH RO1 HL 16152 and a grant from the Maine Affiliate of the American Heart Association.

DISCUSSION

Dr. H. ter Keurs: It looks like the propagating wave has a very much more uniform pattern than you would expect if the wave would be led by sparks that are travelling forward. Did you do any analysis of these propagating waves?

Dr. L. Cleemann: We do not expect to see that with the resolution and frame rate used here. It has been recorded with line scan that waves have a tendency to jump by some kind of saltatory motion [*Cheng H, Lederer MR, Lederer WJ, Cannell MB. Calcium sparks and [Ca²⁺]ᵢ waves in cardiac myocytes. Am J Physiol 1996;270:C148–C159*] but we have not analyzed that.

Dr. J. Downey: Is the wave caused by calcium activation? Is this a non–buffered cell?

Dr. L. Cleemann: Yes.

Dr. J. Downey: It looks like the back of the wave follows very closely behind the front. Does that mean that the cell is never fully activated at once?

Dr. L. Cleemann: The waves move typically at a speed of 100 μ/sec. It takes a full second for the wave to move down a cell. On the other hand, the increase in calcium activity during a calcium wave lasts only a few hundred milliseconds. We often see that the cell becomes quiet after the wave front has passed, so that sparking activity will stop for a short time and then come back. Thus, you get the impression that sparking does not occur unless the sarcoplasmic reticulum is filled with calcium and ready to release it. You might argue that sparks do not occur unless you have at least some modest degree of calcium overload, but that has not been settled as yet.

Dr. H. ter Keurs: Your measurements with the TIRFM machine is limited to the superficial 100 nm of the cell and the cell is required to attach to a glass plate on which it is lying. What is the effect of the limitation of the diffusion space in that glass plate on what you see? Suppose, for example, that calcium entry through the DHP receptor is necessary in order to activate sparks. How does the physics and the chemistry of that surface layer influence your conclusions?

Dr. L. Cleemann: We are clearly not seeing the diadic junctions deep inside the cells. Perhaps we see diadic junctions which are close to the surface or we may see some kind of surface couplings. One type of experiment you may want to do is to look at atrial cells which have been reported to have many more junctions to the surface membrane. Another thing you might focus on is the possible difference between calcium signals at the surface and in the middle of the cell. You could combine this technique with measurements of calcium from the whole cell and you could pose the question whether the calcium channels which you measure in cell–attach patches are more closely related to the superficial calcium signals or to the deeper calcium signals. It has not been completely settled that the calcium channels measured with a cell attached patch are necessarily those relevant to calcium release and excitation–contraction coupling.

Dr. M. Morad: Dr. ter Keurs' is worried that the attachment is so close that you may have confined spaces between the cells and the bottom of the chamber, so that you will not have enough calcium to diffuse into myocytes. This is unlikely to be a problem because in cell cultures we often have growing cells which are completely attached and the calcium channels in neurons or heart cells on their attached side work perfectly well on the bottom as well. When you change solutions, the solutions change all around the cell.

Dr. L. Cleemann: You can also say that you see calcium sparks not just at the periphery of adhesions. You also see them at the center. So there is no real indication that calcium is not getting in through the calcium channels where the sparks are occurring, or that the cell exterior is starved for calcium to enter channels. But obviously it is a concern.

REFERENCES

1.   Fabiato A. Time and calcium dependence of activation and inactivation of calcium–induced release of calcium from the sarcoplasmic reticulum of a skinned canine cardiac Purkinje cell. *J Gen Physiol* 1985;85:215–267.
2.   Rose WC, Balke CW, Wier WG, Marban E. Macroscopic and unitary properties of physiological ion flux through L–type Ca^{2+} channels in guinea–pig heart cells. *J Physiol* 1992;456:267–284.
3.   Rousseau E, Smith JS, Henderson JS, Meissner G. Single channel and $^{45}Ca^{2+}$ flux measurements of the cardiac sarcoplasmic reticulum calcium channel. *Biophys J* 1986;50:1009–1014.
4.   Tinker A, Williams AJ. Divalent cation conductance in the ryanodine receptor channel of sheep cardiac muscle sarcoplasmic reticulum. *J Gen Physiol* 1992;100;479–493.
5.   Page E. Quantitative ultrastructural analysis of cardiac membrane physiology. *Am J Physiol* 1978; 235:C147–C158.
6.   Sun XH, Protasi F, Takahashi M, Takeshima H, Ferguson, DG, Franzini–Armstrong C. Molecular architecture of membranes involved in excitation–contraction coupling of cardiac muscle. *J Cell Biol* 1995;129:659–671.
7.   Cheng H, Lederer WJ, Cannell MB. Calcium sparks: elementary events underlying excitation–contraction coupling in heart muscle. *Science* 1993;262:740–744.
8.   Lipp P, Niggli E. Modulation of Ca^{2+} release in cultured neonatal rat cardiomyocytes: insight from subcellular release pattern revealed by confocal microscopy. *Circ Res* 1994;74:979–990.

9. Cannell MB, Cheng H, Lederer WJ. Spatial non–uniformities in [Ca] during excitation contraction coupling in cardiac myocytes. *Biophys J* 1994;67:1942–1956.

10. Lopez–Lopez JR, Shacklock PS, Balke, CW, Wier, WG. Local stochastic release of Ca^{2+} in voltage clamped rat heart cells: visualization with confocal microscopy. *J Physiol* 1994;480:21–29.

11. Adachi–Akahane S, Cleemann L, Morad M. Cross–signaling between L–type Ca^{2+} channels and ryanodine receptors in rat ventricular myocytes. *J Gen Physiol* 1996;108:435–454.

12. Lipp P, Niggli E. Submicroscopic calcium signals as fundamental events of excitation–contraction coupling in guinea–pig cardiac myocytes. *J Physiol* 1996;492:31–38.

13. Klein, MG, Cheng H, Santana LF, Jiang Y–H, Lederer WJ, Schneider MF. Two mechanisms of quantized calcium release in skeletal muscle. *Nature* 1996;379:455–458.

14. Stern MD. Theory of excitation–contraction coupling in cardiac muscle. *Biophys J* 1992;63:497–517.

15. Santana LF, Cheng H, Gomez AM, Cannell MB, Lederer WJ. Relation between the sarcolemmal Ca^{2+} current and Ca^{2+} sparks and local control theories for cardiac excitation–contraction coupling. *Circ Res* 1996;78:166–171.

16. Cleemann L, DiMassa G, Morad M. Distribution of "Ca^{2+} sparks" in cardiomyocytes recorded with rapid confocal microscopy. *Biophys J* 1996;70: A273.

17. Truskey GA, Burmeister JS, Grapa and Reichert WM. Total internal reflection fluorescence microscopy (TIRFM) II. Topographical mapping of relative cell/substratum separation distances. *Cell Science* 1992;103:491–499.

18. Axelrod D, Thompson NL, Burghardt TP. Total internal fluorescence microscopy. *J Microscopy* 1982;129:19–28.

19. Mitra R, Morad M. A uniform enzymatic method for dissociation of myocytes from hearts and stomachs of vertebrates. *Am J Physiol* 1985;249:H1057–H1060.

20. Stratton JA. *Electromagnetic Theory.* McGraw–Hill Book Company, New York, 1941; 497–500.

CHAPTER 6

UNCOUPLING OF G–PROTEIN COUPLED RECEPTORS *IN VIVO*: INSIGHTS FROM TRANSGENIC MICE

Howard A. Rockman[1]

ABSTRACT

Heart failure is a problem of increasing importance in medicine. An important characteristic of heart failure is reduced agonist–stimulated adenylyl cyclase activity (receptor desensitization) due to both diminished receptor number (receptor down regulation) and impaired receptor function (receptor uncoupling). These changes in the β–adrenergic receptor (β–AR) system, may in part account for some of the abnormalities of contractile function in this disease. Myocardial contraction is closely regulated by G–protein coupled β–adrenergic receptors through the action of the second messenger cAMP. The β–AR receptors themselves are regulated by a set of specific kinases, termed the G–protein–coupled receptor kinases (GRKs). The study of this complex system *in vivo* has recently been advanced by the development of transgenic and gene targeted ("knockout") mouse models. Combining transgenic technology with sophisticated physiological measurements of cardiac hemodynamics is an extremely powerful strategy to study the regulation of myocardial contractility in the normal and failing heart.

INTRODUCTION

Heart failure is a problem of increasing importance in cardiovascular medicine with 400,000 new cases diagnosed annually in the US [1]. The prognosis is poor with an overall 5 year survival of 50% and a 1 year survival of less than 50% in patients with severe symptoms [1]. Plasma norepinephrine levels which reflect sympathetic nervous system activity are universally elevated in patients with symptomatic and asymptomatic left ventricular (LV) dysfunction [1], and are directly related to mortality in chronic heart

---

[1]Department of Medicine, University of California at San Diego, School of Medicine, La Jolla, CA, USA

failure [2]. Data from V–HeFT II demonstrate the importance of neuroendocrine activation on worsening survival chances, i.e., patients with the highest levels of plasma norepinephrine are at the greatest mortality risk [3]. Although the clinical course can be modified by treatment with angiotensin converting enzyme inhibitors, a progressive rise in plasma norepinephrine still results over time. An important characteristic of heart failure, possibly related to chronic sympathetic activation, is reduced agonist–stimulated adenylyl cyclase activity (receptor desensitization) due to both diminished receptor number (receptor down regulation) and impaired receptor function (receptor uncoupling) [4]. These changes in the β–AR system, may in part account for some of the abnormalities of contractile function in this disease. To begin to unravel the complex process of β–AR signaling and desensitization *in vivo*, we have utilized transgenic technology to target the heart and selectively overexpress various molecules involved in β–AR signal transduction. Here we provide an overview of our current understanding of β–AR function and highlight potential future directions.

EXPLORING THE β ADRENERGIC RECEPTOR

β–AR Signaling in the Failing Myocardium

In chronic human heart failure, decreased β–AR density is limited to the β_1–AR subtype [5]. Steady state levels of β_1–AR mRNA are reduced while β_2–AR mRNA is unchanged in patients with both nonischemic and ischemic cardiomyopathy [6]. Although abnormalities in Gsα have not been documented as assessed by either ADP ribosylation, reconstitution or functional assays, there is good evidence for an increase in both the amount and activity of the inhibitory G–protein (Gi), indicating an increase in the activity of the inhibitory adenylyl cyclase pathway in the failing heart (for review see [7–9]). In contrast, activation of the catalytic subunit appears to be intact indicating that the Gsα–adenylyl cyclase interaction is unaltered in human heart failure [7–9].

Alterations of βARK in Heart Failure

High levels of circulating catecholamines in heart failure may also act to desensitize remaining β–AR's, possibly through GRK mediated mechanisms. In this regard, mRNA levels for βARK1 and phosphorylation activity of βARK have recently been shown to be elevated in tissue samples taken from the LV of failing human hearts [6,10]. In an experimental porcine model of heart failure βARK activity correlated with the level of β–receptor activation in that βARK activity decreased following treatment with the selective β_1–AR blocker bisoprolol [11]. Myocardial levels of βARK2 and both β arrestin isoforms appeared to be unchanged in human heart failure [10].

To date, the level of GRK5 in chronic heart failure has not been determined. Taken together, this suggests that elevated activity of βARK in failing myocardium may be an important mechanism for β–AR desensitization through enhanced receptor phosphorylation and subsequent receptor uncoupling from G–protein. The consequence of this pathologic process would lead to one of the characteristic observations found in chronic heart failure: reduced functional responsiveness to β–AR stimulation [8, 12].

Use of Transgenic Technology to Delineate β–AR Signal Transduction *In Vivo*

We have recently generated and characterized the phenotype of transgenic mice created from several different constructs, including the human β_2–AR [13,14], the bovine βARK1 [15], a peptide inhibitor of βARK1 that competes for Gβγ binding [15], and GRK5 [16]. Detailed molecular, biochemical and physiologic analyses have been performed and provided important insights into the function of the β–receptor system in the heart *in vivo*.

Targeted Overexpression of the β_2–AR Receptor

To determine whether an increase in receptor number would lead to greater G–protein–coupling, transgenic mice with cardiac targeted overexpression of the human β_2–AR were generated [13]. With the transgene driven by the α–MHC promoter, these mice showed a marked increase in myocardial β–AR density (> 100–fold) associated with a two–fold increase in adenylyl cyclase activity [13]. The physiologic phenotype created by targeted cardiac overexpression of the β_2–AR was one of markedly enhanced myocardial contractility and relaxation, which was unresponsive to further isoproterenol stimulation [13, 17]. These data suggest that a marked overexpression of the β_2–AR can result *in vivo* in a signaling pathway which is maximally activated [13, 17].

An important principal learned from these transgenic animals is evidence supporting the concept that, *in vivo*, β–AR's can couple to G–protein and stimulate adenylyl cyclase even in the absence of agonist [18]. Since a small proportion of β–AR will spontaneously isomerize to the active confirmation, overexpression of an abundance of receptors results in a greater number in the active state, which can then generate a physiological response.

A second principal learned from these transgenic mice was evidence for the existence of compounds which, *in vivo*, can shift the receptor equilibrium towards an inactive receptor conformation. Ligands which shift the equilibrium from an active to inactive conformation are termed inverse agonists or negative antagonists [18]. Administration of an inverse agonist to the β_2–AR overexpressing mice resulted in a dramatic fall in contractile function, whereas no change was observed when the inverse agonist was infused into wild type mice, confirming that the myocardium of the transgenic mice contain an elevated number of β–AR in the active conformation [14]. These experiments have important implications with regard to the use of inverse agonists in the treatment of disease states which result from constitutively active receptor mutations [19], since therapy with a neutral antagonist ("classic blocker") would have little impact on the physiological phenotype.

OVEREXPRESSION OF G–PROTEIN–COUPLED RECEPTOR KINASES

To investigate whether alterations in receptor G–protein–coupling can affect contractile function *in vivo*, transgenic mice were generated with cardiac specific overexpression of either βARK1 [15], a peptide inhibitor of βARK1 [15], or GRK5 [16] in murine myocardium. All the transgenes consisted of the α–MHC promoter ligated to either the entire coding region for bovine βARK1, GRK5, or the coding sequence for the peptide corresponding to the carboxyl terminus of βARK1 (which *in vitro* competes for Gβγ binding, a process required for βARK1 activation) [15, 20]. Compared to wild type controls, transgenic mouse lines which overexpressed either βARK1 or GRK5 led to increased mRNA and protein levels for the respective transgene, which was associated with enhanced kinase activity as assessed by rhodopsin phosphorylation. Furthermore, extracts of heart homogenates from the βARK1 and GRK5 transgenic animals showed decreased adenylyl cyclase activity both at baseline and in response to isoproterenol.

To assess the physiological phenotype, transgenic mice underwent cardiac catheterization using a high fidelity micromanometer inserted into the LV. Compared to litter mate control mice, overexpression of both βARK1 and GRK5 showed a significant blunting of the inotropic and chronotropic response to β–AR stimulation [15, 16]. In contrast, a striking phenotype was observed in the βARK inhibitor animals which showed a significant increase in basal contractility with preserved isoproterenol responsiveness [15].

To determine whether overexpression of βARK1 and GRK5 would desensitize other G–protein–coupled receptors, cardiac catheterization was used to measure the physiologic response to angiotensin II infusion. Stimulation of angiotensin II receptors resulted in a similar rise in LV pressure for both transgenic mouse lines (βARK1, GRK5) and controls. However, only mice which overexpressed βARK1 demonstrated a blunted contractile response with angiotensin II infusion [16].

Since baseline contractility in response to sympathetic stimulation can be altered by general anesthesia, hemodynamic evaluation was performed in chronically instrumented mice in the conscious state. As expected, recovery from anesthesia was associated with a marked increase in LV pressure, LV dP/dt_{max}, and heart rate in wild type mice. Enhancement of contractile function following recovery from anesthesia with GRK5 overexpression was significantly blunted, demonstrating the marked uncoupling of β–AR's in these animals, even in the presence of an integrated autonomic nervous system [16].

Taken together, these results suggest that *in vivo*, both β–adrenergic and angiotensin II receptors are targets for βARK1 mediated desensitization, whereas selective desensitization of G–protein–coupled receptors occurs with GRK5 overexpression. Furthermore, the demonstration of opposite phenotypes i.e., reduced β–AR desensitization (βARK inhibition) and enhanced β–AR desensitization (βARK1 overexpression), suggests that βARK1 is a critical modulator of myocardial function.

CONCLUSION

Understanding cardiac contractility is essential for advances in the treatment of cardiac diseases, particularly heart failure. Future research will combine transgenic and gene targeting technologies, which allow for the targeted and selective manipulation of candidate molecules, with models of clinically important diseases such as hypertrophy and heart failure [21,22]. Monitoring the physiological phenotype in these models will provide an extremely powerful approach to the understanding of disease processes where normal regulatory mechanisms have failed.

Acknowledgments

Drs. R. J. Lefkowitz and W. J. Koch are gratefully acknowledge for their contributions to this work. This work was supported in part by the National Institutes of Health Grants HL56687 (H.A.R.).

DISCUSSION

Dr. N. Alpert: In some of these situations where you get a change in phospholamban, do you also get a change in the other calcium cycling, such as SERCA–II or ryanodine receptor, or is this a change in one protein only. It would seem strange if it were.

Dr. H. Rockman: The mouse is a little different from other species. In the mouse with pressure overload, especially in the model of the pulmonary artery banding, the right ventricle dilates with a decrease in function. Phospholamban is dramatically down but the sarcoplasmic reticulum calcium ATPase is barely down, if at all. We have looked at both the protein and the mRNA levels. In fact, in the β–2 adrenergic transgenic mice, phospholamban is also down, but SERCA–II is not. So it is a little different.

Dr. H. ter Keurs: What about MLP in the contractile cell?

Dr. H. Rockman: This is an interesting question. MLP is a positive regulator of myogenic differentiation associated with the actin–based cytoskeleton. It appears to act as a molecular adapter to promote protein assembly.

Dr. H. Strauss: Could you tell us more about the Ras–oncogene overexpressed mice? They obviously are a very interesting model of hypertrophy, but there may be a lot of other proteins that are turned on by this oncogene because it is fairly important in cell signalling. What other proteins are turned on in this model?

Dr. H. Rockman: The ones that have been looked at were markers of the hypertrophic response. In transgenic animals, markers such as ANF, BNP, ANP, the immediate early genes are all turned on. We have not looked systematically at every protein. These transgenic mice have cavity obliteration, myocytes disarray, but they are not desensitized, although relaxation is abnormal.

Dr. M. Morad: You suggest that relaxation was not changed in the mice that hypertrophied so dramatically. Did you look at relaxation on the isolated myocyte level, or on a whole heart level?

Dr. H. Rockman: Relaxation is abnormal, both in the hypertrophied animals that were banded (pressure overload) and in the Ras mice. Relaxation is abnormal as measured in the intact animal.

Dr. M. Morad: Since SERCA–II and phospholamban have not changed, do you suggest that this is a mechanical issue of the whole heart hypertrophy?

Dr. H. Rockman: Yes.

REFERENCES

1. Cohn JN. Plasma norepinephrine and mortality. *Clin Cardiol* 1995;18(Suppl):I–9–I–12.
2. Cohn JN, Levine B, Olivari MT, Garberg V, Lura D, Francis GS, Simon AB. Plasma norepinepherine as a guide to prognosis in patients with chronic congestive heart failure. *N Engl J Med* 1984;311:819–823.
3. Francis GS, CCohn JN, Johnson G, Rector TS, Goldman S, Simon A. Plasma norepinephrine, plasma renin activity and congestive heart failure. *Circulation* 1993;87[suppl]:VI40–VI48.
4. Brodde OE. Beta–adrenoceptors in cardiac disease. *Pharmac Ther* 1993;60:405–430.
5. Bristow MR, Minobe WA, Raynolds MV, Port JD, Rasmussen R, Ray PE, Feldman AM. Reduced β_1 receptor messenger RNA abundance in the failing human heart. *J Clin Invest* 1993;92:2737–2745.
6. Ungerer M, Parruti G, Bohm M, Puzicha M, DeBlasi A, Erdmann E, Lohse MJ. Expression of β–arrestins and β–adrenergic receptor kinases in the failing human heart. *Circ Res* 1994;74:206–213.
7. Feldman AM. Experimental issues in assessment of G–protein function in cardiac disease. *Circulation* 1991;84:1852–1861.
8. Bristow MR, Hershberger RE, Port JD, Gilbert EM, Sandoval A, Rasmussen R, Cates AE, Feldman AM. β–adrenergic pathways in nonfailing and failing human ventricular myocardium. *Circulation* 1990;82:(suppl I)I12–I25.
9. Bohm M. Alterations of β–adrenoreceptor–G–protein–regulated adenylyl cyclase in heart failure. *Mol Cell Bioche* 1995;147:147–160.
10. Ungerer M, Bohm M, Elce JS, Erdman E, Lohse MJ. Altered expression of β–adrenergic receptors in the failing human heart. *Circulation* 1993;87:454–463.

11.   Ping P, Gelzer–Bell R, Roth DA, Kiel D, Insel PA, Hammond HK. Reduced β–adrenergic receptor activation decreases G–protein expression and β–adrenergic receptor kinase activity in porcine heart. *J Clin Invest* 1995;95:1271–1280.

12.   Bristow MR, Ginsburg R, Minobe W, Cubicciotti RS, Sageman WS, Lurie K, Billingham ME, Harrison DC, Stinson ED. Decreased catecholamine sensitivity and β–adrenergic–receptor density in failing human hearts. *N Engl J Med* 1982;307:205–211.

13.   Milano CA, Allen LF, Rockman HA, Dolber PC, McMinn TR, Chien KR Johnson TD, Bond RA, Lefkowitz RJ. Enhanced myocardial function in transgenic mice overexpressing the β2–adrenergic receptor. *Science* 1994;264:582–586.

14.   Bond RA, Johnson TD, Milano CA, Rockman HA, McMinn TR, Apparsunndaram S, Kenakin TP, Allen LF, Lefkowitz RJ. Physiologic effects of inverse agonists in transgenic mice with myocardial overexpression of the β_2–adrenoceptor. *Nature* 1995;374:272–275.

15.   Koch WJ, Rockman HA, Samama P, Hamilton R, Bond RA, Milano CA, Lefkowitz RJ. Reciprocally altered cardiac function in transgenic mice overexpressing the β–adrenergic receptor kinase or a βARK inhibitor. *Science* 1995;268:1350–1353.

16.   Rockman HA, Choi DJ, Rahman NU, Akhter SA, Lefkowitz RJ, Koch WJ. Receptor–specific *in vivo* desensitization by the G–protein–coupled receptor kinase–5 in transgenic mice. *Proc Natl Acad Sci USA* 1996;93:9954–9959.

17.   Rockman HA, Hamilton R, Milano CA, Mao L, Jones LR, Lefkowitz RJ. Enhanced myocardial relaxation *in vivo* in transgenic mice overexpressing the β_2–adrenergic receptor is associated with reduced phospholamban protein. *J Clin Invest* 1996;97:1618–1623.

18.   Lefkowitz RJ, Cotecchia S, Samama P, Costa T. Constitutive activity of receptors coupled to guanine nucleotide regulatory proteins. *Trends Pharmacol Sci* 1993;14:303–307.

19.   Schipani E, Langman CB, Parfitt AM, Jensen GS, Kikuchi S, Kooh SW, Cole WG, Juppner H. Constitutively activated receptors for parathyroid hormone and parathyroid hormone–related peptide in Jansen's metaphyseal chondrodysplasia. *N Engl J Med* 1996;335:708–714.

20.   Koch WJ, Inglese J, Stone WC, Lefkowitz RJ. The binding site for the βγ subunits of heterotrimeric G–proteins on the β–adrenergic receptor kinase. *J Biol Chem* 1993;268:8256–8260.

21.   Rockman HA, Ross RS, Harris AN, Knowlton KU, Steinhelper ME, Field L, Ross J Jr, Chien KR. Segregation of atrial–specific and inducible expression of an atrial natriuretic factor transgene in an *in vivo* murine model of cardiac hypertrophy. *Proc Natl Acad Sci USA* 1991;88:8277–8281.

22.   Rockman HA, Ono S, Ross RS, Jones LR, Karim M, Bhargava V, Ross J Jr, Chien KR. Molecular and physiological alterations in murine ventricular dysfunction. *Proc Natl Acad Sci USA* 1994;91:2694–2698.

II. THE CONTRACTILE MECHANISM AND ENERGETICS

CHAPTER 7

Molecular Control of Myocardial Mechanics and Energetics: The Chemo–Mechanical Conversion

Amir Landesberg[1]

ABSTRACT

Energy consumption in the cardiac muscle is characterized by two basic phenomena: 1) The well known linear relationship between energy consumption by the sarcomere and the mechanical energy it generates, and 2) the ability to modulate the generated mechanical energy and energy consumption to the various loading conditions, as is manifested by the Frank–Starling Law and the Fenn effect. These basic phenomena are analyzed here based on coupling calcium kinetics with crossbridge (Xb) cycling. Our previous studies established the existence of two feedback mechanism: 1) a positive feedback mechanism, the cooperativity, whereby the affinity of the troponin for calcium, and hence Xb and actomyosin–ATPase recruitment, depends on the number of force generating Xbs, and 2) a mechanical feedback, whereby the filaments shortening velocity, or the Xb strain rate, determines the rate of Xb turnover from the strong to the weak conformation. The cooperativity mechanism determines the force–length relationship (FLR) and the related Frank–Starling Law. It also provides the basis for the regulation of energy consumption and the ability of the muscle to adapt its energy consumption to the loading conditions. The mechanical feedback regulates the shortening velocity and provides the analytical solution for the experimentally derived Hill's equation for the force–velocity relationship (FVR). The mechanical feedback regulates the generated power and provides the linear relationship between energy consumption and the generated mechanical energy, i.e., the external work done and the liberated heat. Thus, the two feedback mechanisms that regulate sarcomere

[1]Heart System Research Center, Julius Silver Institute, Department of Biomedical Engineering, Technion–IIT, Haifa 32000, Israel

dynamics, and determine the FLR and FVR, also regulate the energy consumption and the mechanical energy generated by the muscle.

INTRODUCTION

One of the most interesting aspects of muscle physiology is the regulation of energy consumption and the generated mechanical energy. Extensive experimental studies [1] at the global left ventricle (LV) level have established the existence of a linear relationship between oxygen consumption (V_{O_2}) and the generated mechanical energy, which is quantified by the pressure–volume area (PVA) in the LV pressure–volume plane:

$$V_{O_2} = a \cdot PVA + b \qquad (1)$$

where the PVA corresponds to the mechanical energy generated by the Xbs and utilized by the actomyosin ATPase; a and b are constants [1], where b represents the energy consumed by the Ca–ATPase, the Na–K pumps and the basal metabolic energy consumption. The mechanical energy, PVA, is the sum of the external work (EW) done by the LV and the mechanical potential energy (PE), i.e.,

$$PVA = EW + PE \qquad (2)$$

where the potential energy (PE) is defined as the elastic energy generated during the contraction and stored at the end systole in the LV wall [2].

Using ferret papillary muscle fibers, Hisano and Cooper [2] have shown that the force–length area (FLA), the cardiac fiber analog of the ventricular PVA for the mechanical energy, is also closely correlated with oxygen consumption (V_{O_2}), i.e.:

$$V_{O_2} = a^* \cdot FLA + b^* \qquad (3)$$

where a^* and b^* are constants. The FLA is quantitatively defined, similar to the ventricular PVA, as the sum of the external work and the potential energy. This linear relationship between the FLA and oxygen consumption at the level of the muscle fiber (Eq. (3)) suggests that the linear relationship between PVA and V_{O_2} at the LV level (Eq. (1)) is an integrated result of the basic characteristics of the myocytes.

The second basic feature of the control of energy consumption and the generated mechanical energy is the dependence on the prevailing loading conditions and the ability of the cardiac muscle to modulate energy consumption; The generated pressure and ejected volume, and hence the mechanical energy, depend on the preload, as defined by the Frank–Starling law. The dependence of energy consumption on the afterload is best described by the Fenn effect [3], which was originally discovered in the frog sartorius muscle by Fenn in 1923 [4]: the cardiac muscle and the skeletal muscle mobilize energy more than the amount needed for activation and the equivalent isometric contraction during shortening, and the excess energy accounts for the work and dissipation of energy accompanying the work process [5]. The cardiac muscle, like the skeletal muscle, can adjust its energy cost to the prevailing mechanical constrains, after the stimulation, during the contraction [3, 5]. The questions that arises: How does the LV adapts its energy consumption to the loading conditions? What is the mechanism that sustains the linear relationship between energy consumption and the generated mechanical energy?

The control of the generation of mechanical energy and the regulation of energy consumption by the actomyosin–ATPase are analyzed here by utilizing our earlier suggested control mechanisms [6–10] of the sarcomere. These control mechanisms are based on biochemical studies of calcium kinetics and Xb cycling. Our previous studies have established the existence of two intracellular feedback mechanisms: a positive feedback, i.e., the cooperativity mechanism [7], and a negative feedback, i.e., mechanical feedback [8].

The *cooperativity mechanism*, originally based on the analysis of the force–length–free calcium relationship in skinned cardiac fibers [7], was recently validated at the LV level by utilizing the strain–stress–free calcium relationship obtained from isolated tetanized ferret hearts [10]. The cooperativity mechanism relates the affinity of troponin for calcium to the number of Xbs in the strong, force generating, conformation. It determines the amount of bound calcium to troponin, and hence the rate of force generation and energy consumption. The cooperativity mechanism explains the FLR and the related Frank–Starling law [6, 7]; it also explains [9] the linear relationship between the energy consumption and the force–time integral (FTI) [2, 11], as well as the linear relationship between energy consumption and the FLA [2] for isometric contraction. Moreover, the cooperativity is an adaptive feedback mechanism that enable the muscle to modify energy consumption according to the prevailing loading conditions.

The *negative mechanical feedback* [8] assures that the rate of Xb weakening, i.e., the rate of transition from the strong, force generating conformation to the weak, non–force generation conformation, is linearly dependent on the filament shortening velocity. This mechanism is substantiated [8] by the analytical derivation of the force–velocity relationship (FVR), in agreement with the well established, experimentally derived, Hill's equation. A detailed description of the dependence of the shortening velocity on various physiological parameters as the rate of Xb cycling, internal load, calcium kinetics, sarcomere length, the time during the contraction, are given elsewhere [8], in agreement with experimental studies [12, 13]. The negative mechanical feedback determines the generated power [6, 8] and is the key element in understanding the regulation of energy conversion from biochemical to mechanical energy: this mechanical feedback provides the analytical solution for the general equation of energy conversion in the muscle, and the linear relationship between energy consumption and mechanical energy, i.e., the liberated heat and external work.

THE PHYSIOLOGICAL MODEL

The basic assumptions underlying the model are detailed elsewhere [6, 8] and only the most relevant ones are briefly summarized here for coherency and convenience.

1) The regulatory unit is a single regulatory troponin–tropomyosin complex, with the fourteen neighboring actin molecules, and the adjacent heads of the myosin.

2) The Xb cycles between the weak non–force generating conformation and the strong force generating conformation due to nucleotide binding and release. The hydrolysis of ATP occurs as the Xb turns from the weak to the strong conformation [14, 15]. Thus, energy consumption is proportional to the total amount of Xb turnover from the weak to the strong conformation.

3) The individual Xb act like a Newtonian viscoelastic element: the FVR of a single Xb is linear [12], based on simultaneous measurements of the generated force, shortening velocity and the dynamic stiffness.

4) Calcium binding to the low affinity troponin sites regulates the actomyosin ATPase activity [16] and the rate of phosphate dissociation from the myosin–ADP–P complex, which is required for the transition of the Xbs to the strong conformation [15].

Thus, calcium binding to troponin regulates Xb recruitment and the energy consumption by the sarcomere.

        To couple calcium binding and dissociation from troponin and Xb cycling between the weak and the strong conformation, the troponin regulatory units are divided into four different states, as is depicted in Fig. 1. State R_s represents the rest state; the Xbs are in the weak conformation and no calcium is bound to the troponin. Calcium binding to troponin leads to State A_s. State A_s denotes regulatory units "activated" by calcium binding, but the adjacent Xbs are still in the weak conformation. Thus, State A_s represents the level of the mechanical activation, i.e., the number of available Xbs in the weak conformation that can turn to the strong, force generating, conformation (see below). Xb turnover from weak to strong conformation leads to State T_s where calcium is bound to the low affinity sites and the Xbs are in the strong conformation. Calcium dissociation at State T_s leads to State U_s, in which the Xbs are still in the strong conformation but without bound calcium.

THE MATHEMATICAL MODEL

The State Variables

        We define $\bar{R}_s$, $\bar{A}_s$, $\bar{T}_s$, $\bar{U}_s$ as the densities of the four troponin states existing within the single–overlap region. For example, $\bar{R}_s = R_s/L_s$, where L_s is the length of the single–overlap. The transitions between the density state variables within the single–overlap region are given by:

$$
\begin{pmatrix} \dot{\bar{R}}_s \\ \dot{\bar{A}}_s \\ \dot{\bar{T}}_s \\ \dot{\bar{U}}_s \end{pmatrix} = \begin{pmatrix} -K_\ell & \kappa_{-\ell} & 0 & g_0+g_1V \\ K_\ell & -f-\kappa_{-\ell} & g_0+g_1V & 0 \\ 0 & f & -(g_0+g_1V)-\kappa_{-\ell} & K_\ell \\ 0 & 0 & \kappa_{-\ell} & -(g_0+g_1V)-K_\ell \end{pmatrix} \cdot \begin{pmatrix} \bar{R}_s \\ \bar{A}_s \\ \bar{T}_s \\ \bar{U}_s \end{pmatrix}
\tag{4}
$$

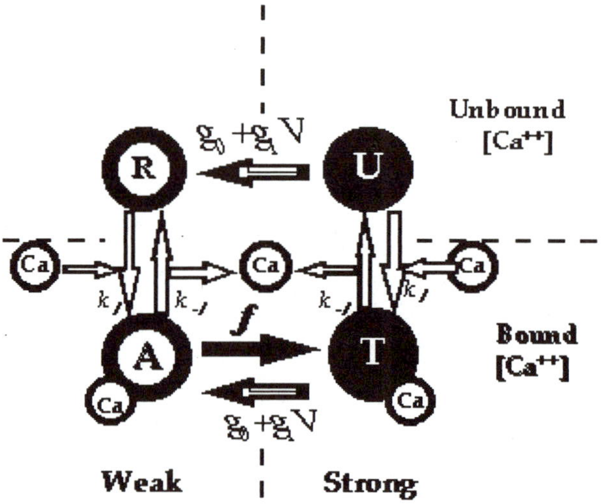

Figure 1. The transitions between the four–states of the troponin regulatory units are defined by calcium kinetics and crossbridge cycling rates.

where $K_\ell = \kappa_\ell \cdot [Ca]$; $[Ca]$ denotes the free calcium concentration. The rate coefficients κ_ℓ and $\kappa_{-\ell}$ represent the rate constants of calcium binding to, and calcium dissociation from, the low affinity sites of troponin. Note that the rate coefficient $\kappa_{-\ell}$ is not constant since the cooperativity mechanism dictates the dependence of this coefficient on the state variables [7, 10]. Xb cycling is described by f, g_0 and g_1; f is the rate of Xb turn–over from the weak to the strong conformation and g_0 is the rate of Xb weakening in the isometric contraction regime. g_1 is the magnitude of the mechanical feedback; it describes the effect of the filament shortening velocity on the rate of Xb weakening and has the units of $[1/m]$. V is the sarcomere shortening velocity.

The force (F) generated by the sarcomere is the product of the number of force generating Xbs in the single–overlap region, $(T_s + U_s)$, and the average force generated by each Xb. According to Assumption 3:

$$F = L_s \cdot (\overline{T}_s + \overline{U}_s) \cdot (\overline{F} - \eta V) \tag{5}$$

where $\overline{F}$ is the unitary isometric force developed by each regulatory unit and η represents the viscous element property of the Xb.

The Activation Level, Force Generation and Energy Consumption

Ford (9) has defined the mechanical activation level as the ability of the muscle to generate new force–producing Xbs. The number of force generating Xbs $(T_s + U_s)$, in the single overlap region, is given by:

$$\frac{d(T_s + U_s)}{dt} = f \cdot A_s - (g_0 + g_1 \cdot V) \cdot (T_s + U_s) \tag{6}$$

The ability of the muscle to generate new force–producing Xbs is determined by state A_s. Therefore, the equivalent definition here for the activation level is the number of available Xbs in the weak conformation that can turn to the strong force generating confor–mation, i.e., State A_s. Moreover, the transition from State A_s to State T_s describes Xb cycling from the weak to the strong conformation, which requires one ATP hydrolysis and phosphate release [14, 15] per each Xb turnover from the weak to the strong confirmation. Thus, the rate of ATP hydrolysis by the actomyosin–ATPase, $\dot{E}$, is determined by the amount of available Xbs in the weak conformation that can turn to the strong conformation, i.e., state A_s, and by the rate of Xb turnover, f, from the weak to the strong conformation:

$$\dot{E} = A_s f \tag{7}$$

Thus, the activation level, State A_s, defines the rate of force generation as well as the rate of energy consumption.

RESULTS

Isometric Contractions and the Cooperativity Mechanisms

The FTI is the integral of the force over the time duration of the twitch. For isometric contraction, where V=0, the average unitary force $\overline{F}$ generated by each Xb is constant, and the force (Eq. (5)) is proportional to the number of Xbs in the strong conformation. The FTI is obtained by utilizing Eqs. (5) and (6):

$$FTI = \int_0^T F(t) \cdot dt = \overline{F} \cdot \int_0^T \{T_s(t) + U_s(t)\} \cdot dt = \overline{F} \cdot \frac{f}{g_0} \cdot \int_0^T A_s(t) dt = \frac{\overline{F}}{g_0} E \qquad (8)$$

Equation (8) states that the FTI is proportional to E, the energy consumption by the Xbs at isometric contraction. This theoretically derived linear relationship between FTI and E was experimentally shown by Alpert et al. [11] and Hisano and Cooper [2]. Moreover, The energy consumption at isometric contraction also correlates with the FLA [2]. The total amount of energy consumed by the Xbs at isometric contraction is given by

$$E = N_{Xb} \cdot \overline{E}_{Xb} \qquad (9)$$

where N_{Xb} is the amount of Xbs that were in the strong conformation during the twitch, and $\overline{E}_{Xb}$ represents the average energy consumption per single Xb at isometric contraction.
Combining Eqs. (3) and (9) for a differential length change, dL, yields the relationship between the increase in the number of cycling Xbs, dN_{Xb}, and the increase in the sarcomere length [9]:

$$\frac{dN_{Xb}}{dL} = \frac{a*}{\overline{E}_{Xb}} \cdot F_M(L) \qquad (10)$$

where F_M is the peak isometric force.
The experimentally derived linear correlation between the FLA and the energy consumption [8, 10] suggests that the change in Xb recruitment depends on the prevailing number of force generating Xbs. This conclusion is in accordance with the previously suggested cooperativity mechanism [6, 10], whereby calcium affinity, and hence Xb recruitment, depend on the magnitude of the generated isometric force, i.e., on the number of force generating Xbs.
The four state model can not describe the linear correlation between the FLA and energy consumption without the cooperativity mechanism [9], as in that case, the coefficients (k_ℓ, $k_{-\ell}$, f and g_0) in Eq. (4) are constants, and State A_s, and the energy consumption according to Eq. (6), are independent of the sarcomere length. Thus, without a cooperativity mechanism there is a dissociation between energy consumption and the generated force and mechanical energy: the energy expenditure is constant and independent of the muscle length while the force is length dependent [9].
The effect of incorporating the cooperativity mechanism is shown in the simulations of isometric contractions of cardiac fibers at various sarcomere lengths (Fig. 2). Figure 2A depicts the time course of the force at various sarcomere lengths. Figure 2B depicts the FLA and the FTI against the energy consumption at the different sarcomere lengths. The cooperativity mechanism provides the tight linkage between the energy consumption and the FLA or the FTI (Fig. 2B) at isometric contractions.

Shortening Beats and the Mechanical Feedback

During the isotonic contraction (dF/dt = 0) the shortening velocity reaches steady state (dV/dt = 0), and Eqs. (4) and (5) reduce to Hill's equation for the FVR:

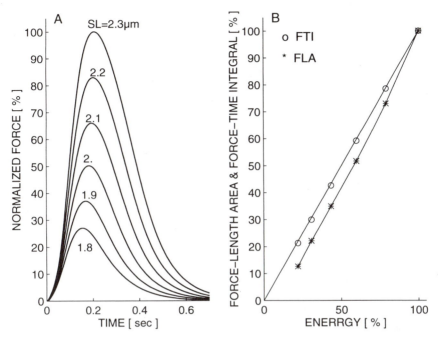

Figure 2. Simulated isometric contraction at various sarcomere lengths, accounting for the cooperativity mechanism. **A)** Time course of force development. **B)** The relation between force–length area, *, or the force–time integral (o), and the energy consumption by the Xbs.

$$V = b_H \frac{F_M - F}{F + a_H} = \frac{g_0(F_M - F)}{\left\{ \left(g_1 + \frac{1}{L_s} \right) F + \frac{g_0 F_M}{V_u} \right\}} \tag{11}$$

where V_u is the unloaded shortening velocity, and Hill's constants are given by:

$$a_H = \frac{g_0}{g_1 + L_s^{-1}} \cdot \frac{F_M}{V_U} = b_H \cdot \frac{F_M}{V_u} \qquad\qquad b_H = \frac{g_0}{g_1 + L_s^{-1}} \cong \frac{g_0}{g_1} \tag{12}$$

Equation (11) provides the physiological meaning for the experimentally derived Hill's constants a_H and b_H.

Figure 3 describes the FVR and the power load relationship for three different amplitudes of the mechanical feedback. The power output depends on the curvature of the FVR, and thus on the mechanical feedback.

As described by Alpert *et al.* [11], the curvature of the FVR is determined by the ratio a_H/F_M. The increase in the power output is consistent with the increase in the ratio a_H/F_M. However, Eq. (12) suggests that the ratio a_H/F_M is a function of the mechanical feedback g_1, since $a_H/F_M = g_0/g_1 \cdot V_u$. Thus, the smaller the mechanical feedback, g_1, the smaller the curvature of the FVR and the higher the power as a function of the load.

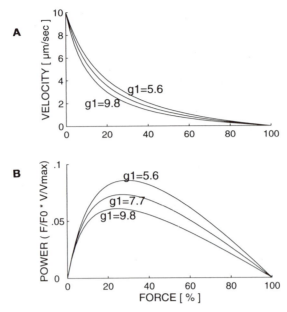

Figure 3. The curvature of the force–velocity relationship (FVR) and the generated power output depends on the magnitude of the mechanical feedback g_1.

The energy consumption and the generated mechanical energy are calculated from the amount of Xbs that participate in the Xb cycle during contraction. The general equation for energy conversion is obtained by solving Eq. (6):

$$\int_0^T f A_s(t) \cdot dt = \frac{g_0}{\overline{F}} \int_0^T F(t) dt + \frac{1}{\overline{F}} \left(g_1 + \eta \frac{g_0}{\overline{F}} \right) \cdot \left[\int_0^T F(t) V(t) dt + \int_0^T \frac{F(t) V(t)^2}{V_U - V} dt \right] \tag{13}$$

Multiplying both sides of the equation by $\overline{F}/(g_1 + \eta g_0/\overline{F})$ gives:

$$\rho \cdot E = PE + W + Q\eta \tag{14}$$

where:

$$W = \int_0^T F(t) V(t) dt \quad ; \quad Q\eta = \int_0^T \frac{F(t) V(t)^2}{V_U - V} dt \quad ;$$

$$PE = \frac{g_0}{g_1 + \eta \dfrac{g_0}{\overline{F}}} \int_0^T F(t) dt \quad ; \quad \rho = \frac{\overline{F}}{g_1 + \eta \dfrac{g_0}{\overline{F}}} \tag{15}$$

E is the ATP consumption during the twitch (Eq. 7), W is the external work. The potential energy is proportional to the FTI for the isometric contraction. $Q\eta$ represents energy

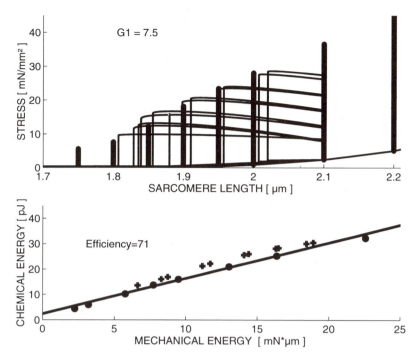

Figure 4. (Top) Isometric contraction at different sarcomere lengths (bold curve) and physiological contraction, starting from the same preload but with different afterloads. **(Bottom)** The linear relationship between energy consumption and the generated mechanical energy, for both the isometric contractions (dots) and shortening beats (+).

dissipation due to the viscoelastic property of the Xb ([15], Assumption 3). Qη represents the viscous component since it is the integral over the force multiplied by the square of the velocity, (and by even higher degree of the velocity). ρ is the efficiency of the biochemical to mechanical energy conversion.

Figure 4 (top) depicts one set of isometric contraction at different sarcomere lengths, and one set of physiological contractions, starting from the same preload but with different afterloads. The afterload is described by the Windkessel model. A linear relationship is obtained between energy consumption and the generated mechanical energy (Fig. 4, bottom). Note that the mechanical energy was calculated here by the FLA (i.e., without the viscous term) according to Suga [1]. The calculated efficiency is 71%.

DISCUSSION

As shown here, the two feedback mechanisms that regulate sarcomere dynamics and determine the FLR and FVR, also regulate the energy consumption and the generated mechanical energy of the muscle. The cooperativity mechanism determines the FLR [6, 7] of the cardiac muscle fiber, and the stress–strain relationship at the LV level [10]. This describes the dependence of the affinity of troponin for calcium on the number of Xbs in the strong conformation, and is the dominant feedback mechanism that regulates calcium binding to troponin [6, 10]. This mechanism is responsible for the "length dependent calcium sensitivity", i.e., the increase in calcium sensitivity with increasing sarcomere length [7]. Thus, the cooperativity mechanism determines the FLR and suggests the basic intracellular mechanism for the Frank–Starling Law.

Calcium binding to troponin regulates Xb recruitment [16] and determines the amount of the activated actomyosin ATPase. Xb cycling from the weak to the strong conformation requires the hydrolysis of ATP. Hence, the cooperativity mechanism, which determines calcium affinity, regulates both the generated force [6, 10] and the energy consumption [9]. Moreover, it provides the linear correlation between energy consumption and the generated mechanical energy, defined either by the FLA or the FTI, in isometric contraction. The cooperativity mechanism provides the feedback loop whereby the afterload and changes in the loading conditions, as quick releases can affect the kinetics of calcium binding to troponin, the amount of the bound calcium, and the energy consumption. This explains the ability of the muscle to adapt to loading conditions.

The mechanical feedback, required by energetic considerations, originates from the biochemical studies of Eisenberg and Hill [15], who have suggested that the filament sliding velocity affects the rate of Xb weakening. The magnitude of the mechanical feedback is described by the parameter g_1, which determines the effect of the filament shortening velocity on the rate of Xb weakening. The existence of this mechanism was substantiated previously [6, 8]. The analytically derived Hill's equation for the FVR (Eq. (11)) strengthens the notion of the capability of the mechanical feedback to describe muscle mechanics. Hill's parameters a_H and b_H are inversely dependent on the mechanical feedback, g_1. The mechanical feedback regulates the generated power, and this simple mechanism provides the linear relationship between energy consumption and the generated mechanical energy (Eq. (14)).

Campbell *et al.* [18] have studied the short time response of the LV pressure to quick and small amplitude changes in the volume, at various flow rates and various volumes. They have fitted their data to a two state model of pressure generators, and have found that the rate of turnover from the strong to the weak state increases with the increase in the velocity of shortening. Moreover, the rate of weakening depends only on the flow rate and was independent of the magnitude of the volume changes i.e., the rate of weakening depends only on the shortening velocity and is independent of the displacement itself. The results are in agreement with the mechanical feedback suggested here.

The mechanical feedback mechanism predicts that the energy consumption is linearly related to the mechanical energy, where the mechanical energy is defined as the sum of the external work, potential energy and energy dissipation as heat due to the viscous property of the Xbs. The efficiency, ρ, of the biochemical to mechanical energy conversion (Eq. (15)) is inversely proportional to the magnitude of the mechanical feedback.

Note that energy dissipation due to the viscous element is not included in the commonly accepted PVA model [1], where the mechanical energy is defined only as the sum of the work and the potential energy. Indeed, the contribution of the viscous element is relatively small at slow shortening velocities. However, it is not negligible when the shortening velocity approach the unloaded velocity.

The potential energy in the present model is determined by the FTI. The term "potential energy" is derived in analogy to the potential energy term in the elastance model [1]. According to the elastance model, no external work is done in isometric contraction, and all the energy consumption is stored as potential energy. At isometric contraction, the energy consumption is also proportional to the FTI. Hence, the FTI is equivalent to the potential energy, defined by Suga [1], for isometric contraction. Note that there are no conserving fields here, and the term "potential energy" differs from the classical physical definition in a conservation field. The "potential energy" used here is consumed during the contraction for force generation and can not be converted to an equal amount of work.

According to the elastance model, or an isometric contraction and an isometric contraction wherein a quick release is imposed at the time of peak force, have identical PVAs, and should have the same energy consumption. However, it was shown that quick releases imposed after end–systole at isometric contraction reduced the oxygen consumption [2]. This finding contradicts the elastance theory and the stipulation that the potential energy is stored in the elastic component till end–systole. Moreover, this also implies that energy is also consumed during the relaxation phase of the isometric contraction, which can not be described by the PVA concept, but is well described by the FTI. The potential energy here describes the energy consumption for force development, during contraction, and only part of it can be utilized for generation of external work.

The mechanical feedback in the present model describes the ability of the muscle to generate power, whereas the cooperativity mechanism determines the FLR and provides the cellular basis for the Frank–Starling law [6, 7]. Therefore, the LV performances and the related, commonly used, term "contractility" are determined by the interplay between the loading conditions and the intracellular control mechanisms: i.e., the mechanical feedback and the cooperativity [6].

The present description of the regulation of energy conversion, based on the intracellular control mechanism which couples calcium kinetics with Xb cycling, has other advantages which were not described here: it explains the Fenn effect [3, 13], and provides the cellular parameters that determine the efficiency and the economy of muscle contraction. These important features are presently under study.

CONCLUSIONS

The biochemical based intracellular control model which describes the basic mechanical properties of the cardiac muscle, i.e., the FLR and the FVR, is extended here to describe the control of energy consumption and mechanical energy generation.

The cooperativity mechanism and the mechanical feedback play a key role in the regulation of energy consumption and the generated mechanical energy. The cooperativity mechanism regulates energy consumption and provides the linear relationship between the energy consumption and the FTI or the FLA, for isometric contractions. Moreover, it explains the effect of changes in the loading condition on energy consumption. The mechanical feedback that determines the FVR, regulates the generated power and provides the linear relationship between energy consumption and the generated mechanical energy.

The analysis shows that the generated mechanical energy is made up of three components: the external work, and energy dissipation as heat due to the viscoelastic property of the Xbs the "potential energy" PE which is determined by the FTI. The contribution of the viscous term is relatively small, unless the shortening velocity approaches the unloaded velocity.

The present analysis provides insight into physiological observations, and describes cardiac muscle function based on better understanding of the intracellular interactions in the myocardium.

Acknowledgments

Particular thanks are due to Professor S. Sideman for his continuous support and generous advice. This study was initiated by the Levi–Eshkol Fellowship of the Ministry of Science and Arts, and by fellowship from the American Physician fellowship for Medicine in Israel. This work was financed by a Grant from the Germany–Israel Foundation (GIF).

DISCUSSION

Dr. Y. Lanir: I wonder about the rational of dividing the extra energy (on top of the work done) to viscoelastic heat loss and potential energy. It puzzles me since in your potential energy expression you have a purely viscous term (η). How were you able to separate between the two? Potential energy expression should not have any viscous effect in it.

Dr. A. Landesberg: The term potential energy (PE) used here is misleading, as there is no conservation of energy here. The term potential energy was borrowed from the commonly accepted concept of the PVA. Suga has defined the potential energy as the elastic energy stored in the LV wall at the end of systole. But the quick release experiments contradict this concept. The potential energy here is the energy cost for the force generation, which is proportional to the FTI. This energy can turn to heat or to work. The rate of energy turnover to heat is determined by g_0, while the maximal rate of energy turnover to work is defined by g_1 and the maximal shortening velocity. The maximal shortening velocity is limited by the viscoelastic properties of the Xbs. Therefore the so called potential energy is a function of the FTI, g_0, g_1 and η.

Dr. L. Cleemann: I understand that the elegance of your model is that it makes very few assumptions. One of them, however, troubles me. I have a hard time imagining your g_1 in molecular terms. Do you have any special molecular model in mind?

Dr. A. Landesberg: Not really. A clue to the molecular model can be obtained from the analysis of the relationship between g_0 and g_1 in various slow and fast muscle fibers. These parameters regulate the interplay between efficiency and economy of the muscle. One thing should be noted. The concept that the rate of weakening depends on the shortening velocity implies that the muscle can generate multiple stroke work steps per hydrolysis of one ATP.

Dr. H. ter Keurs: If I understand your model correctly, force development by the muscle is dictated by f, $g_0 + g_1 V$, where g_1 means the effect of shortening on the rate of Xbs going to the weak state. That means that if you would lengthen the muscle, you would make that term negative and you would be able to reach the maximal number, T+U. If you use your numbers, what is the predicted maximal force that you could achieve with lengthening the muscle? You could test that experimentally, because if you make the load higher than that, you break the Xbs off from the actin and the maximal load should be predictable by you.

Dr. A. Landesberg: The mechanical feedback can not predict the maximal generated force during lengthening, since it depends also on the average force generated by each crossbridge during lengthening. However, I can predict what should be the velocity at which the maximal force is obtained, and this velocity is equal to g_0/g_1, which is approximately equal to the tenth of the maximal shortening velocity ($0.1 * V_U$). It should be tested experimentally.

REFERENCES

1.   Suga Y. Ventricular energy. *Physiological Rev* 1990;70:247–277.
2.   Hisano G, Cooper IV. Correlation of force–length area with oxygen consumption in ferret papillary muscle. *Circ Res* 1987;61:318–328.
3.   Mommaerts WFHM, Seraydarian I, Marechal G. Work and mechanical change in isotonic muscular contractions. *Biochem Biophys Acta* 1962;57:1–12.

4. Fenn OW. A quantitative comparison between the energy liberation and the work performed by the isolated sartorious muscle of the frog. *J Physiol London* 1923;58:175–203.
5. Rall JA. Sense and nonsense about the Fenn effect. *Am J Physiol* 1982;242:H1–H6.
6. Landesberg A. End systolic pressure–volume relation based on the intracellular control of contraction. *Am J Physiol* 1996;270:H338–H349.
7. Landesberg A, Sideman S. Coupling calcium binding to Troponin–C and Xb cycling kinetics in skinned cardiac cells. *Am J Physiol* 1994;266(*Heart Circ Physiol* 35):H1261–H1271.
8. Landesberg A, Sideman S. Mechanical regulation in the cardiac muscle by coupling calcium binding to troponin–C and Xb cycling. A dynamic model. *Am J Physiol* 1994;267(*Heart Circ Physiol* 36): H779–H795.
9. Landesberg A, Sideman S. Regulation of energy consumption in the cardiac muscle; analysis of isometric contractions. *Am J Physiol* 1997; submitted.
10. Landesberg A, Burkhoff D, Sideman S. Calcium binding affinity based on stress–strain and free-calcium data from isolated ferret heart. *Am J Physiol* 1997; submitted.
11. Alpert NR, Mulieri LA, Hasenfuss G, Holubarsch C. Optimization of myocardial function. In: Burkhoff D, Schaefer J, Schaffner K, Yue DT, editors, Myocardial Optimization and Efficiency: Evolutionary Aspects and Philosophy of Science Considerations. Springer–Verlag: New York, (Basic Research in Cardiology, vol. 88, suppl. 2) 1993, pp. 29–41.
12. De Tombe PP, ter Keurs HEDJ. An internal viscous element limit unloaded velocity of sarcomere shortening in rat myocardium. *J Physiol Lond* 1992;454:619–642.
13. Daniels M, Nobel MIM, ter Kerus HEDJ, Wohlfart B. Velocity of sarcomere shortening in rat cardiac muscle: relationship to force, sarcomere length, calcium and time. *J Physiol* 1984;355;367–381.
14. Brenner B, Eisenberg E. Rate of force generation in muscle: correlation with actomyosin ATPase activity in solution. *Proc Natl Acad Sci* 1986;83:3542–3546.
15. Eisenberg E, Hill TL. Muscle contraction and free energy transduction in biological system. *Science* 1985;227:999–1006.
16. Chalovich JM, Eisenberg E. The effect of troponin – tropomyosin on the binding of heavy meromyosin to actin in the presence of ATP. *J Biol Chem* 1986;261:5088–5093.
17. Ford EL. Mechanical manifestations of activation in cardiac muscle. *Circ Res* 1991;68:621–637.
18. Campbell KB, Sharff SG, Kirkpatrick RD, Short time scale left ventricle systolic dynamics. *Circ Res* 1991;68:1532–1548.

CHAPTER 8

Myocardial Cell Energetics

Helmut Kammermeier[1]

ABSTRACT

Energy transformation at the main energy consuming processes of the myocardium takes place with high efficiency, i.e., with relatively small differences between the free energy level provided and the free energy level required for the two coupled processes. Thus, the free energy of ATP is only moderately higher than that of various ATP dependent processes. Under energy deficiency caused by hypoxia, free energy of ATP can drop to a level that critically affects subsequent steps. Detailed evaluation of cell energetics was carried out with the following approach: Cell shortening, oxygen consumption and intracellular calcium transients of isolated rat cardiomyocytes which were investigated under the influence of inotropic interventions. Increased extracellular Ca^{2+} and isoproterenol reduced the economy of contraction (contraction amplitude/$\dot{V}O_2$), whereas Ca−sensitizing agent EMD 57033 did not. This seems to be a consequence of the increased costs of ion cycling under the effect of Ca^{2+} and isoproterenol. Our current investigation suggests that alterations of ion transport processes and crossbridge kinetics have substantial impact on myocardial energetics.

INTRODUCTION

Energy flow through a myocardial cell can be considered from different points of view. Taking the point of view of input and output, according to the scheme in Fig. 1 representing average data, about 70% of energy available from substrate oxidation are preserved in the synthesis of ATP, the remainder being dissipated as heat. The main ATP consuming processes are the ion transport processes and the activity of the contractile system. Ion transport, mainly that of calcium, requires about 20 to 30% of ATP consumed

[1]Institute of Physiology, Faculty of Medicine, RWTH, Pauwelsstrasse 30, D 52057, Aachen, Germany

Analytical and Quantitative Cardiology
Edited by Sideman and Beyar, Plenum Press, New York, 1997

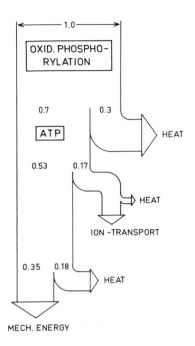

Figure 1. Energy flow through a myocardial cell.

and the contractile system about 70%. This results in an overall (maximum) efficiency of about 35%. Note that the efficiency in all these intermediate steps, i.e., the energy preserved in each downstream step, is above 70%.

This high efficiency can be considered from another point of view. The calculated energy provided from oxidation of 1 mol glucose available to synthesize one (out of 38) mole of ATP is 74 to 75 kJ (Fig. 2). Free energy of ATP hydrolysis depends on the ratio of $[ADP][P_i]/[ATP]$, i.e.:

$$\Delta G_{ATP} = \Delta G^{0'} + RT\ln \frac{[ADP][P_i]}{[ATP]} \tag{1}$$

and amounts to about 60 kJ/ mol in well oxygenated hearts [1, 7], and

$$\Delta G_{ion} = RT\ln \frac{[I_i]}{[I_e]} + zF\psi \tag{2}$$

where R = universal gas constant, T = absolute temperature, $[I_i]/[I_e]$ = ion concentration intra-/ extracellular, z = charge, F = Faraday constant, ψ = membrane potential [7], $\Delta G^{0'}$ = standard free energy of ATP (30.5 kJ/mol), ΔG_{ion} = free energy required (provided) to translocate (from translocation) (of) one mol of ions.

The energy demand of the ATP driven ion transport processes depends on the ion gradients, the electrical potential across the plasma and SR membranes, as well as on the stoichiometric ratios. It amounts to 41 to 54 kJ/ mol. It is interesting to note that for

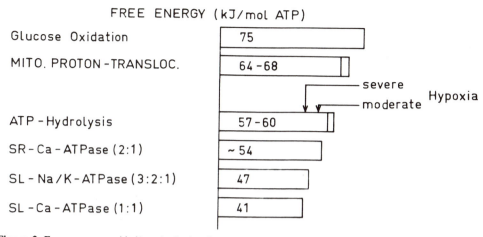

Figure 2. Free energy provided/required of various steps in free energy dependent processes calculated from cytosolic concentrations [1, 7].

thermodynamic reasons the sarcolemmal (SL)–Ca–transporter can only translocate one Ca^{2+} ion (even if it was a $Ca^{2+}/2H^+$ exchanger) as compared to two Ca^{2+} of the SR, since other– wise the energy required would exceed that available from ATP–hydrolysis. The energy requirement of the contractile system cannot be calculated directly, but the crossbridge cycle appears to take place with a fixed stoichiometry, and estimates of efficiency indicate a relatively high requirement of free energy, about 45 kJ/mol/ crossbridge cycle.

The relatively small steps between available and required free energy, together with the fixed stoichiometry, does not allow to utilize more ATP if its free energy is too low. This implies that ATP–dependent processes can fail, or be altered, and ion gradients and/or membrane potential cannot be maintained if the free energy of ATP is substantially reduced as, for instance, in hypoxia or ischemia (Fig. 2). This phenomenon has also recently been demonstrated for the SR/ Ca–accumulation in hypoxia [2].

The small steps in free energy, which occur with high efficiency, and the free energy dependence of the respective process are characteristic of the dominating energy transformation processes. This characteristic implies reversibility of the process under very special conditions, e.g. ATP–synthesis by the SR–Ca^{2+}–ATPase, if ion gradients are experimentally manipulated in a way that the energy required exceeds that of ATP substantially [3]. On the other hand, many other cellular processes hardly depend on the free energy level, since the free energy step is very large and free energy of ATP is sufficient, even if rather low. Many phosphorylation processes and reactions of protein synthesis occur through this type of energy transformation. Consequently, these processes can also take place under conditions of severe energy deficiency.

CHARACTERIZING CELL ENERGETICS

An attempt to characterize the energetics of myocardial cells in more detail was made with the following methodological approach: We developed a chamber which allows simultaneous measurement of oxygen consumption and a detailed evaluation of cell shortening of electrically stimulated isolated cardiomyocytes. Moreover, samples of the cell suspension can be ejected for investigation of sarcolemmal transport processes. Cell shortening is recorded from image processing of 10 to 30 consecutive images with stepwise increase of stimulation–flash exposure–delay. The technical details are given elsewhere [4]. It was also our aim to record shortening of a representative number of cells for correlation with $\dot{V}O_2$ of whole cell suspension of several 100,000 cells.

RESULTS

Experimental recordings of cell shortening and calcium transients are shown in Fig. 3, demonstrating the characteristic changes induced by inotropic interventions. Representative results obtained in measuring PO_2 are shown in Fig. 4. The slope of PO_2 in the chamber medium decreases in proportion to increased stimulation rate. One particular advantage of the isolated cell preparation is the possibility to stimulate at physiological frequencies.

Relating contraction amplitude to $\dot{V}O_2$ results in interesting differences between the various inotropic agents (Fig. 5). The relative increase in $\dot{V}O_2$ is substantially higher than the increase in contraction amplitude under the influence of isoproterenol and increased extracellular calcium. In contrast, upon addition of the presumed calcium–sensitizer EMD 57033, the increase in $\dot{V}O_2$ is equal or lower relative to the increase in the contraction amplitude. Note that the contraction, i.e., the shortening, is in principle an auxotonic contraction against the elastic forces of the cytoskeleton. Thus, the relative work performed against this elastic system with an assumed linear characteristics can be calculated in analogy to work performed via a spring.

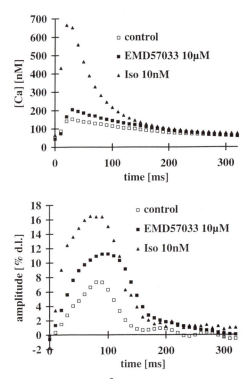

Figure 3. Course of contraction and cytosolic Ca^{2+} (Fluo 3) of isolated cardiomyocytes under the influence of positive inotropic interventions (isoproterenol, EMD 57033).

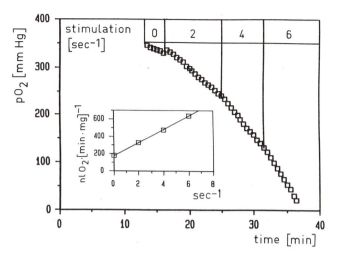

Figure 4. Medium PO_2 of a suspension of isolated rat cardiomyocytes and $\dot{V}O_2$ calculated from rate of PO_2-change as influenced by different stimulation rates (see [4] for method).

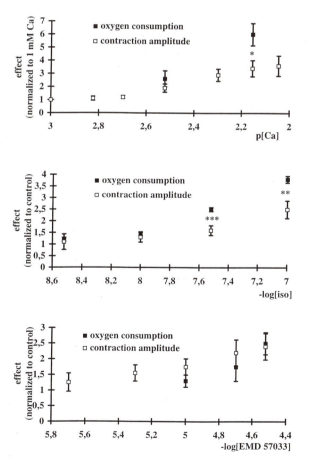

Figure 5. Concentration dependence of increase in contraction amplitude and $\dot{V}O_2$ of isolated cardiomyocytes under the influence of positive inotropic interventions.

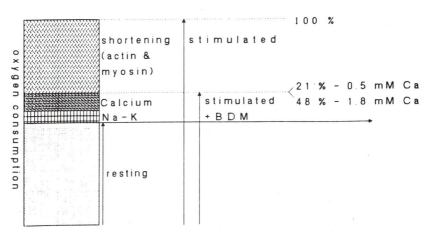

Figure 6. Oxygen consumption attributable to various processes of energy metabolism separated by stimulation and inhibition of actomyosin ATPase by BDM.

We have also attempted to investigate in detail the processes contributing to energy "consumption", e.g. those involved in ion transport. Energetic costs of ion transport can be estimated by selective blocking of the contractile activity. We did this by administration of butanedionemonoxime (BDM). Since BDM in high concentrations also affects ion exchange, we can reach the state of complete inhibition of the actomyosin ATPase from theprevailing effects of partial inhibition of contraction by increasing the concentrations of BDM. The oxygen consumption attributable to ion transports in our model with unloaded shortening cells amounts to 20 to 40%, depending on the extracellular calcium concentration (Fig. 6). We may assume that in loaded cells, or in the myocardium, this fraction will be lower owing to the increase in the fraction of energy consumption attributable to the external work performed.

DISCUSSION

The results shown above are in line with the notion of EMD being a calcium sensitizer. This could also be demonstrated directly by measuring the cytosolic calcium gradients (Fig. 3), where isoproterenol increases the contraction amplitude as well as the cytosolic calcium transients and EMD increases only the contraction amplitude.

In the simplest case, calcium sensitivity is reflected by the affinity of a calcium binding regulatory protein, such as troponin C. However, the kinetics of crossbridge cycling are also considered to be calcium dependent [5]. Thus, drugs such as EMD may act by influencing crossbridge kinetics, resulting in an apparent change of calcium sensitivity. Detailed evaluation of the course of contraction, as presented elsewhere [6], suggests changes of crossbridge cycling kinetics under the influence of EMD 57033.

Our present aim is to evaluate the impact of altered crossbridge kinetics on energy utilization. Following Brenner [5], the contractile process can be described by crossbridges being either in a force producing strong binding state S or in a non−force producing weak binding state W and by the transition kinetics of W → S (f) and S → W (g). Assuming a constant contribution to force of each crossbridge in the strong binding state, the force generation F is given by:

$$F \sim \frac{f}{f+g} \tag{3}$$

As one ATP is supposed to be hydrolysed during each crossbridge cycle, the energy turnover, or cycling rate, P is given by

$$P \sim \frac{fg}{f+g} \tag{4}$$

and the economy of force generation E

$$E \sim \frac{\text{Force}}{\text{Energy turnover}} \sim \frac{1}{g} \tag{5}$$

Thus, modulating g should have an impact on the economy. However, f and g change rapidly in a twitch contraction, relative to the time resolution possible by measuring $\dot{V}O_2$. Steady state conditions can be achieved by tetanic contraction caused by blocking the SR by ryanodine [8]. We are presently studying this model and hope to be able to determine the metabolic impact of alternating g, and the factors influencing g, in the near future.

DISCUSSION

Dr. N. Alpert: With regard to using g for the economy, if g represents the detachment rate, and that is related to the attachment time of the crossbridge, you are assuming that the unitary force and duty cycle are unchanged. But both the unitary force and the duty cycle might be changed; how can you account for that? The unitary force is the force that a single crossbridge develops. The attachment time is the length of time that it stays on; the duty cycle is the attachment time divided by the cycling time. The average force that you get in the muscle is the unitary force times the duty cycle. Somehow or other, you have to reconcile all those things with simply using g to determine the economy.

Dr. H. Kammermeier: We cannot exclude changes of the unitary force due to pharmacological interventions, which would indeed change the economy. However, as the dependence of f and/or g, and thus of the duty cycle (=f/(f+g)) on shortening velocity seems to be substantiated, I merely mentioned implications of that dependence on twitch contractions. We are trying to tackle this problem by measuring under twitch as well as under tetanus conditions.

Dr. A. Landesberg: The economy is used only for isometric contraction. If the definition of economy is the force–tension integral divided by the tension–dependent heat, it is very accurate for isometric contraction. For shortening contraction the question of economy is very complex? During shortening we expect that there will be changes of the duration of the crossbridges in the strong conformation. Eisenberg and Hill [*Eisenberg E, Hill TL. Muscle contraction and free energy transduction in biological system. Science 1985;227:999–1006*] showed a shortening velocity effect on the duration of the crossbridge in the strong conformation.

Dr. L. Cleemann: Could you tell us what fraction of the ion cycling energy goes into removal of calcium via the SL and the SR?

Dr. H. Kammermeier: We did not separate the two processes. I believe there are major species differences, where SR dominates in the rat heart, but we did not differentiate.

Dr. M. Morad: I know it is very fashionable to measure single myocytes, but why was it necessary to use single myocytes instead of an isometric type of measurement that you could very easily have in your chamber?

Dr. H. Kammermeier: It is not that simple. For trabeculae, you can get metabolic signals in the form of heat, but you don't have oxygen consumption, i.e., total energy turnover. There is quite a significant difference between heat liberation and oxygen consumption. We started with this chamber primarily to investigate transport processes. However, the preparations have much improved since we started, so it is time now to proceed with very small preparations, such as are made available in human preparations.

Dr. H. ter Keurs: How many cells do you need for calcium transport measurements and metabolic measurements?

Dr. H. Kammermeier: The metabolic measurements for oxygen consumption we did also for glucose and fatty acid transport. You need, say, 30% of what you get from a heart. That means millions of cells. Contraction measurements are done with a few cells, not only one.

Dr. H. ter Keurs: That limits the use of trabeculae because they are on average 5000 cells.

Dr. H. Kammermeier: Yes, maybe one can do it with a very small chamber.

REFERENCES

1.   Kammermeier H. Meaning of energetic parameters. *Basic Res Cardiol* 1993;88:380–384.
2.   Tian R, Ingwall JS. Energetic basis for reduced contractile reserve in isolated rat hearts. *Am J Physiol* 1996;270:H1207–H1216.
3.   Hasselbach W, Oetliker H. Energetics and electrogeneity of sarcoplasmic reticulum calcium pump. *Annu Rev Physiol* 1983;45:335–339.
4.   Rose H, Strotmann KH, Pöpping S, Fischer Y, Kulsch D, Kammermeier H. Simultaneous measurement of contraction and oxygen consumption in cardiac myocytes. *Am J Physiol* 1991;261:H1329–H1334.
5.   Brenner B. Effect of Ca^{2+} on cross–bridge turnover kinetics in skinned single rabbit psoas fibers. Implications for regulation of muscle contraction. *Proc Natl Acad Sci USA* 1988;85:3265–3269.
6.   Pöpping S, Mruck S, Fischer Y, Kulsch D, Ionescu I, Kammermeier H, Rose H. Economy of contraction of cardiomyocytes as influenced by different positive inotropic interventions. *Am J Physiol* 1996;271:H357–H364.
7.   Kammermeier H, Schmidt P, Jüngling E. Free energy change of ATP–hydrolysis a causal factor of early hypoxic failure of the myocardium. *J Mol Cell Cardiol* 1982;14:267–277.
8.   Landesberg A. Private communication. 1996.

CHAPTER 9

HUMAN HEART FAILURE:
DETERMINANTS OF VENTRICULAR DYSFUNCTION

Norman R. Alpert and Louis A. Mulieri[1]

ABSTRACT

Thin muscle strips were obtained from non–failing (NF) and failing (dilated cardiomyopathy (DCM)) hearts, using a new harvesting and dissection technique. The strips were used to carry out a myothermal and mechanical analysis so that contractile and excitation coupling phenomena in the NF and failing (DCM–F) preparations can be compared. Peak isometric force and rate of relaxation in DCM–F were reduced 46% ($p < 0.02$) while time to peak tension was increased 14% ($p < 0.03$). Initial, tension dependent, tension independent and the rate of tension independent heat liberation were reduced 62–70% in DCM–F ($p<0.03$). The crossbridge force–time integral (FTI_{XBr}) was calculated from these measurements and was shown to increase 40% while the amount and rate of calcium cycled per beat was reduced 70%. As a result of these changes in the contractile and excitation–contraction coupling systems in DCM–F, the force–frequency relationship was significantly blunted while the power output was markedly reduced. These fundamental alterations account for the substantial ventricular dysfunction found in the dilated cardiomyopathic failing heart.

INTRODUCTION

Congestive heart failure continues to be a major health problem with an unacceptably high morbidity and mortality. The available therapeutic interventions do not markedly improve the long term survival of patients with heart failure secondary to mitral

---

[1]Department of Molecular Physiology and Biophysics, University of Vermont College of Medicine, Burlington, Vermont 05405 USA

regurgitation or dilated cardiomyopathy. In this presentation we show that the compromised cardiac output and inadequate response of the failing heart to increased demand is directly related to alterations in the contractile and excitation–contraction coupling systems. Muscle strips from dilated cardiomyopathic human hearts (DCM–F), obtained at the time of transplant, are compared with epicardial strips from non–failing (NF) hearts using a mechanical–myothermal analysis to provide information about the myosin crossbridge cycle and beat to beat calcium cycling.

METHODS

Experimental Tissues

The experimental plan calls for the use of human heart tissue free from ischemic damage or fibrosis. Accordingly, tissue strips were chosen from the hearts at the time of transplant and from NF hearts that met these criteria. DCM–F were made available at the time of transplant, thus allowing the selection of muscle strips free of ischemic insult and with no visible scarring. Epicardial strips from NF hearts, consisting of longitudinally coursing fibers with no ischemic or fibrotic damage, were obtained at the time of coronary artery by–pass surgery (1.5 x 1.5 x 12 mm) [1, 2]. The seven non–failing strips came from patients with normal left ventricular function, no signs of failure and an average ejection fraction of $67 \pm 2\%$. The six patients with end–stage dilated cardiomyopathy, whose hearts were used in this study, had an ejection fraction of $13 \pm 1\%$ and a functional classification NYHA IV [3]. Tissue from the failing and NF hearts was quickly placed in the BDM protective solution (Krebs Ringer containing 30 mM 2, 3–butanedione monoxime, bubbled with 95 5 O_2–5 CO_2, and (in mM) Na^+–152; K^+–3.6; Cl^-–135; HCO_3^-–25; Mg^{++}–0.6; $H_2PO_4^-$–1.3; SO_4^-–0.6; Ca^{++}–2.5; glucose–11.2; insulin–101 U/I [1, 2]. Very thin muscle strips are prepared by placing the excised tissue in the BDM protective solution and, after a 60 min recovery period, sculpting strips approximately 0.2 mm diameter [1, 4]. Loops of 4–0 noncapillary braided silk, previously wired with 25 μm diameter platinum stimulating electrodes, were attached to the ends of the muscle strips with silk ligatures.

The muscles were allowed to recover for an additional 30 min. At that point the muscle was then mounted on the thermopile, positioned so that the flat end of the muscle was apposed to the hot junctions of the pile, with the top end of the muscle attached to a force transducer and the bottom end fixed to a stationary hook as previously described [5, 6].

Myothermal and Mechanical Measurements

The techniques for carrying out mechanical and myothermal measurements have been described in detail elsewhere [5, 6]. After the muscle is appropriately positioned on the thermopile, the muscle and thermopile are incubated in normal Krebs for 90 min to thoroughly wash out the BDM. After replacing the washout solution the muscle is stimulated while being stretched in small increments (0.05 mm) until the length is reached at which maximum active force is developed (l_{max}). The chamber with the muscle and thermopile is then drained of solution and the measurements of force and heat production are made. All measurements are carried out at 37°C.

Analysis of Mechanical and Myothermal Data

When a muscle is stimulated, isometric force is developed (Fig. 1, bottom) and there is a rapid evolution of heat resulting from force development, relaxation and recovery processes (Fig. 1, top). This heat output is the total activity related heat production (T_A). The muscle heat production is liberated in two phases, a rapid initial phase and a secondary slower phase. The secondary slower phase is liberated at a monoexponentially decreasing rate and thus can readily be extrapolated to zero time. This is the recovery heat production (R) and represents the heat output associated with the mitochondrial resynthesis of ATP from ADP produced during contraction and relaxation. Subtracting the recovery heat from the total activity related heat results in the initial heat (I) (Eq. (1), Fig. 1).

$$I = T_A - R \tag{1}$$

The initial heat can be partitioned into a tension dependent heat (TDH) component associated with crossbridge cycling and a tension independent heat (TIH) component associated with the excitation–contraction coupling phenomena (Eq. (2), Fig. 1).

$$I = TDH + TIH \tag{2}$$

This is accomplished by incubating the muscle strip in a BDM Krebs solution (@ 5 mM) which eliminates force and TDH, leaving a triggerable heat that represents TIH. TIH is then subtracted from I to give the TDH [7]. The TDH and the isometric force–time integral (FTI) of the muscle (FTI_{muscle}) can be used to calculate the average crossbridge FTI (FTI_{XBr}). The rationale is that FTI_{muscle} is the sum of FTI_{XBr} that occur in a half sarcomere during contraction and relaxation. Thus, FTI_{XBr} can be obtained by dividing FTI_{muscle} by the number of crossbridge cycles that occur in a half sarcomere during contraction and relaxation (N_{XBrCyc}) (Eq. (3)).

$$FTI_{XBr} = FTI_{muscle} / (N_{XBrCyc}) \tag{3}$$

The number N_{XBrCyc} is obtained by dividing the TDH per half sarcomere ($TDH_{half\ sarc}$) by the enthalpy for hydrolyzing one high energy phosphate bond (56 pnJ) (Eq. (4)).

$$(N_{XBrCyc}) = (TDH_{half\ sarc}) / 56\ pnJ \tag{4}$$

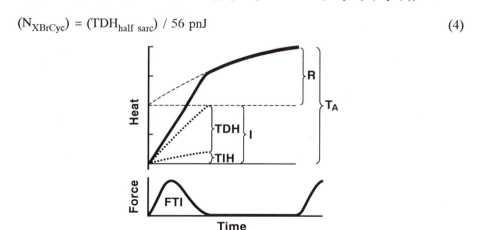

Figure 1. The time course of isometric force development (bottom) and heat production.

TIH can be used to calculate the amount of calcium cycled per gram of muscle during each contraction relaxation cycle (Eq. (5)).

$$Ca^{++}/gram-cycle = (TIH/gram)/(34 \text{ kJ/mole}) [Ca^{++}:CrP \text{ coupling ratio} \cdot K] \quad (5)$$

The Ca^{++}:CrP coupling ratio is assumed to be 2 for the sarcoplasmic reticulum transport [8] while K is a factor that takes into consideration contributions other than the sarcoplasmic reticulum to TIH (K = 0.75) [7]. A detailed discussion of the rationale and background for these calculations has been presented elsewhere [7, 9].

Statistical Significance

The difference between groups was assessed by use of an unpaired t test where $p < 0.05$ was considered to be significant.

RESULTS

Mechanical and Thermal Measurements

Table 1 summarizes the mechanical and myothermal data from the NF and DCM–F hearts. The isometric force (P_0), time to peak tension (TPT) and rate of relaxation (–dP/dt) in the NF preparations were 25.9 ± 3.9 mN/mm^2, 189 ± 9 msec and 148 ± 23 mN/mm^2–sec, respectively. P_0 and –dP/dt in the DCM–F hearts were reduced by 47% ($p < 0.02$) and 46% ($p < 0.02$) while TPT was increased by 14% ($p < 0.03$) (Table 1) [3]. The initial, TDH and TIH for NF hearts are 3.89 ± 0.66, 3.39 ± 0.66 and 0.51 ± 0.13 mJ/g–beat, respectively. These are reduced by 62% ($p < 0.005$), 61 % ($p < 0.01$) and 69% ($p < 0.03$) in DCM–F. The rate of TIH liberation in the strips from NF hearts is 0.82 ± 0.24 mW/g–beat and this is reduced by 70% in DCM–F. An increase in force is expected when the stimulus frequency is increased. This is seen for the NF preparations in Fig. 2 where the frequency at which peak force is developed is 175 beats per minute. In DCM–F hearts this frequency treppe is substantially blunted (Fig. 2) [1].

Table 1. Mechanical and myothermal data from nonfailing (NF) and dilated cardiomyopathic failing (DCM–F) hearts. P_0 –isometric peak active force; TPT – time to peak tension; –dP/dt – rate of isometric relaxation; I – initial heat; TDH – tension dependent heat; TIH – tension independent heat; dTIH/dt – tension independent heat rate.

Parameter	NF	DCM–F	p value
P_0 (mN/mm^2)	25.9 ± 3.9	13.9 ± 2.0	p<0.02
TPT (msec)	189 ± 9	216 ± 8	p<0.03
–dP / dt (mN/mm^2–sec)	148 ± 23	80 ± 13	p<0.02
I (mJ/g–beat)	3.89 ± 0.66	1.50 ± 0.26	p<0.005
TDH (mJ/g–beat)	3.39 ± 0.66	1.34 ± 0.22	p<0.01
TIH (mJ/g–beat)	0.51 ± 0.13	0.16 ± 0.05	p<0.03
dTIH (mW/g–beat)	0.82 ± 0.24	0.25 ± 0.09	p<0.03

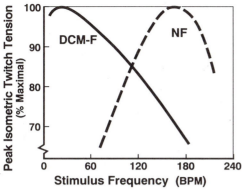

Figure 2. Peak isometric twitch tension as a percent of maximum peak twitch tension (P_0, NF 25.9 ± 3.9, DCM–F 13.9 ± 2.0 mN/mm^2) versus stimulus frequency (redrawn from [1]).

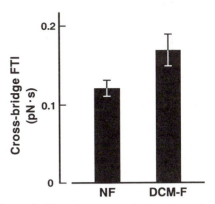

Figure 3. The average crossbridge force–time integral (FTI_{XBr}) for nonfailing (NF) and dilated cardiomyopathic failing (DCM–F) hearts.

Derived Crossbridge and Excitation–Contraction Coupling Parameters

An FTI_{XBr} is developed when a crossbridge head, attached to actin, changes from a weak to a strong binding state, undergoes a conformational transformation developing force and then returns to the weak binding state. The FTI_{XBr} can be calculated from Eqs. (3) and (4) [7, 9]. The average FTI_{XBr} for NF muscle is 0.12 ± 0.01 pNs (pico–Newton seconds). This parameter is increased in failing muscle strips by 40% (p < 0.04) (Fig. 3). This means that more FTI per high energy phosphate hydrolyzed is developed in the failing preparation. Thus, the economy for isometric force development is greater in DCM failure than in NF hearts. The calcium cycled per beat and the rate of calcium removal can be calculated from the TIH and the TIH rate (Eq. (5)) [7]. In NF hearts the calcium cycled and the rate of calcium removal is 21.9 ± 5.6 nmoles/g–beat and 35 ± 8.7 nmoles/g–sec. These values are reduced 69% (p < 0.01) and 70% (P < 0.03), respectively, in DCM failure.

DISCUSSION

Peak Isometric Force

There are significant changes in the mechanical and myothermal properties of failing heart muscle (Table 1). Peak isometric force is reduced by 47%. At the same time, the increased FTI_{XBr} would lead one to believe that the muscle force might be increased. However, if one examines the amount of calcium removed from the cytosol per beat, which is equivalent to the calcium cycled per beat, it is clear that the marked diminution in this quantity (69% reduction) results in incomplete activation of the contractile system. This is readily seen when the peak isometric force is plotted against the calcium uptake per beat (Fig. 4).

Myocardial Power Output

The increase in the FTI_{XBr} results in an increase in isometric economy of contraction (Economy = FTI_{muscle}/unit ATP hydrolyzed) and has consequences with regard

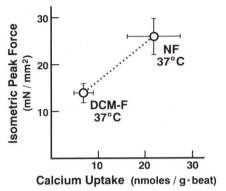

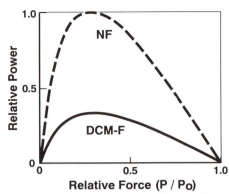

Figure 4. Peak isometric force versus calcium uptake in nonfailing (NF) and failing (DCM–F) hearts.

Figure 5. Relative power in nonfailing (NF) and failing (DCM–F) preparations.

to the velocity of shortening. From myofibrillar ATPase and *in vitro* motility assay data we know that the velocity of shortening in the failing hearts is markedly reduced [10, 11, 12]. Since the velocity of shortening is reduced and the isometric force is reduce, there is a shift of the force velocity curve to the left, with the failing preparation exhibiting a lower V_{max} and P_0. If that power is the rate at which work is carried out, multiplying the force by the velocity for any point on the force velocity curve provides a measure of the power output of the heart. The relative power developed by the failing preparations (DCM–F) is markedly reduced with this reduction resulting from a decrease in force as well as velocity (Fig. 5).

Time to Peak Tension and Rate of Isometric Relaxation

The time to peak tension is increased in DCM–F hearts (Table 1). A possible explanation for this result is that the calcium released during depolarization of the sarcolemma is removed from the cytosol more slowly in the failing heart preparation. From measurements of the rate of TIH liberation (Table 1) and calculation of the rate of calcium removal, it would appear that the decreased rate of isometric relaxation is causally related to the altered calcium kinetics (Fig. 6).

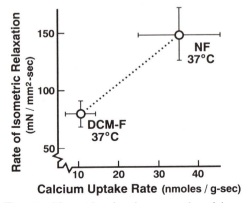

Figure 6. The rate of isometric relaxation versus the calcium uptake rate.

Factors influencing the Altered FTI_{XBr} in DCM Heart Failure

Isoform shifts from V_1 to V_3 myosin can alter the FTI_{XBr} in small mammals [13]. However, in large mammals such as the human virtually all of the ventricular myosin is of the V_3 type. Since in failing hearts there was a decrease in myofibrillar ATPase activity [11, 12] with no change in myosin ATPase activity [12] it seemed appropriate to consider alterations in the thin filaments as a possible cause of this phenomenon. There have been a number of recent reports documenting a change in the TnT4 isoform relative to total TnT and showing a correlation of this change with myofibrillar ATPase activity [14, 15]. The shift in the troponin T isoforms may alter the availability of the surface of the actin during activation so that the actin binding site of myosin attaches differently in the failing than in the normal NF heart muscle.

Factors Altering Calcium Kinetics in DCM Heart Failure

The marked depressions in TIH and TIH rate (dTIH/dt) found in DCM−F hearts are interpreted to indicate marked changes in calcium cycling. It is also apparent that there are mechanical correlates associated with the depressed calcium cycling (P_0 and −dP/dt) (Figs. 4 and 6). The replacement of healthy myocytes with connective tissue and myocyte death might explain the decrease in TIH liberation per gram of muscle. We attempted to minimize this possibility by choosing strips that were free of fibrous tissue and scarring. Furthermore, we never found a reduction in myosin content greater than 20% in any of the tissue samples examined while TIH and dTIH/dt were depressed almost 70% [3, 13]. There have been a number of studies of mRNA and proteins associated with calcium cycling that indicate major changes in DCM−F. The sarcolemmal sodium−calcium exchange protein and mRNA are increased in failing hearts [16, 17]. Calsequestrin remains unchanged while SERCA−2a, phospholamban and the ryanodine receptor are all decreased [18−24]. These alterations in calcium cycling proteins may well account for the differences observed in the TIH measurements. In addition, there are important physiological counterparts of the changes in protein and message. A direct correlation was found between the mRNA for SERCA−2a and the peak for the force−frequency relation found in failing hearts (Fig. 2) [16]. Furthermore, calcium transients are prolonged in failing hearts [25, 26] which could readily be explained by the change in calcium cycling proteins and which might easily account for the prolongation in TPT and the decrease in −dP/dt (Table 1). The general idea is further supported by the decrease in calcium uptake rates by sarcoplasmic reticulum isolated from failing hearts [23, 27, 28].

CONCLUSION

The phenotypic changes found in DCM failing human hearts have profound effects on the crossbridge cycle and on the quantity and kinetics of calcium cycling. The changes are believed to involve shifts in the Troponin T isoform from TnT_3 to TnT_4. With regard to calcium cycling, the increase in the sarcolemmal Na^+-Ca^{2+} exchange protein and the decrease in the sarcoplasmic reticulum SERCA−2a calcium pump, phospholamban and the ryanodine receptor profoundly change excitation−contraction coupling. The results are depressed isometric mechanics, a blunted force−frequency relation and a decrease in power output. These deficiencies account for the major portion of deficit in ventricular function found in the failing myocardium.

Acknowledgements

Supported in part by USPHS grants #PO1 HL 28001−13 and 1 RO1 HL 55641−01.

DISCUSSION

Dr. H. Kammermeier: The shift of calcium pumping from the SR towards the sarcolemma is accompanied with decreased efficiency because in one case you have the stoichiometry of two calcium per ATP, and in the sarcolemma you have one calcium per ATP. Does it have a major influence?

Dr. N. Alpert: Yes. We use a rough approximation. Instead of assuming an average of two calciums per ATP, we multiplied that value by 0.7 to take into consideration what percentage we thought was sarcolemmal and what percentage we thought was sarcoplasmic reticulum. We do not know whether that number is equally accurate for both the normal and failing preparation. Since we found such an enormous reduction in calcium cycling down to 7.5 nmoles/gm/beat from 22 nmoles/gm/beat, we felt that, qualitatively, there is clearly a depression in the calcium cycle per beat in these hearts. Since that correlated very well with the alterations in the calcium cycling proteins, we felt comfortable in believing that there is a decrease in the amount of Ca^{++} cycled. I should add one caution: These preparations are not ischemic and the tissue that we selected was very special healthy tissue from the failing hearts and from the non−failing hearts. Basically, there was no scar tissue and no other visible changes that we could see.

Dr. P. Hunter: How much shortening occurs in the center of your papillary muscle, or center of your trabeculae, even though it is overall isometric? As your conclusions are based on it being an isometric preparation, then there is a question if you have got contraction in the center.

Dr. N. Alpert: The reason that I think that there is no problem in the center of our papillary muscle preparation is that we have used what is called a Paradise test on every preparation. What that test does is to reduce the oxygen tension from 95% to 80%. Then, if you get absolutely no change in the mechanical characteristics, we assume that the center region is not being affected by the oxygen.

Dr. P. Hunter: How much shortening do you get at the center of your fiber?

Dr. N. Alpert: I assume we get about 5% shortening from the damaged ends. After that these are isometric contractions.

Dr. P. Hunter: Given the shift from TnT−3 to TnT−4, have you got any thoughts on how that leads to a more efficient ATP utilization? Why does the heart not use that normally?

Dr. N. Alpert: Our hypothesis is that shifting from TnT−3 to TnT−4 changes how the tropomyosin is moved when calcium activates the system. This, in turn, leaves a different surface of the actin exposed to the actin binding region of the myosin and that effects the mechanics of the crossbridge cycle.

Dr. H. ter Keurs: I wonder about the role of the sarcoplasmic reticulum that you applied in the negative force frequency relation. You suggest a reduced calcium uptake rate by the sarcoplasmic reticulum, and that force decreases with increasing frequency in the DCM muscles. When you increase the frequency, do you see an increase basal force level? If that is the case, do you account for that in your heat measurements?

Dr. N. Alpert: The diastolic force level goes down when we increase the frequency, until after the optimum is reached. Then it starts going up. So you go over the optimum about 20% in terms of frequency and then the diastolic force starts to go up. But before that, the diastolic force falls as you increase the frequency, and this happens in both the failing and nonfailing preparations.

Dr. H. Rockman: Other studies have shown no difference in phospholamban or SERCA in human heart failure. How do you put it all together when some groups show differences in phospholamban and calcium pump and others do not?

Dr. N. Alpert: It is a question of the preparation that people are using. Most of the people are finding a depression in sarcoplasmic reticulum SERCA-2 and a depression in phospholamban; there is a controversy about the ryanodine receptors. Some find a depression, some find no change, and some people actually find an increase in that. There is also a controversy about the sodium–calcium exchange protein, although lately more people are finding that protein goes up than no change or down. It depends on the preparations that you have and how you treat the preparations once you get them. I can not say anything about the measurements that other people make. These are the measurements that we made.

Dr. A. Landesberg: Your measurement of economy relates to isometric contraction and measuring the force–time integral divided by the tension dependent heat for isometric contraction. This means that isometric contraction in cardiomyopathy is more economical. What happens in shortening contraction. What should we expect?

Dr. N. Alpert: I do not know.

Dr. M. Morad: The issue of creating heart failure is fascinating. Dr. Alpert has shown that SERCA-2 activity goes down and the total calcium metabolism seems to be compromised, and yet the sodium–calcium exchanger is overexpressed, which would eventually lead to further emptying of the SR, unless something happens to the calcium exchanger to force it to bring calcium in.

How do we come to some kind of reasonable explanation for this phenomenon? It is clear from a number of models that the exchanger is overexpressed. It is also clear that SERCA-2 is downexpressed and the relaxation of the muscle is slowed. The heart will kill itself this way; it will go into even more failure, if you like.

Dr. N. Alpert: However you explain it, it seems very clear that you have less calcium released in each beat in these preparations. That is true for dilated cardiomyopathy and it is true for failure secondary to mitral regurgitation. There is less calcium released, less activation, and the force–frequency relationship is blunted in all of those preparations. The other important point is that half the people do not die from pump failure, but die from arrhythmias. This is a very serious problem. Understanding arrhythmias is as important as understanding pump failure.

Dr. D. Noble: I am puzzled about the role of the Na^+–Ca^{2+} exchanger in heart failure. What are the expected outcomes of the up and down regulation of the sodium–calcium exchanger? There is a similar question relating to the generation of arrhythmias. Is it best to inhibit the exchanger and so stop the current that generates the arrhythmia, or is it better to go in the other direction and get more calcium out, so delaying or preventing the calcium overload in the first place? This shows that we badly need to integrate together our electrical and metabolic modeling, and this is partly what we are doing (Chapter 24). Until we get answers, we are going to keep on raising these questions.

Dr. H. Strauss: The microdomains are probably very important with regard to cell function. The disparity in calcium concentrations between different domains, particularly as we start upregulating and downregulating proteins, may become much greater than we have conceived. It is probably no longer reasonable to try and estimate the effect of calcium levels averaged across a cell on the function of a particular current system.

Dr. H. ter Keurs: One observation that is not taken into account is that of increasing force in between stimuli at a high stimulus rate. We have observed in trabeculae taken from rats with right sided heart failure as a result of a gigantic infarct in the left ventricle, that with increased stimulus frequency the cells in the trabeculae start to develop spontaneous activity much more easily than in control hearts, as an expression of spontaneous calcium release. Calcium uptake rate, certainly in the intact cell, is only the net uptake rate which is influenced both by the uptake rate of the pump itself, and by a spontaneous calcium release through ryanodine receptor. This process has spontaneous activity made by itself, and contributes to the arrhythmias.

Dr. D. Noble: It is difficult to be certain about all the functional roles in these complex situations. David Eisner [*Personal Communication*], for example, has presented arguments recently to say that the spontaneous release is actually a mechanism that very effectively gets more calcium out of the cell than would otherwise be the case, so that it acts to delay the growth of calcium overload. If you can put up with the arrhythmias, it seems that you may be doing a good thing by having them, if you see what I mean, or if you see what he means!

Dr. H. ter Keurs: The point is that spontaneous activity is a big contributor to reduced force development of a contraction that is activated by synchronized activation of the membrane.

Dr. M. Morad: If in fact the recirculation fraction of calcium is very low, then Dr. Eisner may have a point. But when SERCA−2 is downregulated, it is not downregulated to the levels where he would have liked it. Because even when SERCA−2 is significantly downregulated, it still can beat the sodium−calcium exchanger in the rate by which it can transport Ca^{2+}.

Dr. H. Rockman: More and more information is systematically available using targeted overexpression or gene knockouts. For instance, the phospholamban knockout does not produce heart failure; it produces a hypercontractile state. Overexpression of SERCA−2, as you would expect, increases calcium uptake. It is probably an integrated mechanism involving many different calcium proteins, and probably involves not only the SR and SR−calcium relationship, but perhaps cell surface molecules that, in an integrated manner, combine to form the phenotype.

Dr. N. Alpert: There is a recent paper [*Fazio et al. New England J Med 1996;334:809*] dealing with a group of patients who had dilated cardiomyopathy and very severe heart failure. These patients were given growth hormone for three months. During that period of time, the patients felt better, their exercise tolerance went up, their heart rate went down, and the myocardial efficiency at rest and during exercise went up. What that says to me is that the protein synthetic machinery in the failing preparation has somehow been put into a positive feedback cycle where the calcium pump, phospholamban and ryanodine receptors are not expressed adequately. When catecholamines are up, they accentuate the inadequate expression of these proteins. The addition of growth hormone counteracted the deleterious changes in those patients.

Dr. M. Morad: One other thing that surprised me in looking at the sodium−calcium exchanger overexpressed mice was that in previous studies of cardiac myopathy in hamsters we have seen that the overexpression of the exchanger goes together with the down regulation of the SERCA−2. We were surprised to find that in these mice the overexpression went hand−in−hand together with the over activity of the calcium pump. We do not know whether the Ca^{2+}−pump protein was overexpressed or whether just the activity of the pump had increased to compensate for the increase in the exchanger activity. I feel that there may be some molecular signaling that takes place in heart failure that is quite unique and different than if one overexpresses these molecules in a normal heart.

Dr. H. Strauss: A lot of very worthwhile information has come from the study of patients with end−stage heart disease. Clearly, one does not want to do things to patients without having adequate justification. But this is really the end of the road for a lot of these people and you are dealing with an irreversible problem at that point. It might be worthwhile to start gathering information about patients earlier on in the course of their heart failure. Clearly, you are trying to prevent progression. If events such as apoptosis and other irreversible events are occurring early in the disease process, it obviously would be better to find them out and to establish what they are and determine their cause so that one can intervene and, if not arrest, then certainly slow down that ultimate deteriorating spiral.

REFERENCES

1. Mulieri LA, Leavitt BJ, Hasenfuss G, Allen PD, Alpert NR. Contraction frequency dependence of twitch and diastolic tension in human dilated cardiomyopathy (Tension–Frequency relation in cardiomyopathy) In: Hasenfuss G, Holubarsch Ch, Just H, Alpert NR, eds. *Cellular and Molecular Alterations in the Failing Human Heart* Steinkopf Verlag Darmstadt 1992; 199–212

2. Mulieri LA, Hasenfuss G, Ittleman F, Blanchard EM, Alpert NR. Protection of human left ventricular myocardium from cutting injury with 2, 3–butanedione monoxime. *Circ Res* 1989;65:1441–1444.

3. Hasenfuss G, Mulieri LA, Leavitt BJ, Allen PD, Haeberle JR, Alpert NR. alterations in contractile function and excitation–contraction coupling in dilated cardiomyopathy. *Circ Res* 1992;70:1225–1232.

4. Mulieri LA, Hasenfuss G, Leavitt BJ, Allen PD, Alpert NR. Altered myocardial force–frequency relation in human heart failure. *Circulation* 1992:85;1743–1750.

5. Mulieri LA, Luhr G, Treffry J, Alpert NR. Metal–film thermopiles for use with rabbit right ventricular papillary muscles. *Am J Physiol* 1977:233;C146–156.

6. Alpert NR, Mulieri LA. Increased myothermal economy of isometric force generation in compensated cardiac hypertrophy induced by pulmonary artery constriction in rabbit. *Circ Res* 1982;50:491–500.

7. Alpert NR, Blanchard EM, Mulieri LA. Tension independent heat in rabbit papillary muscles. *J Physiol (Lond)* 1989;414:433–453.

8. Weber A. Energized calcium transport and relaxing factors. *Current Topics in Bioenergetics* 1966; 1:203–254.

9. Alpert NR, Mulieri LA, Hasenfuss G. Myocardial chemo–mechanical energy transduction. In: Fozzard et al., eds. *The Heart and Cardiovascular System* New York:Raven Press 1992; 111–128.

10. Harris DE, Work SS, Wright RK, Alpert NR, Warshaw DM. Smooth, cardiac and skeletal muscle myosin force and motion generation assessed by cross–bridge mechanical interactions in vitro. *J Molec Res Cell Motility* 1994;15:11–19.

11. Alpert NR, Gordon MS. Myofibrillar adenosine triphosphatase activity in congestive heart failure. *Am J Physiol* 1962;202:940–945.

12. Pagani ED, Alousi AA, Grant AM, Older TM, Dziuban Jr SW, Allen PD. Changes in myofibrillar content and Mg–ATPase activity in ventricular tissue from patients with heart failure caused by coronary artery disease, cardiomyopathy or mitral valve insufficiency. *Circ Res* 1988;63:380–385.

13. Hasenfuss G, Mulieri LA, Blanchard EM, Holubarsch Ch, Leavitt BJ, Ittleman F, Alpert NR. Energetics of isometric force generation in control and volume–overload human myocardium: Comparison with animal species. *Circ Res* 1991;68:836–846.

14. Anderson PAW, Grieg A, Mark TM, Malouf NN, Oakeley AE, Ungerleider RM, Allen PD, Kay BK. Molecular Basis for human cardiac troponin T isoforms in the developing, adult and failing heart. *Circ Res* 1995;76:681–686.

15. Mesnard L, Logeart D, Taviaux S, Diriong S, Mercadier JJ, Samson G. Human cardiac troponin T. Cloning and expression of new isoforms in normal and failing heart. Circ Res 1995;76:687–692.

16. Hasenfuss G, Reinecke I, Struder R, Pieske B, Holtz J, Holubarsch Ch, Just H. functional consequences of altered expression of SR–Ca^{2+} ATPase and Na^+–Ca^{2+} exchanger in failing human myocardium. Circulation 1993;88(4. Part 2):401–407.

17. Struder R, Reinecke H, Bilger J, Eschenhagen T, Bohm M, Hasenfuss G, Just H, Holtz J, Drexler H. Gene expression of cardiac Na^+–Ca^{2+} exchanger in end–state human heart failure. *Circ Res* 1994;75:443–453.

18. Arai M, Alpert NR, Periasamy M. Cloning and characterization of the gen encoding rabbit cardiac calsequestrin. *Gene* 1991;109:275–279.

19. Arai M, Alpert NR, MacLennan D, Barton P, Periasamy M. Alterations in sarcoplasmic reticulum gene expression in human heart failure: A possible mechanism of alterations in systolic and diastolic

properties of the failing myocardium. *Circ Res* 1993;72:463–469.

20. Mercadier JJ, Lompre AM, Duc P, Boheler KR, Fraysse JB, Wisnewski G, Allen PD, Kokajda M, Schwartz K. Altered sarcoplasmic reticulum Ca^{2+}–ATPase gene expression in human ventricle during end–state failure. *J Clin Invest* 1990;85:305–309.

21. Nagai R, Zarain–Herzberg A, Brandl CJ, Fujii J, Tada M, MacLennan DH, Alpert NR, Periasamy M. Regulation of myocardial Ca^{2+}–ATPase and phospholamban mRNA expression in response to pressure overload and thyroid hormone. *Proc Natl Acad Sci USA* 1989;85:2966–2970.

22. Feldman AR, Ray PE, Silan CM, Mercer JA, Minobe W, Bristow MR. Selective gene expression in failing human heart: quantification of steady state levels of messenger RNA in endomyocardial biopsies using polymerase chain reaction. *Circulation* 1991;83:1886–1872.

23. de la Bastie D, Levitsky D, Rappaport L, Mercadier JJ, Marotte F, Wisnewski C, Brovkovich V, Schwartz K, Lompre AM. function of the sarcoplasmic reticulum and expression of its Ca^{2+} ATPase gene in pressure overload induced cardiac hypertrophy in the rat. *Circ Res* 1990;66:554–564.

24. Takahashi T, Allen PD, Lacro RV, Marks AR, Dennis AR, Schoen FJ, Grossman W, Marsh JD, Isumo S. Expression of dihyropyridine receptor (Ca^{2+} channel) and calsequestrin genes in the myocardium of patients with end–stage heart failure. *J Clin Invest* 1992;90:927–935.

25. Guathmey JK, Copelas L, MacKinnon R, Schoen F, Feldman MD, Grossman W, Morgan JP. Abnormal intracellular calcium handling in myocardium from patients with end–stage heart failure. *Circ Res* 1987; 61:70–76

26. Morgan JP, Emy RE, Allen PD, Grossman W, Guathmey JK. Abnormal intercellular calcium handling, a major cause of systolic and diastolic dysfunction in ventricular myocardium from patients with heart failure. *Circulation* 1990;81:(Suppl III) III 21–32.

27. Limas CJ, Olivari MT, Goldenberg IF, Levine TB, Benditt DG, Simon A. Calcium uptake by cardiac sarcoplasmic reticulum in human dilated cardiomyopathy. *Cardiovasc Res* 1987;21:601–605.

28. Siri FM, Kreuger J, Nordin C, Ming Z, Aronson RS. Depressed intracellular calcium transients and contraction in myocytes from hypertrophied and failing guinea pig hearts. *Am J Physiol* 1991;261:H514–530.

III. Cardiac Mechanics and Flow Dynamics

CHAPTER 10

HOW CARDIAC CONTRACTION
AFFECTS THE CORONARY VASCULATURE

Nicolaas Westerhof, Pieter Sipkema, and Martijn A. Vis[1]

ABSTRACT

We modeled the influence of cardiac contraction on maximally dilated coronary blood vessels, whether single or in juxtaposition, taking into account the nonlinear material properties of both the vascular wall and the myocardium. We calculated pressure–area relations of single, embedded coronary blood vessels, and used these relations to calculate diastolic and systolic coronary pressure–flow relations in a model of the coronary vasculature. The model shows that the change in myocardial material properties during contraction can explain the decrease in coronary vessel area and coronary flow generally observed in experiments. The model also shows that arterioles can be protected from the compressive action of the cardiac muscle by the presence of accompanying venules, which is favorable for coronary blood flow.

INTRODUCTION

Coronary arterial inflow is impeded during cardiac contraction [1]. Several hypotheses exist to explain this flow impediment [2–8]. The earlier reports suggested that ventricular pressure played the major role [2–4], but we showed that the impediment is mainly the result of the time–varying mechanical properties of the cardiac muscle [5–8]. In the isolated Langendorff perfused rabbit and cat heart, under conditions of constant perfusion pressure and maximal vasodilation, similar flow impediment was observed in both isovolumic and isobaric contractions [5, 6]. Also changes in ventricular pressure

---

[1]Laboratory for Physiology, Institute for Cardiovascular Research (ICaR–VU), Van der Boechorst straat 7, 1081 BT Amsterdam, The Netherlands

obtained by changes in ventricular filling had little effect on flow impediment, while changes in cardiac contractility did [8]. Later, we showed that in the isolated perfused papillary muscle coronary inflow impediment did not change with muscle length and different afterloads [9].

We have found, in the blood perfused isovolumically beating rat heart, that vasomotor tone affects the systolic and diastolic flow in a similar proportion, leaving the relative impediment the same [10]. However, we have also found in that preparation that ventricular pressure contributes to flow impediment [11], a finding which differs from our earlier observations in rabbit [5] and cat [6–8], but is in line with the findings of Kouwenhoven *et al.* [12].

Since not all of the findings could be explained on the basis of the time–varying elastance concept, and the interpretation was based on qualitative reasoning and lacking a quantitative description, we decided to describe the time–varying elastance concept in a quantitative way using a modeling approach. In the model, we have studied pressure–area relations of arterioles and venules embedded in a piece of cardiac muscle, and calculated pressure–flow relations in diastole and systole using a coronary vascular network. Furthermore, arteries and arterioles are often accompanied by one or two veins or venules, forming a triad. Therefore, we have also studied the effects of contraction on vessels that are in juxtaposition in the myocardium.

METHODS

Material Properties

Myocardium. The myocardial tissue (muscle fibers + collagen) was assumed to be incompressible, homogeneous and nonlinearly elastic in diastole and in systole. The papillary muscle was used as a representation of the ventricular myocardium. Because the fibers in the papillary muscle run predominantly in the longitudinal direction [13], the fibers in the model were assumed to run in parallel. Accordingly, the myocardial tissue was assumed to be transversely isotropic [14, 15]. Static uniaxial (i.e., in fiber direction) force–length relations of papillary muscle in diastole and systole were obtained in our laboratory [16]. These relations were converted to Cauchy stress–strain relations and fitted with an empirical two–parameter exponential relation proposed for diastolic muscle [17], to which a three–parameter exponential relation was added for developed force [18]. The relations fitted the experimental data well [19].

Recent studies show that active stress is not developed only in the muscle fiber direction, but also in the cross–fiber direction [20–22]. On basis of data reported in the literature [14, 15, 20, 22], the stress–strain relations in the transverse (cross–fiber) direction could be derived from their longitudinal counterparts for diastole and systole. These relations depend on muscle length. They were worked out for two lengths: slack length and 90% of maximum muscle length (Lmax) [16]. Details are presented by Vis *et al.* [19].

Vessels. Pressure–area relations for an isolated, maximally dilated, arteriole and an isolated, maximally dilated venule were taken from the literature [23, 24] and were fitted with an empirical arctangent relation, modified from [25]. These relations fully contain the nonlinear material properties of the vascular wall, for the *in vivo* muscle length. The vascular wall was assumed to be incompressible. The space between the vessels and the surrounding myocardium was assumed to be filled with a constant amount of (incompressible) interstitial fluid.

Geometrical Considerations

The following geometrical considerations hold for both the case of single vessels and the case of juxtaposed vessels.

Vessels and muscle fibers were assumed to run in parallel, as is predominantly the case in the papillary muscle [13]. Vessels were assumed to be cylindrically shaped and to remain so during the cycle. It was assumed that the cavity of the muscle at slack length, and in diastole, had an internal diameter equal to the external diameter of the vessel at zero transmural pressure. The muscle cavity pertaining to the blood vessels was also assumed to have a circular cross–section, for single vessels as well as for vessels forming a triad. This assumption allowed relatively easy calculations of cardiac muscle deformation and was estimated to induce no major quantitative errors [26]. Note that, because the vessels run in parallel to the muscle fibers, the myocardial material properties in the cross–fiber direction, thus not in fiber direction, determine the interactions between the vessels and the cardiac muscle. The pressure–area relations of a cavity in the cardiac muscle can be calculated from the transverse stress–strain relations in diastole and systole. This was done by numerical calculation of the finite deformation of a thick–walled cylinder of myocardial tissue. It is noted that the myocardium contributing to the pressure–area relation of a cavity amounts to about three times the internal radius of the cavity.

Single Vessels in Cardiac Muscle in Diastole and Systole

The pressure–area relation of a maximally dilated vessel in the cardiac muscle is calculated from of the summation of the pressure–area relation of the vessel and the muscle cavity in which it is located. Details have been presented earlier [19, 26, 27].

As it is not clear how cardiac contraction influences the intravascular pressure, we have assumed constant arteriolar (35 mmHg) and venular pressures (17 mmHg) during the cardiac contraction. Vascular internal diameters in diastole are 39 and 48 μm for the arteriole and venule, respectively.

Coronary Pressure–Flow Relations in Diastole and Systole

Using the data reported in the literature on morphometry of the coronary vasculature [28–31], a symmetrical, maximally dilated, coronary arterial system was generated by a bifurcation process down to diameters of 7 μm. The venous system was modeled by mirroring the arterial tree. The venous diameters were taken as √1.5 times larger than the arterial diameters and the number of venules and veins at any level was taken as twice the number of their arterial counterparts. Flow through this network was calculated as a function of pressure, utilizing Poiseuille's law. The pressure in the middle of the entrance artery, with a diameter of 200 μm, was varied around the physiological control value of 60 mmHg. The pressure in the middle of the largest veins was set at 10 mmHg. Viscosity of the crystalloid perfusion medium was set at 1 mPa.s. Flow was expressed in ml/min/g by assuming 6.10^6 capillaries per gram tissue (3000 per mm^2).

Juxtaposed Arterioles and Venules in the Cardiac Muscle in Diastole and Systole

To calculate the influence of cardiac contraction on juxtaposed blood vessels, we modeled one arteriole (internal diameter 39 μm at a pressure of 35 mmHg in diastole), accompanied by two larger, equally sized venules (internal diameter 48 μm at a pressure

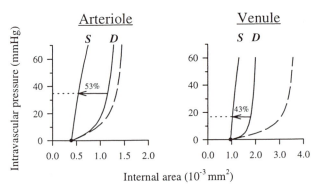

Figure 1. Pressure–area relations of a thick–walled arteriole and thin–walled venule in isolation (dashed lines) and when embedded in myocardium (solid lines). 'D' and 'S' denote diastole and systole, respectively.

of 17 mmHg in diastole) assuming intravascular pressures to remain constant during contraction.

We have also calculated the influence of cardiac contraction on the resistance of a vascular system consisting of one arteriole in series with two parallel venules, with these vessels taken either as singles or in a triad arrangement.

RESULTS

Single Vessels

Pressure–area relations of an arteriole and a venule in the cardiac muscle in diastole and systole at muscle slack length are given in Fig. 1. It may be seen that the arteriolar wall properties contribute in diastole and systole to the pressure–area relations of the embedded vessel. The pressure–area relation of the isolated venule is at such a low level that it does not contribute to the pressure–area relation of the embedded vessel. The relations depend somewhat on muscle length [19].

Coronary Pressure–Flow Relations

Pressure–flow relations were derived for the coronary vascular network. The pressure distribution along the arterial and venous system is found to be close to data presented in the literature [27]. Pressure–flow relations at two muscle lengths are given in Fig. 2. It may be seen that muscle length has little influence on the systolic relation while there is an effect in diastole.

Vessels in a Triad

Arteriolar and venular diameters in static diastole and systole were calculated for single vessels or in a triad. The results are presented in Table 1. It can be seen that arterioles are strongly protected by the accompanying venules.

Using the values in Table 1, it can be calculated that flow through a vascular system consisting of one arteriole in series with two parallel venules decreases by 73% during contraction when these vessels are single, but decreases by only 49% when these vessels are in a triad arrangement. This shows the hemodynamic advantage of vessels running closely together in the contracting muscle.

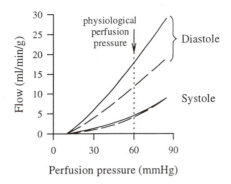

Figure 2. Perfusion pressure–flow relations of the coronary network for two muscle lengths: slack length (solid lines) and 90% of Lmax (dashed lines).

Table 1. Vascular diameters (in μm) in static diastole and static systole for the cardiac muscle fixed at slack length, and kept at their physiologic pressur of 35 mmHG for the arteriole and 17 mmHg for the venule.

Vessel	Single Vessels		Vessels in a Triad	
	Diastole	Systole	Diastole	Systole
Arteriole	39	28	39	38
Venule	48	36	48	31

DISCUSSION

We have found that the time–varying properties of the myocardium have an effect on the pressure–area relations of arterioles and venules, so that cardiac contraction affects the coronary pressure–flow relation. We have also shown that when arterioles are accompanied by (two) venules the arteriole is "protected" from the effects of cardiac contraction. Here we show only the effect of isometric cardiac contraction on vascular diameter for the muscle at slack length. The effect of cardiac contraction with shortening or isometric contraction at 90% Lmax, is given elsewhere [19, 26].

The calculations were performed in static diastole and systole only. Modeling the dynamic variations of cardiac muscle would be of great interest but has not yet been carried out. We have chosen the maximally dilated vasculature. The smooth muscle is sufficiently slow to allow calculations assuming constant vasomotor tone during the cardiac cycle, and constant vasomotor tone can in principle be modeled as well.

The development of stress in the cross–fiber direction has been shown experimentally [20–22] to exist, but the formalization of the description of the multiaxial material properties, taking into account the cross–fiber stress development, is still very limited.

Data on vascular diameters in the maximally dilated coronary vasculature in static cardiac muscle have been reported by Westerhof et al. [32] for the papillary muscle, and by Goto et al. [33] and Judd and Levy [34] for the whole heart. The data on vessels in the heart wall are not directly comparable with the present data because the ventricular pressure

[10–12] and the different amounts of shortening in subendocardium and subepicardium may play a role as suggested by the findings that vessels at different locations may exhibit rather different responses during contraction [33, 34]. When we compare to the experimental data from papillary muscle, we note that the reported 30% decrease in cross–sectional area of the thin–walled capillaries is not much different from the findings in Table 1 for (thin-walled) venules. The effect of contraction on coronary flow predicted here (Fig. 2) is about twice as much as found in the isolated perfused papillary muscle [9]. However, in these calculations, the juxtaposition of arterioles and venules was not taken into account.

The accompaniment of arterioles and venules serves as a countercurrent exchanger of heat, gasses and small metabolites. This arrangement results in the reduction of heat loss from the extremities and allows for the exchange of vasoactive substances, giving upstream arterioles the possibility to sense what happens distally. We found that there is also an important hemodynamic effect of the juxtaposition of arterioles and venules: arteriolar resistance varies much less during muscle contraction when vessels are in a triad. Because the venules in triads are subject to larger diameter decreases during muscle contraction than single venules, the venous pump is augmented.

The derivations also show that the intramyocardial pressure exists even without reference to the left ventricular pressure [26], in accordance with our earlier predictions [35]. The intramyocardial or interstitial pressure is the result of the varying muscle properties on the one hand and the "load" (i.e., the vessels) on the other hand. This suggests that the pressure just outside a thick–walled arteriole, with high inside pressure, is much higher than just outside a thin–walled venule with low pressure.

CONCLUSIONS

The impediment of coronary flow in the maximally dilated bed can be explained on the basis of the time–varying elastic properties of the myocardium. The adjacent arterioles and venules serve to protect the arterioles from the compressive action of the cardiac muscle, so that coronary arterial inflow is impeded to a lesser extent during systole.

Acknowledgements

This work is supported by the Netherlands Organization for Scientific Research (NWO), Foundation of Life Sciences, grant # 810–406–005.

DISCUSSION

Dr. H. ter Keurs: That is a very interesting concept, but, if I am not mistaken, you need some degree of curvature in the muscle that you are discussing. If you take a ribbon shaped trabeculae, that would generate only forces in a longitudinal direction. Does anything happen to the artery and the vein in that trabeculae? If so why?

Dr. N. Westerhof: It is not the force but the mechanical properties of the muscle. We assume a blood vessel, with negligible pressure inside, to fit exactly in the myocardial tissue with certain elastic properties. When the vessel is filled to physiologic pressure, the volume increase depends on the vessel wall properties and on the elastic properties of the surrounding myocardium. If the muscle properties change, i.e., the myocardial stiffness increases as from diastole to systole, the pressure inside the vessel increases, or at constant pressure, diameter decreases. Thus, it is not the fact that vessels and muscle fibers run in certain directions, or that fibers bend around the vessels, but it is the fibre properties that count.

An analogy that may help understand this phenomenon is the relationship between charge (analogous to volume), voltage (analogous to pressure) and a capacitor (analogous to compliance, i.e., inversely proportional to muscle stiffness). The capacitance prescribes the ratio of charge and voltage. When muscle stiffness increases, as in systole, capacitance decreases and if volume cannot change, the pressure increases. Of course, this only works when there is a charge (volume) and voltage (pressure) at the start of the experiment. This idea was first suggested by Suga *et al.* [*Suga H, Sagawa K, Shoukas AA. Load independence of the instantaneous pressure–volume ratio of the canine left ventricle and effects of epinephrine and heart rate on the ratio. Circ Res 1973;32:314–322*] for the left ventricular pressure–volume relation and we propose this to hold for vascular lumen as well.

The orientation matters for a vessel in a muscle. When the vessel is, as in the papillary muscle, parallel to the muscle fibers it is mainly the mechanical properties of the muscle in the transverse direction that matters. Brenner and Yu [*Brenner B, Yu LC. Characterization of radial force and radial stiffness in C^{2+}-activated skinned fibers of the rabbit psoas muscle. J Physiol 1991;441:703–718*] and later Strumpf *et al.* [*Strumpf RK, Humphrey JD, Yin FCP. Biaxial mechanical properties of passive and tetanized canine diaphragm. Am J Physiol 1993;265:H469–H475*] have shown that the transverse properties of muscle change during contraction. By and large, the transverse properties change like the properties in the fiber direction.

Dr. H. ter Keurs: If there is no shortening in that trabeculae of the sarcomeres adjacent to the vessels, there would be an increase in longitudinal stiffness and an increase in lateral stiffness. But I can not see, if there is no curvature change of the myofibrils containing that sarcomere, how they would affect the artery and the vein.

Dr. N. Westerhof: Consider a cavity like a blood vessel in the muscle, and the vessel is 'blown up', i.e., there is pressure inside, and the muscle tissue surrounding it changes its elastic properties, i.e., it is getting stiffer, pressure increases or volume decreases. Sarcomere stiffness does it. The changes in pressure and volume depend on 'the loading' of the vessel, i.e., can the blood be moved out or not.

Dr. J. Downey: We did a very simple experiment about 20 years ago [*Cardiovasc Res 9:161, 1975*] where we perfused a segment of a coronary artery on a beating dog heart. Then we poisoned the segment with nembutal down that vessel so that the muscle would just be passive but ventricular pressure was unchanged. Removing active contraction had virtually no effect on the systolic impediment. Then we went the other way and put isoproterenol down that vessel and again, the augmented contractility had almost no effect on the extravascular resistance. Would your model predict that? That was what led us to say that the ventricular pressure is the most important factor in the contracting heart.

Dr. N. Westerhof: Yes, but you also showed that the LVP, under certain circumstances, has very little effect on coronary flow. This work was done with Donna van Winkle [*van Winkle DM, Swafford AN, Downey JM. Subendocardial coronary compression in beating dog hearts is independent of pressure in the ventricular lumen. Am J Physiol 1991;261:H500–H505*].

Dr. J. Downey: Yes, that is right. If we decompress the heart and allow it to beat empty, there is still a systolic impediment to flow. We said that the vessel is probably responding to the predominant stress and that if it is beating empty, then the transverse stresses become very important. But if it is beating in a physiological way, where you have a strong radial stress, then that is the major determinant. Is that compatible with your elastance model?

Dr. N. Westerhof: I was talking here only on the papillary muscle, where flow impediment in systole is seen [*Allaart CP, Westerhof N. Effect of length and contraction on coronary perfusion in isolated perfused papillary muscle of rat heart. Am J Physiol 1996;271:H447–H454*]. We also did some modelling on this. We have extended this model to the heart wall and there the situation is much more complex [*Vis MA, Bovendeerd PHM, Sipkema P, Westerhof N. Modeling coronary blood vessels in the ventricular wall: contribution of ventricular contractility, pressure, and circumferential wall stretch. Am J Physiol 1997; in press*]. The calculations show that contractility, ventricular pressure and wall stretch all contribute to coronary resistance, depending on the layer in the wall (sub–epicardial or sub–endocardial) and on the mode of contraction (isovolumic or isobaric).

Dr. E. Ritman: There is a way that you could perhaps evaluate the implications of what you are saying. From your model you can calculate the total blood volume within the papillary muscle. How does that volume change during the contraction and how does that relate to what we know from the literature and can measure with fast CT?

Dr. N. Westerhof: When you have an isolated perfused papillary muscle, there is no LVP, and yet, during contraction you see arterial inflow decrease [*Allaart CP, Westerhof N. Effect of length and contraction on coronary perfusion in isolated perfused papillary muscle of rat heart. Am J Physiol 1996;271:H447–H454*]. This is known in skeletal muscle for many years [*Guyton AC, Hall JE. Textbook of Medical Physiology. Philadelphia, Saunders Comp., 1996, p 253–254*]. Thus, there is no question that contraction of the muscle itself has an effect on flow and that it is not necessary to have a LVP in the lumen of the ventricle, although this may contribute as well. We have not measured vascular volume yet. However, we did measure muscle diameter and we saw that the diameter increases with each contraction when the muscle is not perfused (local shortening and thus local diameter, volume, increase). During perfusion we see a decrease in muscle diameter with each contraction suggesting that muscle volume decreases due to the decrease in vessel volume [*Allaart CP. Interactions between coronary perfusion and myocardial mechanical properties. Ph.D. Dissertation, Free University of Amsterdam, 1995, pp 98–99*]. We estimate basal muscle volume to change 15%. A fluorescent dye could help perhaps, but this measurement may be complicated by the finding that we see indicators squirting out of the Thebesian openings with each contraction, thereby filling the muscle bath with indicator. But it could be possible in principle. We are now trying to measure intramuscular pressures [*Heslinga JW, Allaart CP, Westerhof N. Intramyocardial pressure measurements in the isolated perfused papillary muscle of rat heart. Eur J Morphology 1996;34:55–62*].

Dr. H. Kammermeier: It is frequently not taken into account that venous outflow is increased when systolic inflow is decreased during systole. Does your model describe this phenomenon?

Dr. N. Westerhof: Yes, you see this in the papillary muscle as well. You see flow coming out with every contraction.

Dr. R. Beyar: Do you allow that vessels that do not run in parallel to the fibers may have a different feel of their surrounding? What is really happening in those differently oriented vessels?

Dr. N. Westerhof: We have not done that. We realize that in the heart the situation is much more difficult because the vessels run transmurally and not parallel to the fibers, or not even perpendicular to the fibers, so the situation is much more difficult. It needs very sophisticated modeling to take all this into account, and we have not done it.

Dr. R. Beyar: I completely agree with the idea of increased transverse stiffness during systole. The question is, how much of that is related to the fact that the collagen mesh is stretched because of shortening, on the one hand, and how much of the active force is actually directed in the perpendicular direction? We know that the fibers are not just perfectly perpendicular to each other. We have all these "syncytium" arrangements with the force directions which are not exactly parallel to the fibers, but some of them go in angles. So there is also an active element of force that is in the transverse direction, in addition to the passive force which is generated in the collagen mesh.

Dr. N. Westerhof: Absolutely. We have simply not taken that into account. We wanted to start with a simple model and that was already difficult enough. A sophisticated model should take all of this into account.

Dr. D. Noble: Dr. ter Keurs' point still worries me. Do you agree that if a lot of muscle fibers are arranged independently in parallel with a vessel in between them and the vessel itself does not disturb the arrangement of the fibers, then there is no way in which the contraction of those fibers would deform the vessel? That is Dr ter Keurs' point. It seems to me that the only ways of moving away from that situation are either to have non-uniform contraction of those fibers so that with lateral connections between them they produce lateral displacement, or, the other possibility (and this be the case in the heart generally) is that the alignment of the fibers themselves is affected by the presence of the vessel so that, as they contract, they have to align themselves in a different way. That way, the mere presence of the vessel itself will ensure that the fibers contract in a way that disturbs the vessel.

Dr. N. Westerhof: This is true. It depends on what you call deformation. We assume the vessel with zero internal pressure and the muscle in diastole to fit the muscle cavity exactly. Pressure inside the vessel thus implies deformation.

Dr. H. ter Keurs: I could see that a vessel that does not fit the environment, in a muscle that is organized in a purely unparallel fashion, where there are transverse branches in that muscle, those branches are compressed during longitudinal contraction of that muscle, even if the contraction is completely isometric at the sarcomere level. That would be shape change and not due to stiffness change.

Dr. Y. Lanir: Your data is very convincing. The interpretation raises many questions. For instance, what is the origin of the intramyocardial pressure? You attach importance to the IMP as being the mediator between contraction and flow in the vessels. But where is the origin of it? Do you have any explanation for that?

Dr. N. Westerhof: I mean that changes in muscle properties (stiffness) alone have an effect on the coronary vasculature, but that length changes (stretch) and external pressure changes may also contribute.

Dr. Y. Lanir: Yes, but then Dr. ter Keur's comment should be considered: the LV wall has a curvature over a closed volume. This gives rise to increased pressure. But within the myocardium, there is an array of parallel fibers and there are parallel vessels in between. Contraction should not increase the pressure unless another mechanism is involved.

Dr. N. Westerhof: We have used the servo-null technique with a micropipette to measure IMP in between the fibers. This pipette is not as small as an electropipette, but is about 4 μ diameter. During the contraction of the papillary muscle, and I am not talking about the heart, you see an increase in intramuscular pressure. This means that intramyocardial pressure can arise from changes in muscle stiffness.

Dr. Y. Lanir: What puzzles me is that contractility is the major factor, even under isometric conditions.

Dr. N. Westerhof: This boils down to the same question. If you consider the heart in an isovolumic contraction, pressure in the lumen increases. If you have an isometric contraction of the papillary muscle the muscle properties change but not muscle length. It is the muscle properties that do it.

REFERENCES

1.   Gregg DE. *The coronary circulation in health and disease.* Philadelphia: Lea and Febiger; 1950.
2.   Downey JM, Kirk ES. Inhibition of coronary flow by a vascular waterfall mechanism. *Circ Res* 1975;36:753–760.
3.   Arts MGJ. *A mathematical model of the dynamics of the left ventricle and the coronary circulation.* Ph.D. Dissertation, The Netherlands, State Univ. of Limburg, 1978.
4.   Spaan JAE, Breuls NPW, Laird JD. Diastolic–systolic coronary flow differences are caused by intramyocardial pump action in anesthetized dog. *Circ Res* 1981;49:584–593.
5.   Krams R, van Haelst ACTA, Sipkema P, Westerhof N. Can coronary systolic–diastolic flow differences be related to left ventricular pressure or time–varying intramyocardial elastance? *Bas Res Cardiol* 1989;84:149–159.
6.   Krams R, Sipkema P, Westerhof N. Coronary oscillatory flow amplitude is more affected by perfusion pressure than ventricular pressure. *Am J Physiol* 1990;258:H1889–H1898.
7.   Krams R, Sipkema P, Westerhof N. Varying elastance concept may explain coronary systolic flow impediment. *Am J Physiol* 1989;257:H1471–H1479.
8.   Krams R, Sipkema P, Zegers J, Westerhof N. Contractility is the main determinant of coronary systolic flow impediment. *Am J Physiol* 1989;257:H1936–H1944.
9.   Allaart CP, Westerhof N. Effect of length and contraction on coronary perfusion in isolated perfused papillary muscle of rat heart. *Am J Physiol* 1996;271:H447–H454.
10. Bouma P, Sipkema P, Westerhof N. Vasomotor tone affects diastolic coronary flow and flow impediment by cardiac contraction similarly. *Am J Physiol* 1994;266:H1944–H1950.
11. Bouma P, Sipkema P, Westerhof N. Coronary arterial flow impediment during systole is little affected by capacitive effects. *Am J Physiol* 1993; 264:H715–H721.
12. Kouwenhoven E, Vergroesen I, Han Y, Spaan JAE. Retrograde coronary flow is limited by time–varying elastance. *Am J Physiol* 1992;263:H484–H490.
13. Streeter DD, Bassett DL. An engineering analysis of myocardial fiber orientation in pig's left ventricle in systole. *Anat Rec* 1966;155:503–511.
14. Humphrey JD, Strumpf RK, Yin FCP. Determination of a constitutive relation for passive myocardium: I. a new functional form. *ASME J Biomech Eng* 1990;112:333–339.
15. Humphrey JD, Strumpf RK, Yin FCP. Determination of a constitutive relation for passive myocardium: II. parameter estimation. *ASME J Biomech Eng* 1990;112:340–346.
16. Schouten VJA, Allaart CP, Westerhof N. Effect of perfusion pressure on force of contraction in thin papillary muscles and trabeculae from rat heart. *J Physiol (London)* 1992;451:585–604.
17. Glantz SA, Kernoff RJ. Muscle stiffness determined from canine left ventricular pressure–volume curves. *Circ Res* 1975;37:787–794.
18. Ter Keurs HEDJ, Rijnsburger WH, Van Heuningen R, Nagelsmit MJ. Tension development and sarcomere length in rat cardiac trabeculae: evidence of length–dependent activation. *Circ Res* 1980;46:703–714.
19. Vis MA, Sipkema P, Westerhof N. Modeling pressure–area relations of coronary blood vessels embedded in cardiac muscle in diastole and systole. *Am J Physiol* 1995;268:H2531–H2543.
20. Halperin HR, Chew PH, Weisfeldt ML, Sagawa K, Humphrey JD, Yin FCP. Transverse stiffness: a method for estimation of myocardial wall stress. *Circ Res* 1987;61:695–703.
21. Strumpf RK, Humphrey JP, Yin FCP. Biaxial mechanical properties of passive and tetanized canine diaphragm. *Am J Physiol* 1993;265:H469–H475.
22. Lin DH, Yin FCP. Biaxial mechanical properties of barium–activated left ventricular myocardium. *FASEB J* 1995;9:A559,#3239.
23. Giezeman MJMM. *Static and dynamic pressure–volume relations of isolated blood vessels.* Ph.D. Dissertation, The Netherlands, Univ. of Amsterdam, 1992.
24. Davis MJ and Sikes PJ. Myogenic responses of isolated arterioles: test for a rate–sensitive mechanism. *Am J Physiol* 1990;259:H1890–H1900.
25. Langewouters GJ, Wesseling KH, Goedhard WJA. The static elastic properties of 45 human thoracic

and 20 abdominal aortas *in vitro* and the parameters of a new model. *J Biomech* 1984;17:425–435.

26. Vis MA, Sipkema P, Westerhof N. Compression of intramyocardial arterioles during cardiac contraction is attenuated by accompanying venules. *Am J Physiol* 1997; in press.

27. Vis MA, Sipkema P, Westerhof N. Modeling coronary pressure–flow relations in diastole and systole. *Am J Physiol* 1997; in press.

28. VanBavel E, Spaan JAE. Branching patterns in the porcine coronary arterial tree: estimation of flow heterogeneity. *Circ Res* 1992;71:1200–1212.

29. Kassab GS, Rider CA, Tang NJ, Fung YCB. Morphometry of pig coronary arterial trees. *Am J Physiol* 1993;265:H350–H365.

30. Kassab GS, Fung YCB. Topology and dimensions of pig coronary capillary network. *Am J Physiol* 1994;267:H319–H325.

31. Kassab GS, Lin DH, Fung YCB. Morphometry of pig coronary venous system. *Am J Physiol* 1994;267:H2100–H2113.

32. Westerhof N, Allaart CP, Sipkema P. Effect of contraction on arterial inflow and capillary size of rat papillary muscle. *Heart & Vessels* 1992;suppl. 8:14, KL–25.

33. Goto M, Flynn AE, Doucette JW, Jansen CMA, Stork MM, Coggins DL, Muehrke DD, Husseini WK, Hoffman JIE. Cardiac contraction affects deep myocardial vessels predominantly. *Am J Physiol* 1991;261:H1417–H1429.

34. Judd RM, Levy BI. Effects of barium–induced cardiac contraction on large- and small–vessel intramyocardial blood volume. *Circ Res* 1991;68:217–225.

35. Westerhof N. Physiological hypotheses – intramyocardial pressure: a new concept, suggestions for measurement. *Bas Res Cardiol* 1990;85:105–119.

CHAPTER 11

Dynamic Interaction between Myocardial Contraction and Coronary Flow

Rafael Beyar and Samuel Sideman[1]

ABSTRACT

Phasic coronary flow is determined by the dynamic interaction between central hemodynamics and myocardial and ventricular mechanics. Various models,including the waterfall, intramyocardial pump and myocardial structural models, have been proposed for the coronary circulation. Concepts such as intramyocardial pressure, local elastance and others have been proposed to help explain the coronary compression by the myocardium. Yet some questions remain unresolved, and a new model has recently been proposed, linking a muscle collagen fibrous model to a physiologically based coronary model, and accounting for transport of fluids across the capillaries and lymphatic flow between the interstitial space and the venous system. One of the unique features of this model is that the intramyocardial pressure (IMP) in the interstitial space is calculated from the balance of forces and fluid transport in the system, and is therefore dependent on the coronary pressure conditions, the myocardial function and the transport properties of the system. The model predicts a wide range of experimentally observed phenomena associated with coronary compression.

BACKGROUND

Coronary flow dynamics have been characterized in numerous studies following the development of electromagnetic and ultrasonic techniques to measure phasic blood flow [1, 2]. Methods to measure the dynamics of coronary flow in patients using Doppler ultrasound [3–5] have expanded the accessibility of measurements of coronary flow dynamics to every

---

[1]Department of Biomedical Engineering, Technion–IIT, Haifa 32000, Israel

Analytical and Quantitative Cardiology
Edited by Sideman and Beyar. Plenum Press. New York. 1997

diagnostic or interventional cardiology technique [6, 7]. However, while flow measurements can be easily accomplished today, the understanding of the dynamics of coronary flow is less than complete, with controversial theories trying to explain the clinical and experimental observations. It is generally understood that the dynamics of coronary flow results from multi–level interactions between hemodynamics, myocardial contraction, the structure and function of the epicardial and intramyocardial circulation, and various control mechanisms. Yet, the precise mechanisms by which the coronary flow dynamics is related to the multiple cardiac parameters remain unclear. The parameters that play a major role in modifying the coronary flow signal are highlighted here.

INTERACTING PARAMETERS

*Myocardial compression:*As the myocardium contracts it compresses the intramyocardial circulation and impedes coronary flow [8–14]. While there is no doubt that the intramyocardial circulation is subjected to local compression, many questions are still open. What is the nature of myocardial compression? What parameters interact to impede myocardial flow during systole and what mechanisms are involved in this phenomenon?

Intramyocardial vasculature: The intramyocardial vasculature is rather unique in its structure, with arterioles penetrating the myocardium perpendicular or oblique to the muscle fibers, and capillaries running between the fibers in a parallel pattern. The intramyocardial vasculature is embedded within a collagen matrix between the fibers and muscle fibers bundles and is attached to the myocardial fibers with interconnecting collagen fibers [15].

Epicardial vasculature: The epicardial vasculature lies in the epicardial surface of the heart in regions where compression of the vessels by the muscle cannot occur. This is of utmost importance since these conductance vessels offer minimal resistance to coronary flow under normal conditions. The epicardial capacitance is important in modifying the epicardial flow dynamics, yet it is several orders of magnitude smaller than the intramyocardial compliance [16].

Aortic pressure: The aortic pressure is the driving force in the coronary tree. Since the pressure gradient over the epicardial coronary tree is rather small, the aortic pressure is almost identical to the pressure that enters into the microcirculation under normal conditions. Only under conditions of significant coronary stenosis is the pressure that is felt by the large arterioles different from the aortic pressure.

Autoregulation and control: The coronary circulation regulates the blood–flow response to the myocardial metabolic demand. Tight regulatory functions play a major role in coronary autoregulation [17]. Coronary flow reserve is an important characteristic of the coronary tree as it allows the heart to increase the blood supply five–fold, when this increase is required [18]. Various factors which impede this important function limit the functional reserve of the heart.

Fluid transport: Fluid permeates the heart capillaries and accumulates in the interstitial space. However, unlike other organs which do not contract like the myocardium, fluid transport in the heart is a complex function of the capillary pressure and the dynamic pressure in the interstitial space, which in turn depends on the myocardial contraction. With a rich lymphatic network, the heart keeps its water content within a narrow critical range, which is important for the normal function of the heart [19, 20].

Models of Myocardial Compression

Left ventricular pressure (LVP) has been earlier used in mathematical models of myocardial mechanics as the major parameter in compression [21–28]. However, evidence that coronary compression can occur even when no LVP is generated (e.g. the empty beating heart, [29]), and newer evidence showing coronary compression to be independent of the LVP under constant contractile conditions [9], has led to the search for other theories to explain these observations. One such hypothesis involves linear forces in the muscle fibers that are translated to hydrostatic pressure [21, 22, 30]. This kind of model yields that the pressure between the muscle fibers changes between zero at the epicardium to LVP at the endocardium [31]. Obviously, such models cannot explain coronary compression under zero LVP conditions.

Coronary compression under conditions of zero LVP can be explained [29] when collagen, connected between the muscle fibers in multiple directions, is accounted for [32, 33]. Thus, the observation of Krams *et al.* [9] that coronary compression is independent of the LVP, can be explained by the two phase fluid fibrous skeleton of the myocardium. It is assumed [32] that when the myocardium contracts in the fiber direction, it thickens in the cross–fiber direction. This thickening leads to tension that is developed in the cross fiber collagen, which in turn generates hydrostatic pressure in the fiber–fluid composite material. Such a pressure in the fluid media can indeed develop even under conditions of linear muscle fibers without curvature. In reality, both this mechanism and the curvature of the fibers generating Laplacian pressures contribute to coronary compression.

Westerhof [13] introduced a theory based on an analogy to the time varying elastance of the LV. Accordingly, a piece of myocardium that has a defined myocardial space can be viewed as a time varying elastance chamber that includes the intramyocardial blood vessels. These vessels are in turn compressed by the local changes in myocardial elastance, which in turn can be translated to pressure for a given compartmental volume.

Zinemanas *et al.*[35, 36] have developed a model wherein the transcapillary fluid transport plays a major role in modifying coronary compression. The model is schematically shown in Fig. 1. The model includes three compartments: muscle fibers, interstitial space and the vascular space. Fluid transport at the capillary level occurs between the blood vessel space and the interstitial space. The fluid transport equations describe the transport between the capillaries and the interstitial space. As before [32], the muscle fibers in the

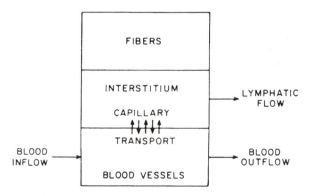

Figure 1. Schematic description of myocardial components and functional relations (reproduced from [36] with permission of the American Physiological Society).

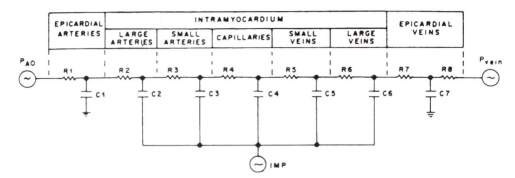

Figure 2. An electrical analog model of the coronary circulation. Each of the right and left values are calculated from the local instantaneous transmural pressure vessel area relationship (reproduced from [36] with permission of the American Physiological Society).

fiber–fluid composite are distributed across the wall according to Streeter's [37] fiber angle distribution. In addition, the collagen fibers are included to account for the stiffness in directions other than the fiber directions. The pressure in the interstitial space, which is an important parameter in fluid transport as well as in coronary compression, is defined as the intramyocardial pressure (IMP). The lymphatic drainage is simulated to account for the flow of excessive interstitial fluid into the venous system. Such a model is then linked to a model of the coronary circulation to test the various hypotheses as to coronary compression as detailed below.

Models of the Intramyocardial Vasculature

Previous models of the intramyocardial circulation have used the waterfall theory to explain flow impedance during systole [25]. According to the waterfall concept, flow within a collapsible tube that is within a pressure chamber is proportional to the pressure difference between the input pressure and the chamber pressure (which is higher than the exit pressure). While this theory can indeed explain systolic flow impedance, this phenomenological model has severe limitations. Its major limitation is the fact that collapse has not been observed within the myocardial vessels, and that various experiments failed to show independence of the flow and of the exit coronary pressure. Yet, it is conceivable that some vessel collapse can occur under certain conditions and the waterfall model may be appropriate under certain circumstances.

An alternative to the waterfall concept has been suggested by describing the myocardial circulation as pressure dependent resistance–compliance compartments [21, 24, 27]. The basic law for each compartment that is embedded within the myocardium is that there is a unique relationship between the transmural pressure and cross sectional area of the compartment. This relationship, which is highly nonlinear, defines the compliance and resistance of each compartment as a function to the instantaneous transmural pressure of that compartment. Models describing the intramyocardial circulation as distributed between arterial microcirculation and venous compartments were used in conjunction with a myocardial compression model to explain the different arterial and phasic waveforms obtained under myocardial contraction [21, 34].

The role of the epicardial vasculature should not be underemphasized. The conductance vessels that run on the epicardial surface are not subject to significant coronary compression. They offer very small resistance to flow under normal conditions, but contribute significantly to flow modification by having a typical coronary capacitance. Wave propagation must be accounted for by precise understanding of the fine details of flow dynamics [38]. The importance of the epicardial vasculature is further enhanced in disease conditions, where coronary stenosis causes a pressure drop over the diseased segment and interferes with the flow and autoregulatory process of the coronary circulation.

The role of aortic pressure in modification of coronary flow dynamics is also of great import and LV contraction causes a reduction in the coronary flow that reflects a mirror image of the compression function under constant perfusion pressure conditions and the aortic pressure interferes with this pattern during ejection. While coronary flow rapidly decreases upon the onset of isometric contraction, it is the opening of the aortic valve and the rapid aortic upstroke that reverses this flow decrease and causes a mid–systolic flow increase in proportion to the pressure increase in the aorta. Later, systolic flow decreases in parallel to the late–systolic decrease in aortic pressure. Immediately after the aortic valve closure, as the LVP falls rapidly and dissociates from the aortic pressure, the coronary flow rapidly increases to its diastolic value and then slowly decays during diastole according the aortic pressure decay.

Taking all the above into consideration, a model was constructed that combines the myocardial fiber–fluid composite model, with a compartmentalized resistance capacity (RC) pressure–dependent coronary circulation model and includes the fluid transport equation [35, 36] (Figs. 1 and 2). In this model, the IMP was calculated, rather than assumed *a priori*, based on the above interacting parameter. As shown, the model could explain most of the reported observations regarding coronary flow under various conditions.

Typical simulation results from the model are shown in Fig. 3. Preload is assumed constant and afterload is described by a three element Windkessel model. The results correspond to a steady state condition under maximum vasodilatation. The net fluid transport is zero, i.e., the transcapillary fluid flux equals the lymphatic flow. Note the aortic pressure (AOP), LVP and the predicted intramyocardial pressure (IMP), which is lower than the LVP. The IMP represents an average value across the wall. A typical flow wave is shown in Fig. 3B. Note the early systolic flow decrease followed by a mid–systolic flow increase, a small late systolic flow decrease and a rapid flow increase during isovolumic relaxation.

Figure 4 demonstrates a simulation where the coronary inflow pressure was gradually increased from 80 to 140 mmHg, allowing for fluid transport equilibration at each pressure. Note that, as expected for a non–autoregulated bed, the coronary flow increases accordingly (Fig. 4B). Note the increase in the mean and end–diastolic IMP, which is also associated with an increase in peak LVP. This may be explained by an increased volume of the interstitial space as well as the vascular space, increasing the IMP, which in turn increase the LVP through an immediate or transport mediated erectile effect. This effect is also evident in an increase in the oscillatory flow amplitude with an increase in coronary pressure, a phenomenon that has been observed by Krams *et al.* [9].

Figure 4 demonstrates a simulation where the coronary inflow pressure was gradually increased from 80 to 140 mmHg, allowing for fluid transport equilibration at each pressure. Note that, as expected for a non–autoregulated bed, the coronary flow increases accordingly (Fig. 4B). Note the increase in the mean and end–diastolic IMP, which is also associated with an increase in peak LVP. This may be explained by an increased volume of the interstitial space as well as the vascular space, increasing the IMP, which in turn increase the LVP through an immediate or transport mediated erectile effect. This effect is also evident in an increase in the oscillatory flow amplitude with an increase in coronary pressure, a phenomenon that has been observed by Krams *et al.* [9].

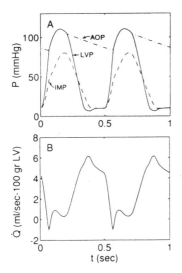

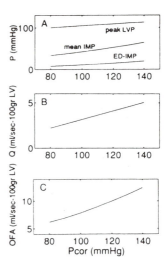

Figure 3. Calculated results using the model shown in Figs. 1 and 2. **A)** The aortic pressure (AOP), LV pressure (LVP) and the predicted IMP. **B)** Typical flowwave (reproduced from [36] with permission of the American Physiological Society).

Figure 4. The effect of coronary pressure (Pcor) on **A)** the IMP and LV; **B)** the coronary flow; **C)** the oscillatory flow amplitude (OFA) (reproduced from [36] with permission of the American Physiological Society).

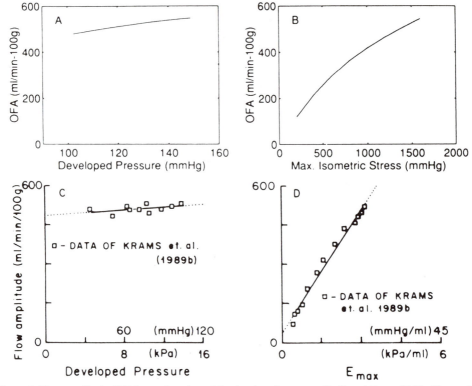

Figure 5. Flow amplitude (OFA) as a function of the developed pressure (**A,C**) and Emax (**B,D**). The model simulation (**A,B**) are compared to the experimental results by Krams *et al.* [9] (reproduced from [36] with permission of the American Physiological Society).

As shown in Fig. 5, the model predicts very well the observations made by Krams *et al.* [9]. As shown experimentally in feline hearts under constant perfusion pressure, the oscillatory flow amplitude, which may be seen as representing coronary compression, depends on the contractility represented by E_{max}, but not on the developed pressure that is achieved by modifying the afterload. This may be seen as a proof that contractility is the main determinant of coronary compression. However, while these experimental and theoretical observations may be true for these conditions, the picture may change under different conditions.

Figure 6 compares a simulation of an actively contracting or a passively pressurized myocardium to the experimental data of Doucette *et al.* [39]. In this experiment, a region of the myocardium was perfused with constant pressure, the flow measured and the contraction process paralyzed by administering lidocaine. The normalized oscillatory flow amplitude (OFA) was again viewed as an index of myocardial compression. Note that while a contracting myocardium is independent of the systolic LVP in its ability to compress the intramyocardial circulation, the pressure in the cavity determines the compressive effects in the paralyzed (by lidocaine) myocardium.

Another way to change the compression pressure is by rapid afterload changes [40], achieved by short transient occlusion of the aorta. As seen in Fig. 7, the model predictions are consistent with the following experimental observations: 1) A negative coronary flow is generated in early systole during the occluded beats (A,D). 2) The LVP is increased

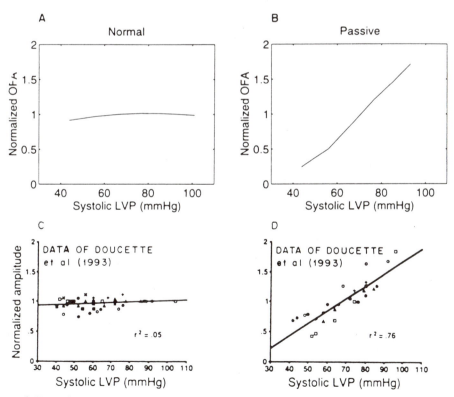

Figure 6. Comparison of the computer simulation (**A,B**) to experimental results (**C, B**) where the oscillatory flow amplitude (OFA) was measured regionally for a normally contracting (**A,C**) or a paralyzed (**B,D**) myocardium (reproduced from [36] with permission of the American Physiological Society).

THEORETICAL   EXPERIMENTAL

DATA OF KOUWENHOVEN
et. al. (1992)

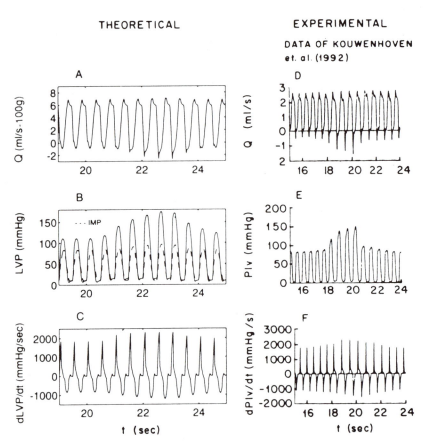

Figure 7. Response to transient aortic occlusion. The model simulation (**A–C**) is consistent with the experimental results (**D–F**). Q is the coronary flow (reproduced from [36] with permission of the American Physiological Society).

acutely as expected (B,E). 3) The derivatives of the LV pressure increase during the occluded beats in both the experimental and model simulations. These can be attributed again to an erectile effect on contractility causing a transient increase in contractility.

CONCLUSIONS

The phasic coronary flow wave signal results from the interactions of many factors which are related to the dynamics of the aortic pressure, the coronary compression and the structure function relationship of the coronary circulation. While the mechanisms of cor-onary compression and the interaction with flow are still debated, it is clear that fluid mass transport is essential for a thorough understanding of coronary dynamics. Comprehensive models that account for the structure and function of the coronary circulation according to the concepts discussed above have shown a fair fit to experimental conditions under a wide range of physiological tests. The ability to obtain relevant information from clinical measurements of the coronary flow waveform is yet limited to coronary flow reserve and some simple indices of flow pulsatility. Future research with more accurately defined hemodynamic conditions may allow to use the coronary waveform in the clinic so as to better understand the relationship between flow and contraction in health and disease.

DISCUSSION

Dr. J. Bassingthwaighte: There is something else you might take into account in the modeling, namely the tethering of vessels to the surrounding tissue. This is demonstrated by an osmotic transient experiment. A step increase in 50 milliosmolar due to sucrose, which remains extracellular and which penetrates the capillary endothelial cleft slowly, results in a decrease in the weight of an isolated perfused heart that is fully vasodilated. What is also seen simultaneously is a diminution of about 50% of the vascular resistance at constant pressure, even down to 20% of the control resistance. That is a huge diminution in resistance in a completely vasodilated preparation. The explanation is capillary tethering to the surrounding myocytes. As the water is sucked out of the myocytes by the increased osmolarity of the perfusate, the cells shrink, and through the tethering, expand the capillaries, resulting in the diminution of resistance.

There is another interesting aspect of these osmotic transient experiments. The transient weight loss is followed by a partial and then a weight regain at a time when there is no chemical driving force. This is due strictly to mechanical restoring forces in the interstitium, expanding the interstitium back toward the control rest level. Do you have that kind of thing in your model?

Dr. R. Beyar: We have not simulated that effect, but we can. The tethering between the muscle is included as the transverse collagen elements. Regarding the osmotic driving force that sucks water out and reduces the resistance, we have not done that experiment, though it may be doable. We have not accounted for direct interactions between muscle and capillaries, which may exist. In the experiment that you are alluding to, it might be that drying up the tissue a little bit pulls the capillaries open. We do not have these parameters in the model because of complexity. We wanted, at least in the initial phase, to keep the model as simple as we can, although it is still very complex.

Dr. Y. Lanir: You have a simple one dimensional model, and then a heart model. What happens in your models under isometric contraction or isovolumic contraction of the whole heart?

Dr. R. Beyar: There is force generated in the fibers in isometric contraction of the whole heart. There is no deformation of the collagen.

Dr. Y. Lanir: Under these conditions, why would contractility affect IMP?

Dr. R. Beyar: Contractility does not affect IMP under these conditions. If you keep the same volume constant as you change contractility, then the force in the fibers, the pressure in the ventricles, and the IMP, all increase in direct relationship to each other. If you try to simulate what Krams has done [9] in his isometric contraction or isovolumic beating heart, then you have a scaled up thing. You increase contractility, you increase pressure. Everything goes up; you cannot keep the same pressure and change contractility, unless you play with the volume.

Dr. H. Strauss: Have you tried to apply the model to other conditions such as end–diastolic hypertension seen in some patients with heart failure or idiopathic hypertropic subaortic stenosis (IHSS) where perturbations in the system would allow you to examine the various factors contributing to modifications in flow?

Dr. R. Beyar: No, we have not reached that point, but we certainly are planning to do that.

Dr. H. ter Keurs: Regarding the transverse fibers that you postulate in the cubical element that you present: You suggest that transverse fibers are stretched when the muscle fibers shorten in that cube.

Why is that? When most fibers shorten, their cross sectional area increases the distance between the muscle fibers decreases and the collagen fibers should be released.

Dr. R. Beyar: No, it is the opposite of that. Take a cross sectional area. You have an extravascular space between the fibers and you have the fibers cross sectional area. When fibers shorten in the longitudinal direction, the area of both the fibers and the extravascular space increase to assure the constancy of the volume, since it shrinks in the other direction. Therefore, distances increase between the fibers.

Dr. H. ter Keurs: But a change in cross sectional area of the muscle is due to a change of cross sectional area of the myofibrils within the cell. How do you make a change in cross sectional area of the structures outside the cell, in addition to that?

Dr. R. Beyar: The principle of incompressibility which holds the fibers (under a very short perturbation of one beat) holds for the extravascular space. Since the extravascular space does not change the volume much, it is relatively constant throughout the cycle. Shortening in the longitudinal direction must be followed by stretch in the transverse direction. That is why the fibers do elongate in the transverse directions during muscle fiber shortening.

Dr. Y. Lanir: What you are saying is different from what Dr. Westerhof is saying. Do you say that increased LVP causes an increase in IMP and it is not the effect of contractility?

Dr. R. Beyar: Contractility is an input into the model. Contractility means the ability to generate force in the fibers. If you increase the force in the fibers and you have a curved sphere, both the pressure in the cavity and the pressure in the interstitial fluid in the myocardium increase to the same extent. That is my understanding and these are the results that we have.

Dr. S. Sideman: The literature in the last few years indicates that we have overcome the stage in which the IMP was a singular property of the LV pressure. Some years back, every paper that dealt with the IMP related it to the LVP, either by a linear relationship between the two or some other function. Eventually, the notion took hold that the IMP is not a singular function of the LVP but is affected by other factors, mainly stresses and strains that come from within the contracting myocardium. We have IMP in the myocardium in the empty heart, when the pressure in the LV cavity is zero. All this leads to the conclusion that we have been too lax in the past with the assumption that IMP is solely related to the LVP.

  We have recently suggested that the IMP is a function of more than one parameter, and that it is affected by the LVP only in the extreme case. In order to explain that, we have defined the IMP as the interstitial fluid pressure, and have shown a large number of examples of correspondence between our theoretical results based on the IMP being a function of the system and not an independent parameter. By adopting this notion, we have made great progress. In our model [*Zinemanas D, et al. An integrated model of left ventricular muscle mechanics, coronary flow and fluid and mass transport. Am J Physiol 1995;268 (Heart Circ. Physiol. 37): H633–H645*] the perfusion, the mechanics of contraction, and the capillary–interstitial mass transfer all affect the IMP. The question is whether the pressure in the interstitial fluid is the true IMP.

Dr. N. Westerhof: Measurement techniques are still a big problem. You can poke a Millar catheter into the heart wall, and people have criticized this, but recently others [*Mihailsecu LS, Abel FL. Intramyocardial pressure gradients in working and nonworking isolated hearts. Am J Physiol 1994;266:H1233–H1241*] have used the servo–null technique, where the tip is only about 4 μ. Still, it does not tell you whether or not you damage the tissue. So this is not a good proof that the measurement of the IMP is correct. If we measure the IMP in the papillary muscle where there is no LVP, and we do it carefully, then we find a clear interstitial pressure increase during contraction. However, if you make a Barium contracture, in other words you wait a long time, then you do not find a sizeable IMP. Apparently, when the heart or the muscle contracts, the interstitial pressure goes up, but then if you leave it contracted, it returns to practically zero, probably because interstitial fluid is removed. If you increase the perfusion pressure, you see an increase in intramyocardial pressure, because apparently you push fluid out of the capillaries and that increases your interstitial volume and thus the IMP. I believe that the IMP is not something we need in modeling but that it is a convenient way to convey the idea to other people [*Vis MA, Sipkema P, Borendeerd PHM, Westerhof N. Modeling coronary blood vessels in the ventricular wall: contribution of ventricular contractility. Am J Physiol, 1997: in press*].

My final remark is that Guyton [*Guyton AC, Granger HJ, Taylor AE. Interstitial fluid pressure. Physiol Rev 1971;51:527–563*] measured a sort of intramuscular or interstitial pressure which was always negative. That may be another problem we have not resolved yet. We never find negative interstitial pressures with the micropipette.

Dr. U. Dinnar: It is known that when you put a pipette, or any kind of a sensor, into a vessel, it pulls fluids around it. What you measure then is the hydrostatic pressure. I expect the same happens when you introduce a pipette into the muscle.

Dr. E. Ritman: This is very reminiscent of arguments 25 years ago about pressure measurements in the pleural space. The great insight that came from that big argument was the so-called swimming pool problem. If you have a swimming pool that is 5 feet deep, you can stand on the bottom. You can measure the water pressure at the bottom of the pool very accurately, but that has little relationship to the pressure between the sole of your foot and the pool bottom. It can have a relationship, but it does not necessarily have one; it depends on how many bricks you have on your head as to what that pressure is. Even if you have a sensor of 1 nm in diameter so that it does not disturb the local tissue, it may still have very little relationship to the pressure that we are interested in. The whole tethering problem comes into this. A blood vessel can be kept open with tethering, so how do you express that in terms of intravascular or extravascular pressure, which will have very little to do with the pressure in the fluid outside the blood vessel that you can measure and that most people probably do measure. This is a complicated problem and you need to talk about the microscopic structure of the tissue you are measuring pressure in.

Dr. A. McCulloch: Whereas Dr Ritman's point is undoubtedly correct, it does not change the fact that the interstitial pressure must contribute to the stress equilibrium of the composite tissue. That is why it is necessary to have a theoretical definition. Beyar and Sideman's choice, if I understand it correctly, is the hydrostatic pressure that arises in enforcing the constraint of incompressibility in the solid phase of the model. In other words, volume is a key element in determining the hydrostatic pressure. The paper that Dr. Westerhof referred to by Mihailescu and Abel [*Am J Physiol 1994;266:H1233–1241*] showed that the measured interstitial pressure depends on intracoronary volume. So my question to Dr. Beyar is: do the changes in IMP with perfusion pressure in your model agree with those measurements?

Dr. R. Beyar: We have compared our prediction to the data of Able and they agree with the transient that they get. But data are relatively limited. People have not probed a lot in venous pressure or in the transport phenomena to be able to do a wide comparison. But the general trend is there. We still need to talk in a coherent manner, and I would stick to the definition that the IMP is the hydrostatic pressure and you can define the pressure in the interstitial fluid. I think that this should be adopted as a consensus. There are measurement artifacts which should not change the definition.

The major question still in my mind is: what compresses the vessels? Is it only the intramyocardial fluid pressure or is it a more complex phenomena involving both hydrostatic pressure and all these structural changes around the vessels with the interconnections between the muscle fibers and the vessels and between the muscle fibers constraining the volume. Obviously, there is a constrained volume there. We need to define our terms appropriately.

Dr. Y. Lanir: There is another aspect which may be of interest. The myocardium is a multi–phasic material. It would be advantageous to learn from the experience in the field of multi–phasic systems. In a porous media, for instance, it is generally accepted that pressure is an average quantity, over some domain which has small spaces which interconnect with each other. Hence, in analogy, IMP is an average quantity. But if one looks at local phenomena, deviations from this average may occur. This is further complicated in the myocardium by the presence of a vascular space which interacts with myocardium.

Dr. U. Dinnar: In engineering, we reserve the term pressure to hydrostatic pressure. When we consider fibers, we relate to the shear as stress and relate the stress to the pressure.

Dr. Y. Lanir: This is the case in uniphasic material in which pressure is defined as average of the three normal stress components. In multi–phasic systems the fluid pressure is independent of the stress in the solid.

Dr. J. Downey: To show how different the stresses and the hydrostatic pressure can be in a multi–phasic system, Arthur Guyton [*ibid*], who was the proponent of the negative tissue pressure, had a model which was simply a plastic bag filled with ping pong balls which he would hook up to a vacuum cleaner. He would invite you to put your hand inside this bag and when he would make the hydrostatic pressure negative, the result was that your hand was crushed by these ping pong balls. You would have a very positive compressive stress by the ping pong balls trying to squeeze your hand, yet the pressure was negative. These things can go in opposite directions, so the hydrostatic pressure can be quite different from what is actually collapsing the blood vessels. It may a bit too simplistic to think only in terms of hydrostatic pressure, especially with what you measure with the fluid pocket vs what you measure with the finite object in myocardium.

Dr. H. Kammermeier: Interstitial pressure from intraventricular pressure, it has to be taken in account that with zero ventricular pressure a heart is in an unphysiological shape where shear of the different layers of the myocardium are occurring. The question: Is this real zero intraventricular pressure or is it zero afterload? In the case of a zero afterload situation one has a certain intraventricular pressure simply owing to the acceleration of the pumped blood.

Dr. H. ter Keurs: Not related to this point, but related to the point that intramyocardial intracellular pressure seems to be very crucial. The measurement of that pressure is equally crucial. If we take a flexible microelectrode, we can penetrate trabeculae endothelial wall and subsequently sarcolemma of the myocyte and measure membrane potential in a stable fashion. If you work with a microelectrode of 0.01 micrometer diameter, that is substantially smaller than intercellular space which is in the range of 200–300 nm in a papillary and trabeculae. I can not quite see that it would be possible to use a 4 μ microelectrode and measure an unperturbed intracellular pressure, even if you use a servo–null technique. When you turn the servo–nulling device on you damage a whole bunch of endocardial cells and a whole bunch of myocytes and that must change the pressure.

Dr. U. Dinnar: What you really measure is a cavity of fluid that is generated within the probe. This kind of represents the interstitial fluids.

Dr. M. Morad: Some 15 years ago we estimated that placing a potassium sensitive electrode of 1 μm in diameter in the ventricular muscle creates a 50 μm pool in the muscle.

Dr. L. Axel: Pushing things apart in order to jam your catheter in the tissue will generate negative pressures. The fluid that you are measuring at the tip of that orifice is seeing many kinds of forces, not simply the transmural hydrostatic forces. There can be local gradients of pressure measured that way and that could well account for discrepancies.

Dr. A. McColloch: Dr Bassingthwaighte suggested [*personal communication*] that although the endothelium was a barrier to metabolite transport, that you thought it was not a barrier to oxygen transport. But there has been some work by Mathieu–Costello [*Mathieu–Costello O. Comparative aspects of muscle capillary supply. Annu Rev Physiol 1993;55:503–525*] and others using comparative physiology type of approaches looking at tissues of a wide range of mitochondrial density and capillary density and capillary tortuosity. As a result of that, they suggest that there is a significant barrier to oxygen transport at the endothelium.

Dr. J.B. Bassingthwaighte: I am not convinced. Historically there is literature stating that there is a barrier for oxygen across the capillary wall. There are reports [*Gayeski TEJ, Honig CR. O$_2$ gradients from sarcolemma to cell interior in red muscle at maximal $\dot{V}O_2$. Am J Physiol 1986;251 (Heart Circ Physiol 20):H789–H799*] in which the authors used optical methods to look at the apparent saturation of hemoglobin vs myoglobin. Those interpretations are totally artifactual because their spatial resolution was much bigger than the cells. To estimate capillary and myocyte pO_2, they changed their choice of reference substance from hemoglobin, when they thought they were over a capillary, to myoglobin, when they thought they were over a cell. The spectral changes between oxygenated and reduced forms of Hb and Mb are similar but the half–saturation pO_2 are 26 and 2.5, respectively; so a shift in choice from Hb to Mb automatically gave an estimated pO_2 of 1/10 of using the Hb as a reference. They have therefore mistakenly reported that there were big gradients in pO_2 across the barriers. Their particular interpretations should therefore be disregarded. I am not familiar enough with the experiments of Mathieu–Costello [*1993; ibid*] to be specifically critical. But I am not convinced that a comparative study gets at the details. If I look at O^{15} in the presence of cyanide which stops metabolism, then $^{15}O_2$ is a flow–limited marker. The shapes of the impulse responses will be hematocrit–dependent, and this is because oxygen's mean transit time volume changes with hematocrit. This is to say that when the hematocrit is low, the relative volume of distribution in the tissue is larger and the mean transit time longer. Carbon monoxide also exchanges so rapidly that you can see, on residue function curves in isolated blood perfused rabbit hearts, a tail of CO binding the myoglobin. From our experiments I would say that oxygen looks to be flow–limited when it is not being consumed. If one does a series of experiments with tracer water, they are also clearly flow limited [*Yipintsoi T, Bassingthwaighte JB. Circulatory transport of iodoantipyrine and water in the isolated dog heart. Circ Res 1970;27:461–477*]. You change the flows and you get similarity scaling between the outflow concentration–time curves scaled with proportion of their mean transit time showing no evidence of barrier limitation. I infer from the similar solubility in lipid membranes between water and oxygen at the end that there should not be any barrier limitation for oxygen.

Dr. A. McColloch: We have also found it very difficult to observe any transmural gradients of capillary density but there is a little bit of theoretical work and some experimental work suggesting that there could be some transmural gradients of vascular capacitance. Of course, the mechanics would suggest that there could be large transmural gradients of whatever the forces are that may affect resistance and capacitance locally.

Dr. J.B. Bassingthwaighte: There is another way of looking at the question of vascular capacitance. An elephant has a much larger fraction of feeder vessels to its myocardium and from its myocardium than does a mouse, simply because it is bigger. Those are capacitances. By the same token, one has to have more capacitance vessel near the epicardium than near the endocardium because it all goes to and comes back to the epicardium. Thebesian vein drainage into the LV is negligible: there are only about 10 or 12 thebesian veins per dog LV cavity, but there are perhaps hundreds in the RV, since all the septum drains into the RV. But basically, most of the capacitance vessels have to be near the epicardium so there must be gradients in capacitance. It cannot be any other way.

Dr. A. McCulloch: Maybe the measurements suggest that the epicardial change in vascular diameter with the change in pressure is actually higher from the endocardium, similar to Yasha Kresh's models.

Dr. J.B. Bassingthwaighte: Yes, I am not sure why that would be. I suppose the compliance of subendocardial arterioles would be higher if the walls were thinner.

REFERENCES

1. Kolin A. Circulatory System, Methods, blood flow determination by electromagnetic methods. in Glasser O (ed) Medical Physics,. Yearbook Publishers. Chicago 3:141–156, 1960.
2. Vatner SF, Franklin D, Van Citters RL. Simultaneous comparison and calibration of Doppler and electromagnetic flowmeters. *J Appl Physiol* 1970;29:907–910.
3. Doucette JW, Corl PD, Payne HM, Flynn AE, Goto M, Nassi M, Segal J. Validation of a Doppler guide wire for intravascular measurement of coronary artery flow velocity. *Circulation* 1992;85:1899–1911.
4. Wilson RF, Laughlin DE, Ackel PH, Chilian WM, Holida MD, Hartley CL, Armstrong ML, Marcus ML, White CAW. Transluminal subselective measurements of coronary artery blood flow velocity and vasodilator reserve in man. *Circulation* 1985;72:82–92.
5. Kern MJ, Donohue TJ, Aguirre FV, Bache RG, Caracciolo EA, Ofili E, Labovitz AJ. Assessment of angiographically intermediate coronary artery stenosis using the Doppler flowwire. *Am J Cardiol* 1993;71:26D–33D.
6. Segal J, Kern MJ, Scot NA, King SB III, Doucette JW, Heuser RR, Ofili E Siegel R. Alternations of phasic coronary artery velocity in humans during percutaneous coronary angioplasty. *J Am Coll Cardol* 1992;20:276–86.
7. Ofili EO, Labovitz AJ, Kern MJ. Coronary flow velocity dynamics in normal and diseased arteries. *Am J Cardiol* 1993;71:3D–9D.
8. Armour JA, Randall WC. Canine left ventricular intramyocardial pressures. *Am J Phys* 1971;220:1833–1839.
9. Krams R, Sipkema P, Zegers J, Westerhof N. Contractility is the main determinant of coronary systolic flow impediment. *Am J Physiol* 1989;257 *(Heart Circ Physiol* 26):H1936–H1944.
10. Panerai RB, Chamberlain JH, Sayers B. Characterization of extravascular component of coronary resistance by instantaneous pressure–flow relationships in the dog. *Circ Res* 1979;45:378–390.
11. Rabbany SY, Kresh JY, Noordergraaf A. Intramyocardial pressure: interaction of myocardial fluid pressure and fiber stress. *Am J Physiol* 1989;257 *(Heart Circ Physiol* 26):H357–H364.
12. Van Winkle DM, Swafford AN, Downey JW. Subendocardial coronary compression in beating dog hearts is independent of pressure in the ventricular lumen. *Am J Physiol* 1991; 261 *(Heart Circ Physiol* 30):H500–H505.
13. Westerhof N. Intramyocardial pressure revisited. In: *Cardiac Electrophysiology, Circulation, and Transport* (Sideman S, Beyar R, editors). Kluwer Academic Publishers, New York 1991; 237–243.
14. Feigl EO, Neat GW, Huang AH. Interrelations between coronary artery pressure, myocardial metabolism and coronary blood flow. *J Mol Cell Cardiol* 1990;22:375–390.
15. Caulfield JB, Borg TK. The collagen network of the heart. *J Lab Invest* 1979;40:364–372.
16. Manor D, Sideman S, Dinnar U, Beyar R. Analysis of the flow in the coronary epicardial arterial tree and intramyocardial circulation. *Med & Biol Eng & Comput* 1994;32(4):S133–S143.
17. Hoffman JIE, Spaan JAE. Pressure–flow relations in coronary circulation. *Physiol Rev* 1990;70:331–390.
18. Gould KL, Kirkeeide, RL, Buchi M. Coronary flow reserve as a physiologic measure of stenosis severity. *J Am Coll Cardiol* 1990;15:459–474.
19. Laine GA, Granger HJ. Microvascular, interstitial & lymphatic interactions in normal heart. *Am J Physiol* 1985;249 *(Heart Circ Physiol* 18): H834–H842.
20. Rodbard S. Capillary Control of Blood Flow and Fluid Exchange. *Circ Res* 1971;28–29 (Suppl. 1):1.51–1.58.
21. Beyar R, Caminker R, Manor D, Sideman S. Coronary flow patterns in normal and ischemic hearts: transmyocardial and artery to vein distribution. *Ann Biomed Eng* 1993;21: 435–458.
22. Beyar R, Guerci A, Halperin HR, Tsitlik JR, Weisfeldt ML. Intermittent coronary sinus occlusion following coronary arterial ligation results in venous retroperfusion. *Circ Res* 1989;65:695–707.
23. Beyar R, Sideman S. Time–dependent coronary blood flow distribution in the left ventricular wall. *Am J Physiol* 1990;252:H417–H433.
24. Bruinsma P, Arts T, Dankelman J, Spaan JAE. Model of the coronary circulation based on pressure

dependence of coronary resistance and capacitance. *Basic Res Cardiol* 1988;83:510–524.

25. Downey JM, Kirk ES. Inhibition of coronary blood flow by a vascular waterfall mechanism. *Circ Res* 1975;36: 753–760.

26. Gordon RJ. A general mathematical model of coronary circulation. *Am J Physiol* 1974;226(3):608–615.

27. Manor D, Beyar R, Sideman S. Pressure–flow characteristics of the coronary collaterals: A model study. *Am J Physiol* 1994;266 (*Heart Circ Physiol* 35): H310–H318.

28. Judd RM, Mates RE. Coronary input impedance is constant during systole and diastole. *Am J Physiol* 1991;260 (*Heart Circ Physiol* 29): H1841–H1851.

29. Baird RJ, Goldbach mm, De La Rocha A. Intramyocardial pressure: The persistence of its transmural gradients in the empty heart and its relationship to the myocardial oxygen consumption. *J Thoracic Cardiovasc Surg* 1970;59:810–823.

30. Arts T, Reneman RS. Interaction between intramyocardial pressure (IMP) and myocardial circulation. *J Biomech Eng* 1985;107:51–56.

31. Beyar R, Sideman S: Computer study of the left ventricular performance based on its fiber structure, sarcomere dynamics, and electrical activation propagation. *Circ Res* 1984;55:358–374.

32. Beyar R, Ben–Ari R, Gibbons–Kroeker CA, Tyberg JV, Sideman S. The effect of interconnecting collagen fibers on LV function and intramyocardial compression. *Cardiovasc Res* 1993;27(12):2254–2263.

33. Chadwick RS, Tedgui A, Michel JB, Ohayon J, Levy BI. A theoretical model for myocardial blood flow. In: *Cardiovascular Dynamics and Models, Proceedings of NIH–INSERM Workshops* (Brun P, Chadwick RS, Levy BI, editors). INSERM, Paris, Vol. 183, 1988; 77–90.

34. Chadwick RS, Tedgui A, Michel JB, Ohayon J, Levy BI. Phasic regional myocardial inflow and outflow: Comparison of theory and experiments. *Am J Physiol* 1990;258: H1687–H1698.

35. Zinemanas D, Beyar R, and Sideman S. Effects of myocardial contraction on Coronary flow: An Integrated model. *Annals Biomed Eng* 1994;22(6):638–652.

36. Zinemanas D, Beyar R, Sideman S. An integrated model of left ventricular muscle mechanics, coronary flow and fluid and mass transport. *Am J Physiol* 1995;268 (*Heart Circ Physiol* 37): H633–H645.

37. Streeter DD, Spotnitx HM, Patel DP, Ross J, Sonnenblick EH. Fiber orientation in the canine left ventricle during diastole and systole. *Circ Res* 1969;24:339–347.

38. Rumberger JAJ, Nerem RM, Muir WW. Coronary artery pressure development and wave transmission characteristics in the horse. *Cardiovasc Res* 1979;13:413–419.

39. Doucette JW, Goto M, Flynn AE, Austin RE Jr, Husseini W, Hoffman JIE. Effects of cardiac contraction and cavity pressure on myocardial blood flow. *Am J Physiol* 1993;265:H1342–H1352.

40. Kouwenhoven E, Vergroesen I, Han Y, Spaan JAE. Retrograde coronary flow is limited by time varying elastance. *Am J Physiol* 1992;263:H484–H490.

CHAPTER 12

THE RELATIONS BETWEEN MICROVASCULAR STRUCTURE AND OXYGEN SUPPLY

Uri Dinnar[1]

ABSTRACT

The current theories of microcirculatory control require a higher command center to maintain tissue homeostasis. The theory of arteriolar vasodilatation generates conflicting results by increasing the flow and the capillary hydrostatic pressures. A new theory, recently suggested to account for local tissue flow control, applies a blinking mechanism of open capillaries, whereby alternating circulatory modes increase flow to specific tissue regions, without inducing a higher control center. The mechanism is evaluated here mathematically by examining the oxygen demand, supply and local tissue concentration of oxygen. It is shown that this theory explains how periods of oxygen debts are compensated by increased flow with changes in the operation mode. The results show that there is a direct relation between the tissue microvascular complexity and the capability of the specific tissue to withstand periods of oxygen deficit.

INTRODUCTION

Our model [1] of the microcirculation has challenged the idea that microcirculatory control is achieved by changing the diameters of the arterioles. If this latter idea is accepted, it is evident that a single cell is incapable to change its oxygen demand. In cases of higher metabolic demand, only a response of multiple cells will change the desired blood flow to yield a higher oxygen supply, which in turn will affect a very large tissue volume. A simple mathematical analysis of pressure distribution and the resulting flow when we eliminate completely the arteriolar resistance, will show that the system is capable to

---

[1]Department of Biomedical Engineering, Technion–IIT, Haifa, 32000, Israel

increase blood flow only by a small fraction of what we observe in reactive hyperemia experiments. Moreover, this small change will deliver the blood to the capillaries with high pressure, much higher than the optimal pressure needed for an optimal oxygen exchange, and will probably cause edema of the tissues. It was shown [1] that the complexity of the microvascular structure, together with a system of capillary enhancement by alternating (blinking) inlet conditions, is capable of changing the regional blood supply by a few hundred percent without significant change in the perfusion pressure and with a negligible increase in the power requirement. The model assumes that only when the entire capillary bed, in a specific region, is at maximal flow conditions, will the "higher levels" of control become operative and the well known changes in arteriolar diameter will take place.

To further investigate the relation between structure and oxygen supply we have studied here the transfer of oxygen from a mesh of capillaries and the changes in oxygen concentrations in the tissues during large metabolic demands and after altering the capillary blood flow. As in the earlier model, we assume here that there is an overlapping supply of vessels in almost every immediate neighborhood of individual cells. The schematic arrangement shown in Fig. 1 is an example of a capillary structure with multiple branches having with two levels of control mechanisms. The first mechanism controls the entire segment by changing the flow in all three branches, while the other mechanism changes flow in each of the individual branches. We will concentrate here on the second control mechanism. Only if this control can not satisfy the requirements for flow supply is the first mechanism to be activated. This specific model is capable to increase blood flow to this segment by 235% without changing pressures. However, a structure with a higher number of branches and a higher overlap will show a much higher capabilities, as they will be able to present a much higher flow value for the blood supply.

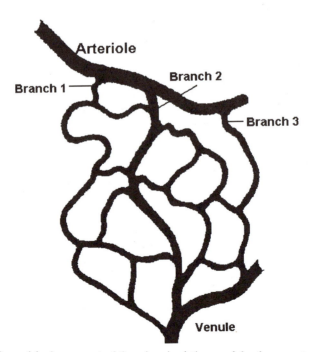

Figure 1. A schematic model of a segment of the microcirculation used for the current study (based on [1]).

The Keogh Cylindrical Model

The oldest and still most common model of blood flow and oxygen exchange in the capillaries is Krogh's cylindrical model, suggested in 1919 [3]. His model assumed a single capillary and formulated the factors governing the rate of diffusion of oxygen from the capillaries into the immediate interstitial space. This two dimensional model neglected longitudinal changes in the oxygen tension of the blood. Keogh obtained a relation between the oxygen tension of the blood, the oxygen consumption of the tissue and the oxygen tension between the capillary and an imaginary boundary that fits the capillary density (Fig. 2). This relationship showed that increased blood flow due to excessive demand by the tissue can be achieved by one of two methods: either by increasing blood flow, which has a weak effect, or by increasing the number of capillaries, which has a strong effect. The idea of capillary recruitment by increasing the capillary count is still controversial 80 years after Krogh's presentation of the model. His model assumed an equilibrium between blood supply and tissue demand and assumes that all body organs are built in the same way, except for the changes in capillary density. To study the changes in the interstitial oxygen tension due to changes in oxygen supply and blood flow, we consider the equations for oxygen concentrations in tissue and capillary blood given by:

$$\frac{\partial C}{\partial t} = D_c \nabla^2 C - V \frac{\partial C}{\partial x} \qquad \text{inside capillaries} \qquad (1)$$

$$\frac{\partial C}{\partial t} = D_t \nabla^2 C - R_t \qquad \text{in tissue} \qquad (2)$$

where $C=C(x,r,t)$ is the oxygen concentration either inside the capillary or in the interstitial space; D_c and D_t are the diffusion coefficients for the capillary and tissues, respectively; V is the velocity of blood in the capillary, and R_t is the oxygen consumption rate per unit volume of tissue.

Equations (1) and (2) are subjected to initial conditions of specified interstitial tissue consumption, arterial oxygen tension at the capillary inlet, conservation of oxygen along the capillary boundaries and circular symmetry.

Numerical solution of Eqs. (1) and (2) yields the oxygen tension distribution shown in Fig. 3. The figure shows that a single capillary can supply only a small volume of tissue

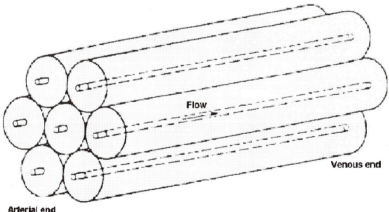

Figure 2. Krogh's classical cylindrical model of tissue microcirculation.

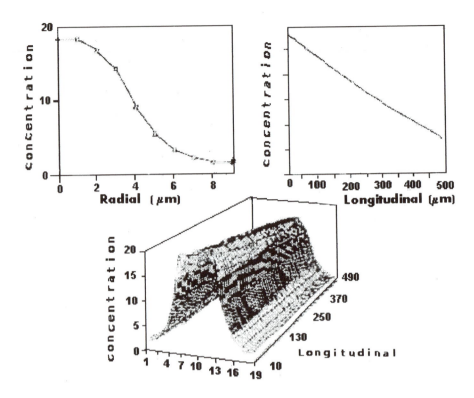

Figure 3. Oxygen tension distribution in the tissue–capillary spaces in the radial (upper left) direction at the middle of the capillary length, at the longitudinal direction (upper right) and the combined cross sectional presentation (lower frame).

and that there is a small, but persisting difference between a region near the capillary inlet and a region further down stream. We assume that the average oxygen tension in the interstitial space can be represented by the average value on the radial line at mid–capillary distance (see below).

The Keogh model was investigated in situations of increased tissue demand for oxygen under conditions of reactive hyperemia. The results agree with reported experimental results [4]. The results presented here are for increased tissue stress and compensation by an increased flow. The tissue demand was increased by two–, three– and six–fold for a duration of 40–200 sec and the rate of increased flow in the hyperemic period was between 1.5 and 10–fold. Tissue stress was determined by the mid–interstitial oxygen tension.

The development of tissue tension with increased metabolic demand, presented in Fig. 4, shows a linear decrease in relative tissue tension which is steeper with increased metabolic demand. This normal decrease mode and the resulting low oxygen tissue tension was the base for metabolic compensation by increased blood flow. It was found that when the stress was maintained for a long period, not every compensation could bring the interstitial space back to normal values. Figure 5 shows the critical value for each compensatory value of increased flow. This value shows the maximal time a tissue can be under excessive oxygen demand before the recovery is ineffective. For example, if the metabolic demand is increased by 300%, and the reactive compensation is 175%, the tissue will suffer irreversible damage within a few seconds. However, if the reactive response is higher than 200%, the duration of oxygen tension stress can be over 50 sec, and still maintain a reversible path. This is not true for a 600% increase in the metabolic demand, were a few minutes are the upper limit.

One can study the effectiveness of compensation by the extended duration of reactive hyperemia required to "pay back" the oxygen debt generated by a period of increased metabolic demand. As expected, it was found that the longer the tissue remains under excessive uncompensated metabolic demand which leads to a tissue stress, the stronger and longer the phenomena of reactive hyperemia.

As seen in Fig. 6, when the excessive metabolic demand continues for a duration of 40 sec and the reactive hyperemia is 200%, then the duration of reactive hyperemia must remain for over 100 sec (two and a half times the stress duration), so as to guarantee a reversible recovery. However, when the compensatory hyperemia is 600%, the required time drops sharply to 10 sec, much shorter than the stress duration.

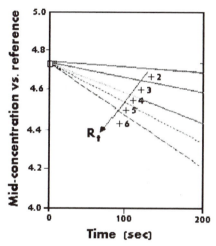

Figure 4. Mid–concentration vs the reference for increased interstitial oxygen demand.

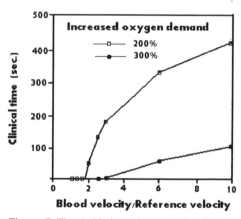

Figure 5. Threshold times for stress duration (in seconds) before reversible compensation can occur.

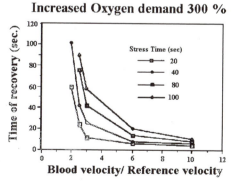

Figure 6. Time of recovery for increments of blood velocities after different times of stress (in seconds). Metabolic demand increased by 300%.

Obviously, the Krogh cylinder is far from a geometric reality. To study a more realistic model we consider the anatomical structure shown in Fig. 1, which has three inlet branches leading from the arteriole to a venule. Note that a structure with fewer inlet branches does not give satisfactory results, while a system with more branches complicates and overloads the mathematical calculations, although its behavior is not different than the present case. Thus, the three branches provide a satisfactory model.

The electrical analog of this structure, shown in Fig. 7, has a purely resistive configuration, since the capillaries are completely covered with collagen fibers which provide rigidity and almost totally eliminate capacitance. Flow is very slow and inertia is usually neglected in capillary flow. Analysis of this circuit using PSPICE program under conditions of alternating (blinking) inlet conditions gives the rate of flow and pressures for each segment and each junctions for different situation of open inlets. A specific section of this complex is shown in Fig. 8. The results of flow rates and pressure distribution for this specific section for specific inlet openings are given in Tables 1 and 2.

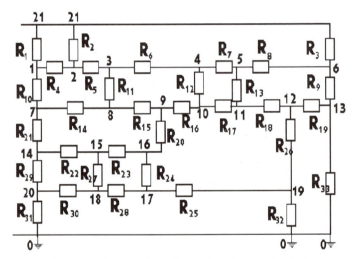

Figure 7. The electric analog of the microvascular bed.

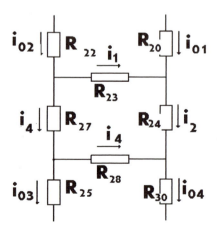

Figure 8. Representation of a single test section by an electric analog.

The oxygen concentration is assumed to decrease with the pressures. This reduction nearly equals the relative distance between arteriole and venule, and is consistent with the notion that the blood releases oxygen along its path; the longer the path, the smaller the oxygen tension in the blood.

Solving the electrical analog yields the inlet pressures and oxygen concentration for the specific tissue element, and allows to solve the differential equations for oxygen concentration within the tissue. For mathematical simplicity we assume a rectangular shape (Fig. 9) in which the tissue region is surrounded by four blood vessels. With conditions of symmetry and uniform plug flow in each blood vessels, Eqs. (1) and (2) become:

$$\frac{\partial C}{\partial t} = D_c \nabla^2 C - V \frac{\partial C}{\partial \ell} \qquad \text{inside capillaries} \qquad (3)$$

$$\frac{\partial C}{\partial t} = D_t \nabla^2 C - R_t \qquad \text{in tissue} \qquad (4)$$

where $C = C(\ell,t)$ and ℓ is the coordinate along the capillary (either X or Y coordinate, respectively). The following boundary conditions are considered:

a. Symmetry along midline of capillaries.
b. Continuity of oxygen saturation values along capillary walls.
b. Equal oxygen flux on both sides of capillary walls.
c. Calculated oxygen saturation values at the entrance to the four entrances of the four capillaries.

Equations (3) and (4) were solved numerically using the Forward Time Centered Space (FTCS) method with a slight variation to account for difficulties arising at the nodes. The new method used the nodes as separate domain with 4x4 grid point, thus avoiding the problems of discontinuity of velocities.

The physiological values were taken from Weibel [5]. The normal value of oxygen reaction coefficient was taken to be 0.0004 ml O_2/100 ml tissue–sec, and the multiplication of this value was used for increased workload.

Table 1. Currents (representing rates of flow) in the test section of the basic element (Fig. 8).

Currents (flow)	Open Inlets:						
	#1	#2	#3	#1 & 2	#1 & 3	#2 & 3	All
I_{01}	0.4007	0.3626	0.2852	0.3795	0.2274	0.0935	0.3389
I_{02}	0.0258	0.0365	0.0282	0.0141	0.0404	−0.0090	0.0239
I_{03}	0.1580	0.1356	0.1193	0.1481	0.0891	0.0452	0.1243
I_{04}	0.2684	0.2636	0.1941	0.2455	0.1786	0.0394	0.2385
I_1	−0.127	−0.1060	−0.0870	−0.1250	−0.0589	−0.0392	−0.1040
I_2	0.1526	0.1428	0.1152	0.1389	0.0993	0.0302	0.1277
I_3	−0.0050	0.0072	−0.004	−0.009	0.0101	−0.0150	0.0034
I_4	0.2739	0.2564	0.1982	0.2546	0.1685	0.0544	0.2350

Table 2. Pressure and oxygen concentration at nodes of the basic element (Fig. 8)

Pressures (above venule)		#1	#2	#3	#1 & 2	#1 & 3	#2 & 3	All
U_1	(mmHg)	11.451	10.121	8.555	10.681	6.690	2.940	9.256
U_2	(mmHg)	9.550	8.526	7.250	8.809	5.806	2.353	7.699
U_3	(mmHg)	7.261	6.384	5.521	6.725	4.316	1.900	5.782
U_4	(mmHg)	7.343	6.275	5.582	6.862	4.163	2.125	5.730
Oxygen concentration								
C_1 (ml O_2/100 ml tissue)		16.290	16.024	15.711	16.136	15.338	14.588	15.851
C_2 (ml O_2/100 ml tissue)		15.910	15.705	15.450	15.762	15.161	14.471	15.540

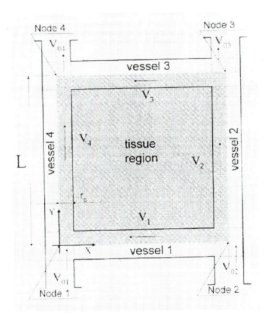

Figure 9. The basic element of mathematical modeling.

RESULTS

For the simple "normal" case we considered the case of one open branch and the other two closed. (Changing any of the three branches will yield a slight negligible modi-fication.) The values for normal loading are shown in Fig. 10, representing steady state conditions with no regions of oxygen stress. A region of oxygen deficit is defined as a region with an oxygen concentration of less than 14 ml O_2/100 ml tissue. In the following figures a darker shade represents oxygen stress at a larger concentration level.

When the oxygen demand is increased five-fold, the supply is not sufficient and a large area, as shown in Fig. 11, will suffer lack of oxygen. As shown, the deprived region is not symmetrical and is shifted in the blood flow direction. At higher oxygen demand values, this region will be mach larger and will cover the entire area [6].

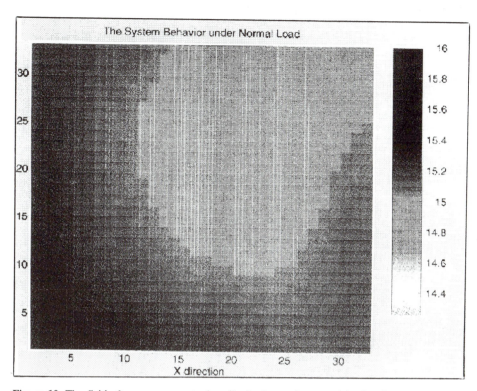

Figure 10. The field of oxygen concentration distribution under normal load and one branch open.

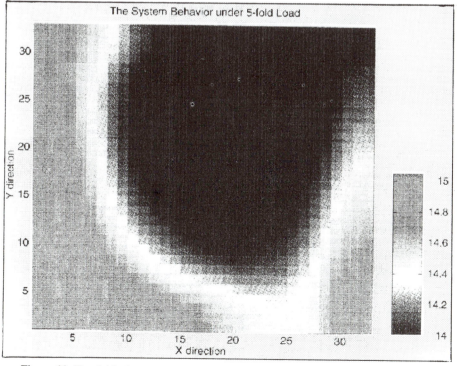

Figure 11. The field of oxygen concentration under five–fold increase in oxygen demand.

Figure 11 represents a steady state solution for a five–fold increase in the oxygen demand. This steady state can not be maintained for a long period of time without some appropriate compensation. However, if we accept the blinking theory, where the branches alternates between open and close, we can change the situation by using this steady state condition as the initial condition for a second stage wherein two branches are now open rather than one. Intervals of 0.5 sec are sufficient to correct the oxygen levels and bring them back to normal. The increased oxygen supply is achieved with no increase in arteriolar flow or variations in capillary pressures.

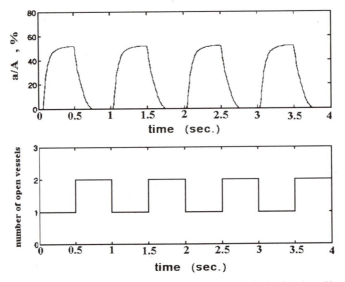

Figure 12. Time dependence of relative oxygen lack area under five–fold load and capillary blinking of 0.5 sec (two mode functioning).

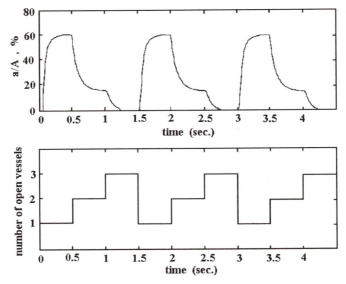

Figure 13. Time dependence of relative oxygen lack area under seven–fold load and capillary blinking of 0.5 sec (two mode functioning).

Note that if the oxygen demand is increased to seven–fold, then any length of the blinking interval by opening of two branches will not supply the lacking oxygen, and only a period of over 0.5 sec with three open inlets alternating with a single opening can maintain and compensate for the oxygen debt generated in the single branch opening.

To facilitate graphical presentation, we relate to the calculated percentage of the oxygen deficit area; a/A, which defines the fraction of tissue area which is under the minimal value of oxygen tension.

Figure 12 shows the results for functioning under a five–fold increase in metabolic demand. The upper panel represents the a/A–parameter as a function of time, while the lower panel shows the periodicity pattern of the blinking mechanism. As seen, the extreme situation where 40% of the area is in oxygen debt is fully recovered in the two open branches period. However, when we increase the demand to seven times the normal value we can see that increasing the supply by opening two inlets is not sufficient to compensate for the oxygen deficit during single branch opening, and there is no complete recovery with two inlet openings. Changing the mode of operation to three modes with additional opening periods where all three branches are open will eliminate this problem (Fig. 13).

DISCUSSION

The calculations can be carried out for any mode of operation, and the results can provide limits as to the capability of a specific tissue to compensate for increased metabolic demand, and the blinking duration needed to fully recover from the periods of oxygen debt. The results show that the complexity of the microvasculature is a key element in the vitality of the cells and the possibility to withstand periods of oxygen lack. It is important to emphasize that his recovery is obtained with minimum demand for increased energy and minimum changes in pressure and flow. It is expected that only when all these local control mechanism fail, will a higher control mechanism, like vasodilation and others, become active.

CONCLUSIONS

It is quite clear that tissue control of oxygen levels at the single cell level can not be governed by arteriolar changes. Such changes will generate high perfusion pressure and excessive edema. There must be a local cellular control which will generate periods of higher perfusion to compensate for the debt brought about by periods of higher demands. The present model suggests such a mechanism, and new measurement techniques must be developed to experimentally study its validity.

Acknowledgments

This research was supported by funds from the Berman Philanthropic Foundation, Michigan U.S.A., The Gerson Family Foundation, Michigan U.S.A. and the Fund for Promotion of Research at the Technion. The Author wish to express his many thanks for those foundations for their continuous support of research at the Technion.

DISCUSSION

Dr. J. Downey: If I understand your model, it is as if you have a ladder with two main channels and rungs. The only way you can really perfuse the rungs is to close off one of the inlets and get a cross–circulation. This gives you better perfusion even though flow is less.

Dr. U. Dinnar: If consider a ladder, then the entire structure can be supplied by one branch of the ladder through the rungs.

Dr. J. Downey: Giving lateral flow through the rungs is more efficient.

Dr. U. Dinnar: If you want more flow then you open both branches and then more flow comes through the entire system.

Dr. J. Downey: Yes, but it is not so efficient.

Dr. U. Dinnar: It is less efficient but there is more flow. This is done without changing the pressure upstream, because if you give the arterioles to change the pressure, then the pressure at the entrance to this level will be much higher for the entire transcapillary exchange. This causes many problems.

Dr. J. Downey: Exactly. If this is really going on, then it ought to be observable by reversal of flow in the network. In other words, any of these small rungs of the ladder ought to flow this way for a while and then that way and we should be able to see that.

Dr. U. Dinnar: How do you observe it? They are very small, to start with. What you observe in reality is that the flow changes in velocity; it goes slow, fast, slow and fast.

Dr. J. Downey: But it never reverses?

Dr. U. Dinnar: In some cases you see a reversed flow, but the reversed flow is very small.

Dr. J. Downey: We are sort of saying that we have a smooth muscle winking on and off to do this. But you bring up another possibility: if you see a leukocyte go through a capillary, it goes so very slowly, and then the flow starts again. Could leukocytes actually contribute to this winking?

Dr. U. Dinnar: Yes. If the leukocytes have the chance of going into a larger vessel or a smaller one, they will choose the larger vessel all the time. But if the vessels are of equal size, then each branch will be blocked for a while.

Dr. J. Downey: Right, so we should be able to detect this by perfusing with neutropenic blood. You should actually see an improved oxygen delivery, that is almost measurable.

Dr. U. Dinnar: I have done some computations where we increased the number of white cells. When we increase the number of white cells, they have no choice, they have to penetrate into the smaller vessel. Then we see a reduction of flow in both vessels. It blinks for a much longer period of time until they pass through. We took this as about 0.5 sec, the time of forming and passing through the capillary.

Dr. J. Downey: But if we actually perfused the heart with neutropenic blood, will it make enough difference so that we could actually measure it with our experimental technique? What does the model predict?

Dr. U. Dinnar: I do not know. This is a mathematical model. We have to look into it.

Dr. H. ter Keurs: Did you ever try changing the stickiness of leukocytes in the capillaries of your endothelium?

Dr. U. Dinnar: We took the equations that we have for added resistance. Our goal is not finding real numbers, but to understand the phenomena. Changing the resistance by increasing it by 5–10% will not change the phenomenon. It will change the blinking time, but it will not change the phenomena.

REFERENCES

1. Dinnar U, Metabolic and mechanical control of the microcirculation. In: Sideman S, Beyar R (eds) *Interactive Phenomena in the Cardiac System.* Plenum Publ.: New York, pp 243–254, 1993.
2. Chambers R, Zweifach BW, Caliber changes of the capillary bed. *Fed Proc* 1942;1:14.
3. Krogh A. The number and distribution of capillaries in muscles with calculation of the oxygen pressure head necessary for supplying. *J Physiol (London)* 1919;52:409.
4. Orion O. Study of flow and transfer of the cardiac microcirculation. *M.Sc. Dissertation*, Technion–IIT, 1993.
5. Weibel ER. The Pathway of Oxygen. Structure and Function in Mammalian Respiratory System. Harvard University Press: Boston, 1984.
6. Mikhailov V. Mathematical analysis of oxygen transport in microcirculation. *M.Sc. Dissertation*, Technion–IIT, 1995.

IV. VASCULAR STRUCTURE AND REMODELING

CHAPTER 13

Endothelial Gene Regulation by Laminar Shear Stress

Nitzan Resnick,[1] Hava Yahav,[1] Levon M. Khachigian,[2] Tucker Collins,[3] Keith R. Anderson,[3] Forbes C. Dewey,[4] and Michael A. Gimbrone, Jr.[3]

ABSTRACT

Endothelial cells, because of their unique localization, are constantly exposed to fluid mechanical forces derived by the flowing blood. These forces, and more specifically shear stresses, affect endothelial structure and function, both *in vivo* and *in vitro*, and are implicated as contributing factors in the development of cardiovascular diseases. We have demonstrated earlier that the shear stress selectively induces the transcription of several endothelial genes, and have defined a shear stress response element (SSRE) in the promoter of platelet–derived–growth–factor B (PDGF–B), that is shared by additional endothelial shear stress responsive genes. Here we further characterize this SSRE and the nuclear factors that bind to it, and imply the possible role of the endothelium cytoskeleton in transducing shear stress, leading to the expression of PDGF–B/SSRE constructs in transfected endothelial cells exposed to shear stress. We also present, yet a new shear stress response element in the Platelet Derived Growth Factor A promoter, that contains a binding site to the transcription factors egr1/sp1. These results further demonstrate the complexity of gene regulation by hemodynamic forces, and support the important part that these forces have in the physiology and pathophysiology of the vessel wall.

[1]Department of Morphological Sciences, Bruce Rappaport Research Institute, Bruce Rappaport Faculty of Medicine, Technion, P.O.Box 9697, Haifa, Israel 31096; [2]Center for Thrombosis and Vascular Research, University of new South Wales, Sydney NSW 2052, Australia; [3]Division of Vascular Biology, Pathology Department, Brigham and Women's Hospital, 221 Longwood Ave. Boston, MA 02115, USA; [4]Fluid mechanics Laboratory, Massachusetts Institute of Technology (MIT), Cambridge, MA 02139, USA

Analytical and Quantitative Cardiology
Edited by Sideman and Beyar, Plenum Press, New York, 1997

INTRODUCTION

Vascular endothelial cells, by virtue of their unique anatomical position, are constantly exposed to the fluid mechanical forces generated by the flowing blood. These hemodynamic forces, which include hydrostatic pressure, cyclic strain and frictional wall shear stress, constitute a special category of physical stimuli that, in addition to better characterized biochemical stimuli, can elicit important biological responses in the cells that compose the blood vessel wall [1]. The non–random distribution of early atherosclerotic lesions observed both in natural disease processes in human and in experimental animal models has long been cited as suggestive evidence for the role these forces play in the pathogenesis of cardiovascular diseases [2, 3]. *In vivo* studies and *in vitro* experiments, using well defined model flow systems, have demonstrated that wall shear stresses can modulate various aspects of endothelial structure and function. Some of these effects appear as a result of modulation of gene expression that occur at the transcription level [4, 5].

We have identified [6] a shear stress response element (SSRE) in the promoter of platelet derived growth factor–B (PDGF–B) chain gene. This element, which does not encode a consensus binding site for known transcription factors, is shared by many endothelial genes that are shear stress responsive and bind to transcription factors that are shear stress inducible [6]. Addition of the SSRE to an SV40 promoter in a hybrid promoter system resulted in the responsiveness of the construct to shear stress. Furthermore, we have demonstrated that the binding to SSRE is also induced in endothelial cells (but not smooth muscle cells) exposed to cyclic strain, suggesting a role for this SSRE in the regulation of endothelial gene expression by several biomechanical forces [7]. We have recently demon-strated [8] that members of the NFkB family p65 and p50 are activated by shear stress and can bind upon activation to the PDGF–B/SSRE through a non–consensus site. The present study demonstrates that NFkB binds functionally to the PDGF–B/SSRE and that mutation of the binding site ablates the responsiveness to shear stress. The possible involvement of the microtubule network in transducing shear stress is suggested based on the regulation of PDGF–B/SSRE containing constructs by nocodazole in transfected endothelial cells.

An additional SSRE, defined in the promoter of PDGF–A gene, is also presented. This promoter does not contain the PDGF–B/SSRE and encodes an element which is a binding site for egr1/sp1 transcription factors, and is important in the regulation of the gene by laminar shear stress.

MATERIALS AND METHODS

Cell Culture

Bovine Aortic Endothelial Cells (BAEC) were prepared as described previously [6]. The cells formed uniformly confluent monolayer and were cultured in Dulbeco Modified Eagle's medium (DMEM – Biological Industries, Beth Haemek, Israel) supplemented with 10% calf serum, 2 mM glutamine, and a mixture of penicillin/streptomycin (100 units/ml and 100 ug/ml, respectively). In all the described experiments, endothelial monolayers were not passaged more than five times.

Shear Stress Apparatus

The modified cone–plate apparatus utilized for generating defined fluid shear stresses is described elsewhere [9]. It consists of a stainless steel cone rotating over a base plate that contains 12 – 1 cm (diameter) – tissue culture coated plastic coverslips, or an insert of a single large 17 cm (diameter) plastic plate. Culture medium within the reservoir (15 ml) was gradually exchanged (0.4 ml/min) without recirculation. The entire apparatus was maintained in 5% CO_2/ 95% air and is thermostatically regulated at 37°C. Fluid mechanical parameters were adjusted to subject the endothelial monolayer to uniform laminar shear stress of 10 dynes/cm^2 . Under these shear stress conditions the endothelial monolayer aligned in the direction of the flow 12–24 hrs. after the onset of flow. Control experiments were incubated under static conditions in a 5% CO_2 incubator.

Transfection Procedure and CAT Assay

BAEC were transfected by the modified calcium phosphate procedure [6]. Briefly, the cells were plated non–confluently (75%) and after 24 hr. transfected with a solution containing BES buffer, calcium phosphate (final concentration 125 mM) and a combination of the tested DNA and a reference plasmid [CMV/βgal or CMV/Luc (Clontech Lab Inc, Palo Alto CA)] in a ratio of 1:1 and a final concentration of 2.5 µg/ml. The transfection mixture was carefully put on the cells in the presence of the growth medium and the cells were incubated over night in a 3% CO_2 atmosphere.

Reporter gene activity was measured 72 hrs after the transfection. CAT activity was normalized to βgal or luciferase activity in order to correct for transfection efficiency.

Nocodazole Treatment

Confluent monolayers were treated with nocodazole (Sigma Chemical Co. St. Louis, MO, USA) to a final concentration of 0.4 µg/ml, 40 min prior to their immunostaining. The cells were fixed in cold methanol for 20 min, treated with a blocking solution (10% goat serum, 0.5% bovine serum albumin, 0.1% glycin in PBS) for additional 20 min, and incubated with the first anti p65 NFkB antibody (Santa–Cruz, San Diego, CA, USA) for additional 60 min. The fixed cells were than incubated with a biotin anti rabbit IgG for 45 min washed and further incubated with Avidin–FITC third antibody. All samples were costained with nuclear stain DAPI.

To study the activation of SSRE containing constructs by nocodazole, 24 hr after their transfection BAEC monolayers were treated for 12 hrs with nocodazole (0.4µg/ml).

Statistical Analysis

The results presented in each table were taken from one representative experiment. All the experiments were repeated three–five times and student's paired t–test was used; $p < 0.05$ was considered significant.

RESULTS

Computer analysis of the PDGF–B/SSRE revealed that this element was not a consensus binding site for any of the known transcription factors. Nevertheless, endothelial nuclear proteins inducible by shear stress did bind to the SSRE as early as 10 min after the exposure of the cells to flow [6, 8].

Several known transcription factors were tested for their activation by shear stress and their potential binding to the PDGF–B promoter in the region containing the SSRE. Immunostaining revealed that NFkB p65 and p50 translocate from the cytoplasm into the nucleus in endothelial cells exposed to laminar shear stress for as little as 10 min (data not shown) as also demonstrated by Lan *et al.* [10]. This time kinetics agreed with both the early activation of PDGF–B by shear stress and the rapid binding of endothelial nuclear proteins induced by shear stress to the SSRE. DNase I footprinting of 300 bp taken from the PDGF–B promoter, in the region of the SSRE, revealed that recombinant heterodimers of p65/p50 were indeed able to bind to the SSRE [8]. Moreover, using mobility shift assays we were able to demonstrate that the SSRE, when used as a probe, formed complexes with nuclear proteins extracted from cells that were either treated with TNFα or exposed to laminar shear stress, and that these complexes were similar to the ones formed with a probe containing an NFkB consensus binding site [8]. Super–shift of these complexes with antibodies to p65 or p50 supported the presence of p65 and p50 in the complexes that were bound to the SSRE [8], and suggested that NFkB heterodimers bind to the SSRE through a non consensus site.

To test whether the binding of NFkB to SSRE plays a role in the induction of genes by laminar shear stress, we have mutated the NFkB binding site both in the context of the PDGF–B chain promoter and in a hybrid promoter system containing the SSRE coupled to the SV40 promoter [7, 8]. The results described in Table 1 clearly demonstrate that mutation of the NFkB site in the SSRE region, either in the context of PDGF–B promoter or in a hybrid promoter construct, ablated the inducibility of these constructs by shear stress, therefore demonstrating the functionality of NFkB binding to the SSRE.

Table 1. Mutation of the NFkB binding site in either PDGF–B promoter constructs or SSRE hybrid promoter constructs ablates their responsiveness to shear stress

Construct	CAT Activity		Fold Induction
	Static	Shear	
1. d17/CAT	17	78	4.6
2. d26/CAT	15	59	3.9
3. md26/CAT	15	18	1.2
4. SV40/CAT	14	13	0.9
5. SSRE/CAT	12	38	3.2
6. mSSRE/CAT	15	17	1.1

The first three constructs are PDGF–B promoter constructs: d17 a 400 bp full promoter construct, d26 the minimal promoter responsive to shear stress that contains the SSRE [6], and md26, a d26 construct in which the SSRE site (CAGAGACCCCC) was mutated into (ACACTGTAGCA). The last three constructs are hybrid promoter constructs: SV40/CAT containing the SV40 promoter backbone without the SSRE, SSRE/CAT containing the SSRE coupled to the SV40 promoter [7], and a mutated SSRE coupled to the SV40 promoter. Recombinant p65/p50 heterodimers were not able to bind to neither md26 nor mSSRE/CAT as shown by mobility shift assays (data not shown).

Activation of NFkB and SSRE Containing Constructs by Nocodazole

It has been recently shown that treatment of HeLa cells with microtubules depolymerization agents, such as nocodazole, lead to the translocation of p65 and p50 into the nucleus and induced expression of NFkB hybrid promoters. It is well documented that rapid cytoskeletal changes occur in endothelial cells exposed to shear stress [11]. We have tested the activation of NFkB by nocodazole in endothelial cells. Both p65 and p50 translocated into the nucleus after treating the cells with nocodazole or colchicine for 40 min (data not shown). This translocation can be inhibited by pretreating the cells with taxol (a stabilizing agent).

To test whether transcriptional regulation via the SSRE is affected by nocodazole, SSRE containing vectors were transfected into BAEC and the cells were treated with nocodazole. Interestingly, CAT activity in cells transfected with either d26 or SSRE/SV40CAT constructs was induced by nocodazole treatment, while the mutated d26 or mSSRE/SV40CAT were not affected (Table 2). These results suggest that indeed in endothelial cells NFkB can be activated by depolymerization of microtubules, and that these changes also lead to overexpression of SSRE containing constructs.

Table 2. Induction of SSRE containing constructs by nocodazole in BAEC

Construct	CAT Activity		Fold Induction
	Control	Nocodazole	
d26/CAT	75,726	293,301	3.8
md26/CAT	127,450	129,876	1.0
SSRE/SV40CAT	45,280	97,767	2.2
mSSRE/SV40CAT	49,160	48,820	1.0

Various constructs containing the SSRE and mutated SSRE sites were transfected into BAEC. 24 hrs after transfection the cells were treated with nocodazole (0.4 µg/ml) for 12 hrs and CAT activity was measured. The results are expressed as CAT activity/microgram protein.

Definition of a SSRE in the PDGF–A chain promoter

PDGF–A gene is also induced in endothelial cells exposed to laminar shear stress, early after the onset of flow [12, 13]. Using run–on analysis we have demonstrated that the induction is transcriptional, although PDGF–A promoter does not contain the PDGF–B/SSRE. To define the element(s) in the promoter responsible for the induction of PDGF–A by shear stress, we have used deletion constructs of the promoter coupled to a CAT reporter gene. The results shown in Table 3 suggest that a region of 50 bp between

Table 3. Definition of the region containing a shear stress responsive element in the PDGF–A promoter

Construct	CAT Activity		Fold Induction
	Static	Shear	
ΔSac (−630 bp)	19	36	1.9
ΔXho I (−260 bp)	15	42	2.8
e33 (−110 bp)	17	44	2.6
f36 (−55 bp)	12	11	0.9

The various deletion constructs [14] were transfected into BAEC and cells were grown under static conditions or exposed to laminar shear stress for 4 hr. CAT activity was measured and normalized to the activity of control plasmid containing the luciferase reporter gene (Clontech Lab. Inc., Palo Alto, CA).

mutations e33 (−110 bp upstream to the initiation site) and f36 (−55 bp upstream to the initiation site) contains the element which is shear stress responsive. This area, which is a GC rich region, contains binding sites for both SP−1 and egr−1 transcription factors. Recently, this region was found to be responsible for the inducibility of PDGF−A gene in endothelial cells treated with PMA (14). In non−treated cells SP−1 constitutively binds to this region, while upon stimulation of the cells with PMA, egr−1 displaces SP−1 binding to the DNA, leading to the induction of egr−1 dependent genes.

DISCUSSION

Hemodynamic forces acting on vascular endothelium play an important role in the structural remodeling of the vasculature and in the development of atherosclerotic lesions [15]. Although the effects of these forces on vessel wall components have been studied both *in vitro* and *in vivo*, the molecular mechanisms mediating these changes are far from understood. In the present study we have focused on two gene models—PDGF A and B chains—and studied the molecular events leading to their induction by physiological levels of laminar shear stress. We have recently shown that PDGF−B chain promoter contains a cis−acting SSRE. This element does not encode a consensus binding site for any known transcription factor and is shared by many genes that are shear stress responsive [6]. Interestingly, SSRE is capable of binding heterodimers of p65/p50, members of the NFkB family, through a non−consensus site [8]. The present study shows that the binding of the NFkB heterodimers is functional, leading to the induction of SSRE containing constructs, but not their mutants, by shear stress. Although, as shown by us and others [4, 10], NFkB is translocated into the nucleus in endothelial cells exposed to shear stress, this activation is not sufficient to induce the expression of all genes containing NFkB consensus binding sites. As shown by Nagel *et al.* [16], several NFkB containing genes such as E−selectin and VCAM−1 are not induced by shear stress, whereas ICAM−1 that encodes for both NFkB consensus binding site and the SSRE is induced. There are several explanations to this phenomenon: 1) The sequence within the binding site might modulate the binding and functional properties of NFkB. 2) More than one transcription factor is involved in the binding; NFkB is known to cooperate with various transcription factors [17–19], and as indeed was shown for VCAM−1, the activation of the gene by cytokines is NFkB dependent, but requires the cooperation with additional factors [20]. Shear stress may alter the activation state or the binding properties of these factors, therefore determining which of the genes that contains NFkB binding site will be induced.

The cellular events leading to the activation of NFkB by biochemical stimuli are well studied, and involve various kinases, phosphatases and proteases. Whether similar steps lead to the activation of NFkB by biomechanical forces is less understood. It has been recently shown that changes in the organization of the cytoskeleton, and more specifically in the microtubule network, lead to the translocation of p65 and p50 into the nucleus. Interestingly, when cells treated with PMA were pretreated with microtubules stabilizing agent such as taxol, the activation of NFkB was not inhibited, suggesting that cytokines and PMA lead to the activation of NFkB through a mechanism that is not cytoskeleton dependent [11].

Shear stress causes rapid changes in the cytoskeleton of endothelial cells [5]. It has been demonstrated that the induction of endothelial genes by shear stress can be inhibited by the reagents which interfere with actin and microtubule organization [21]. In the present study the induced expression of SSRE containing constructs by nocodazole in transfected endothelial cells is demonstrated, induction that can be inhibited by pretreatment with taxol.

Current experiments are carried out to test whether the induction of these constructs by shear stress can be inhibited by pretreatment with taxol.

The characterization of the SSRE in the PDGF–B promoter and the implication of NFkB components in its activation provides a useful experimental model for further investigation, but at the same time raises several interesting issues that demonstrate the complexity of gene regulation by shear stress.

It has been experimentally demonstrated recently that in the case of MCP–1, although its promoter contains the PDGF–B SSRE, an additional site, TRE—a binding site for the transcription factors fos and jun—plays a major role in the activation of the gene by shear stress [22]. PDGF–A gene is transcriptionally regulated by shear stress but its promoter does not contain the PDGF–B SSRE. In the present study we define yet an additional shear stress responsive element, that is located in a GC rich region of the promoter, 55 bp upstream to the initiation of transcription. This region was recently implicated to be involved in the induction of the gene by PMA in endothelial cells [14]. This element is a consensus binding site for two transcription factors, SP–1 and egr–1. While the first occupies constitutively its binding site, upon treatment with PMA, egr–1 is induced in the cells and displaces SP–1 from its binding site, leading to the induced transcription of PDGF–A.

CONCLUSION

The application of simple *in vitro* models has yielded new insights into how fluid mechanical forces act to regulate gene expression in vascular endothelium. In particular, the complex pattern of biological responses elicited by laminar shear stress are now being understood in terms of activation of SSREs in the core promoters of various genes. But the basic question of how frictional force applied to the external surface of the cell is translated into genetic regulatory events in the nuclear compartment remains to be answered. Does the transduction by shear stress, uses well studied receptor activated second messenger cascades, or are novel pathways involving the cytoskeletal elements involved?

It is hoped that as the complexities of endothelial gene regulation by biomechanical forces are unraveled, we will arrive at a better understanding of how the vascular endothelium integrates local biochemical and biomechanical pathological stimuli within the vessel wall. Ultimately, this knowledge may contribute to a better understanding of the pathogenesis of cardiovascular diseases and point to new therapeutic strategies.

Acknowledgements

This study was supported by a grant from the National Institute of Health (M.A.G., PO1–HL30628) and by a grant from the United States–Israel Binational Science Fund (8133801) to N.R.

DISCUSSION

Dr. S. Einav: What is the level of shear stress that begins to affect the gene in your model? Also, you presented continuous steady laminar shear stress. What if it is pulsating shear stress?

Dr. N. Resnick: The level is very low. One dyne is sufficient to induce Intercellular Molecule 1 (ICAM–1) at the transcript level. As for your second question: Pulsatile flow seems to affect endothelial gene expression similarly to steady laminar shear stress, whereas different genes and in different intensities are induced in endothelial cells by disturbed–laminar flow.

Dr. R. Beyar: Shear stress is actually the way that the blood flow within the vessel talks with the surroundings, and probably plays a role not only in the pathology but in the general physiology, and even remodelling, of the artery. For example, if you have suddenly an increased flow in the artery, the artery adapts itself and grows in size. It is not only the endothelium which grows in size, but all the layers, the media and the adventitia. If the endothelium is responding to flow via the shear stress, is there a cross–talk between the endothelium and the other layers? Is there a possibility that the shear stress felt by the endothelium may induce genes at the media, for example?

Dr. N. Resnick: The endothelial cells in all our experiments were moved from static conditions and exposed to flow, which is different from having cells constantly exposed to shear stress. We believe that these experiments represent the effect of changes in the magnitude of shear stress, or a "step-function".

Yes, there is a cross talk between smooth muscle and endothelial cells. Smooth muscles are able to respond to shear stress. Also, there is an induction in the expression of growth and chemotactic factors in endothelial cells which affect the media. Shear stress can affect smooth muscle cells either directly upon the denudation of the endothelium, or indirectly through molecules that are expressed by the endothelium.

Dr. H. Strauss: Are the effects of shear stress on sites similar throughout the vascular system, e.g., the pulmonary artery vs the aorta or the resistance vessels?

Dr. N. Resnick: We are in the process of studying it. This has not been done yet.

Dr. S. Sideman: If you expose endothelial cells to turbulent flow, the cell shape–stress relationship changes back to almost normal for some reason. I do not know why it happens, but the elongation you have in laminar flow does not change from normal back. How would the shear in turbulent flow affect gene expression?

Dr. N. Resnick: We are currently looking at patterns of shear stresses other than laminar shear stress. If you look, for example, at induction of mitosis, while laminar shear stress actually down regulates mitosis in endothelial cells, you get mitosis under turbulence. Why that is, I do not know and there is very little known about it. We do not know how endothelial cells feel the flow and how they feel various patterns of flow, but they do feel various patterns of flow and they respond differently to various patterns of flow.

Dr. S. Sideman: Do we need gene expression for the receptors?

Dr. N. Resnick: I do not know, but I do not think so. The responsiveness to shear stress, if you look at the acute effects, occur seconds after the flow, which is too early for changes in gene expression. For the initial response, you do not need gene expression. But for later responses and maybe for the cross–talk with the media, you do need gene expression.

Dr. M. Morad: When you continue to keep the cells under shear stress, do these genes turn off?

Dr. N. Resnick: Yes. If you keep the cells under flow for more than 8 hours the expression of the genes decreases. But if you increase or decrease the magnitude again, like a step–function, the induction occurs again.

Dr. M. Morad: Do you think something else kicks in after that?

Dr. N. Resnick: I am sure something else kicks in; I am sure hemodynamic forces are not the only parameter. I think it is the combination of changes in shear stress and other things, like cytokines, for example. Several groups are currently studying the combined effects of shear stress and cytokines on endothelial cells.

Dr. H. ter Keurs: How does the endothelial cell first of all detects the stress change, and then translates that into transport of NFkB into the nucleus? If you destroy the cytoskeleton in part, does the process stop?

Dr. N. Resnick: This is one of the things that we are looking at now. There was a manuscript that came out two years ago by Micahel Karin [11] showing that changes in microtubules activated NFkB in HeLa cells. Interestingly, these cytoskeletal changes are not involved in the activation pathway of NFkB by cytokines. We have shown that depolymerization of microtubules in endothelial cells causes an induced expression of SSRE constructs. We are currently testing the effects of various drugs that stabilize the microtubule network, such as taxol, on the induction of NFkB and SSRE constructs by shear stress.

Dr. A. McCulloch: There have been recent reports that the Jun N–terminal kinase (JUNK) is activated by shear stress. Are NFkB or NFATP downstream targets of any of the MAP kinases?

Dr. N. Resnick: Several kinases and phosphatases are involved in the activation of NFkB and NFATp by cytokines. It is not known whether these molecules mediate the activation g NFkB and NFATp by shear stress.

Dr. A. McCulloch: Have you looked at differential effects of gene expression that might result from growing the cells from different matrices?

Dr. N. Resnick: No, we have not.

Dr. H. Kammermeier: There are observations that there are stress dependent ion channels in endothelial cells and that there is some connection between cytoskeleton and ion channels which might be involved in the signal chain.

Dr. N. Resnick: Yes. One very interesting channel, the potassium channel which was found by Peter Davis [5], has not been fully characterized up until now. That is related to the cytoskeleton. Peter Davies is doing a beautiful job testing the immediate changes after the onset of flow that occur in the endothelial membrane, cytoskeleton and focal adhesions and whether changes in each site affect the other sites. We poorly understand the correlation between the opening of ion channels, changes in the cytoskeleton and gene expression in cells exposed to shear stress.

Dr. J. Downey: But in the absence of calcium you do not get this transduction.

Dr. N. Resnick: Calcium is problematic. People have shown that transient levels of calcium are going up, others have shown that they are not.

REFERENCES

1. Frangos JA ed. *Physical forces and the mammalian cell.* Academic Press, San Diego, CA, 1993.
2. Caro CG, Fitz–Gerald JM, Schorter RC. Atheroma and arterial wall shear: Observation, correlation and proposal of shear dependent mass transfer mechanism for atherogenesis. *Proc Natl Acad Sci USA* 1971;177:109–159.

3.   Ku DN, Giddens DP, Zarins CK, Galgov S. Pulsatile flow and atherosclerosis in the human carotid bifurcation: positive correlation between plaque location and low and oscillating shear stress. *Arteriosclerosis* 1985;5:293–302.

4.   Resnick N and Gimbrone MA Jr. Hemodynamic forces are complex regulators of endothelial gene expression. *FASEB J* 1995;9:874–882.

5.   Davies PF. Flow mediated endothelial mechanotransduction. *Physiol Rev* 1995;75:519–560.

6.   Resnick N, Collins T, Atkinson W, Bonthron DT, Dewey FC Jr, Gimbrone MA Jr. Platelet derived growth factor B chain promoter contains a cis–acting fluid shear–stress–responsive element. *Proc Natl Acad Sci USA* 1993;90:4591–4595.

7.   Resnick N, Sumpio BE, Gimbrone MA Jr. Endothelial gene regulation by biomechanical forces. In: Woodford FP, Davignon J, Sniderman A, eds. *Proceedings of the Xth International Symposium on Atherosclerosis.* Montreal, Quebec. Elsevier, NY. 1994;838–843.

8.   Khachigian LM, Resnick R, Gimbrone MA Jr, Collins T. Nuclear factor kB interacts functionally with the platelet derived growth factor B chain shear stress response element in vascular endothelial cells exposed to fluid shear stress. *J Clin Invest* 1995;96:1169–1175.

9.   Bussolari SR, Dewey CF Jr, Gimbrone MA Jr. Apparatus for subjecting living cells to fluid shear stress. *Rev Sci Instrum* 1982;53:1851–1854.

10.   Lan Q, Mercurius KO, Davies PF. Stimulation of transcriptional factors NFkB and AP1 in endothelial cells subjected to shear stress. *Biochem Biophys Res Commun* 1994;201:950–956.

11.   Rosette C, Karin M. Cytoskeletal control of gene expression: depolymerization of microtubules activates NFkB. *J Cell Biol* 1995;6:1111–1119.

12.   Hsieh HJ, Li NQ, Frangos JA. Shear stress increases endothelial platelet derived growth factor messenger RNA levels. *Am J Physiol* 1991;260:H642–646.

13.   Hanlon NJ, Collins T, Gimbrone MA Jr, Resnick N. Regulation of the endothelial PDGF–A gene by shear stress. *Circulation* 1994;IV468 (abstract).

14.   Khachigian LM, Lindner V, Williams AJ and Collins T. Egr–1 induced endothelial gene expression: A common theme in vascular injury. *Science* 1996;271:1427–1431.

15.   Sumpio BE ed: *Hemodynamic Forces and Vascular Cell Biology.* RG Landes Company, Austin, TX, USA. 1993.

16.   Nagel T, Resnick N, Atkinson WJ, Dewey CF Jr, Gimbrone MA Jr. Shear stress selectively upregulates intercellular adhesion molecule 1 expression in cultured human vascular endothelial cells. *J Clin Invest* 1994;94:885–891.

17.   Lewis H, Kaszubska W, Delamarter JF, Whealan J. Cooperativity between two NFkB complexes mediated by high–mobility–group proteins 1(Y) is essential for cytokine–induced expression of the E–selectin promoter. *Mol Cell Biol* 1994;14:5701–5709.

18.   Fujita T, Nolan GP, Gosh S, Baltimore D. Independent modes of transcriptional activation by the p50 and p65 subunits of NFkB. *Genes & Dev* 1992;6:775–787.

19.   Collins T, Read MA, Neish AS, Whitley MZ, Thanos D, Maniatis T. Transcriptional regulation of endothelial cells adhesion molecules: NFkB and cytokine–inducible enhancers. *FASEB J* 1995;9:883–893.

20.   Neish A, Read MA, Thanos D, Pine R, Maniatis T, Collins T. Endothelial interferon regulatory factor –1 cooperates with NFkB as a transcriptional activator of vascular cell adhesion molecule 1. *Mol Cell Biol* 1995;15:2558–2569.

21.   Morita T, Kurihara H, Maemura K, Yoshizumi M, Yazaki Y. Disruption of cytoskeletal structure mediates shear stress–induced endothelin–1 gene expression in cultured porcine aortic endothelial cells. *J Clin Invest* 1993;92:1706–1712.

22.   Shyy Y, Hsieh HJ, Usami S, Chien S. Fluid shear stress induces a biphasic response of human monocyte chemotactic protein 1 gene expression in vascular endothelium. *Proc Natl Acad Sci* 1994;91:4678–4682.

CHAPTER 14

3D Architecture of Myocardial Microcirculation in Intact Rat Heart: A Study with Micro–CT

Patricia E. Beighley, Paul J. Thomas, Steven M. Jorgensen, and Erik L. Ritman[1]

ABSTRACT

The branching geometry of the coronary arterial tree may play a significant role in the observed spatial heterogeneity in myocardial perfusion. To provide more insight into this possibility we used a micro–CT scanner to image the intact rat heart and its opacified coronary arterial tree, for quantitative analysis of the coronary arterial architecture. Results show a consistent pattern of branching throughout the heart wall.

INTRODUCTION

The branching architecture of the coronary arterial tree is of interest for several reasons. One is that the spatial heterogeneity of myocardial perfusion, which is quite stable over extended periods of time, is likely to be in large part due to the branching pattern of the arterial tree [1, 2], even though the regional metabolic influences on perfusion distribution modulate this distribution.

Secondly, as was first shown by Murray [3, 4] in the late 1920s, the branching pattern should reflect an optimization of the tradeoff between the energy expended in making and maintaining a vascular tree versus the energy expended in utilizing the tree, i.e., the cardiac work needed to transport the blood through it. A consequence of Murray's optimization model is that the cube of the diameter of the "mother" branch equals the sum of the cubes of the diameters of the "daughter" branches [5–9].

---

[1]Department Physiology and Biophysics, Mayo Clinic, 200 First Street SW, Rochester, MN 55905, USA

Thirdly, the mechanism involved in achieving and maintaining Murray's optimization of the branching geometry could be nitric oxide–mediated [10–14]. This system involves a feed–back mechanism for maintaining endothelial shear stress within a predetermined magnitude. A consequence of this mechanism is that the same relationship between the cubes of branch diameters should also hold true. Hence, the nitric oxide–based feedback mechanism has as a consequence an optimization of the branching architecture.

Traditional methods for measuring the coronary arterial branching geometry have been greatly limited by the enormous logistic task involved in terms of measuring the dimensions in true anatomic relationship along the length of each vessel and its branches. In addition, there is a more subtle problem (which also results from very practical considerations) which results from the lumping of the dimensions of all vessel segments of the same branching order. This approach destroys information about the hierarchical relationship between specific mother and daughter branch segments [15, 16].

In an attempt to overcome these practical measurement and analysis problems, we present a method, using 3D tomographic imaging at a microscopic level, which provides the 3D geometry of the entire, intact, arterial tree of the rat heart. Application of well established, computer–based, 3D image analysis techniques enabled us to measure the detailed branching anatomy of the intact coronary arterial tree.

METHODS, MATERIALS AND PROCEDURES

The Micro–CT Scanner

Figure 1 is a schematic of the micro–CT scanner's main features. It consists of a spectroscopy X–ray source which has two important features. The overall design of the micro–CT scanner is based on the system developed by Flannery *et al.* [17]. One is that the anode (target) can be selected for the desired energy of the X–ray. While the Molybdenum target best meets our needs (17.5 keV), other targets could be inserted, such as a Silver target for 25 keV and Copper for 8 keV X–rays. Secondly, a selection of thin metal filters can be inserted in the X–ray source to further reduce the bandwidth of the X–ray photon energy. We use a Zirconium foil to preferentially pass the approximately 17.5 keV X–rays. Thirdly, the focal spot of the source is large (12 x 0.4 mm^2) which allows us

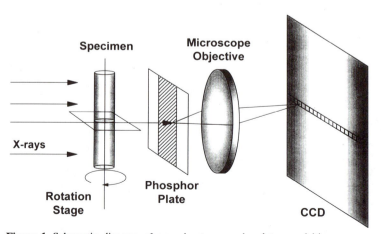

Figure 1. Schematic diagram of our microtomography data–acquisition camera.

to greatly increase the heat load on the target and thereby increase the X–ray flux. This speeds up the scanning process and/or increases the signal–to–noise ratio. The focal spot is rendered more uniform and geometrically symmetrical by orienting the X–ray tube at a 6 degree angle so that the projected focal spot dimension approximately is 0.4 x 0.3 mm^2.

The specimen itself is positioned on computer–controlled precision stages for rotating and translating the specimen during the scanning procedure. The specimen is positioned as close to the X–ray fluorescent crystal plate as possible.

The fluorescing plate is made of Thallium doped Cesium Iodide which is sublimated in a thin layer on a 3 cm x 3 cm square plate of thin aluminum (X–ray side). A microscope objective lens is used to focus the fluorescing image generated in the crystal onto a 1024 x 1024 pixel charge coupled device (CCD) array sensor. Each pixel in the CCD array is a 21 μm on a side square. The lens can be adjusted to vary the magnification from 1 x 1, 4 x 1 and 10 x 1, thereby altering the effective size of the CCD sensors from 21 to 5.2 to 2.1 μm respectively.

The Specimen

The rat is anesthetized and the aorta is cannulated. Heparin, a vasodilator, is infused, followed by infusion of Microfil® (a silicon polymer containing lead chromate) at 100 mmHg pressure. As soon as the Microfil® emerges from the coronary sinus the infusion is stopped and the *in situ* heart is stored in a refrigerator overnight to permit "setting" of the Microfil®. Next the heart is dissected free and progressively dehydrated with increasing concentrations of glycerol. Finally, the specimen is embedded in bioplastic or a low temperature paraffin. Figure 2 is of a typical specimen.

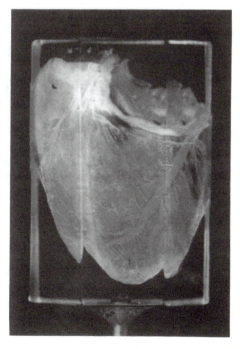

Figure 2. Photograph of a rat heart, embedded in hard plastic, with coronary vessels injected with Microfil®silicon polymer. Specimen approximately 1 cm diameter.

3D Image Generation

The specimen is scanned at approximately 700 angles of view around 360 degrees and tomographic cross sections are computed from these data. The voxel is usually the same dimension as the effective pixel size in the CCD. Thus, a 1 x 1 scan results in 21 μm on–a–side cubic voxels.

Figure 3 shows examples of typical tomographic cross sections of a rat heart with opacified coronary arteries. Such data are not particularly useful for obtaining the measurements desired for this type of study. Hence, we use maximum intensity projections of the 3D image data or volume rendered displays [18] such as shown in Figure 4 and Figure 5.

3D Image Analysis

The first level of analysis is to isolate one major branch of the coronary arterial tree. This is performed with a "connect" function in our image analysis software package [18]. Figure 6 illustrates this capability.

21 μm Voxels   **42 μm Voxels**

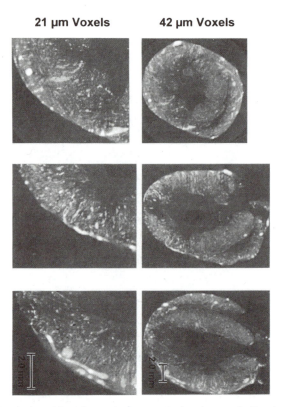

Figure 3. CT images of a single, mid cardiac transverse, sagittal and coronal slice through a rat heart. The white "spots" and "wiggles" are cross sections of coronary vessels filled with Pb CrO_4 containing Microfil®. In right panels data are displayed at 42 μm voxel size and in left panels the same data are displayed at 21 μm voxel size. Scale bar = 2 mm.

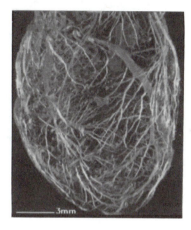

Figure 4. Brightest voxel projection of a 512^3 voxel micro–CT image of contrast–filled coronary arteries of a rat heart.

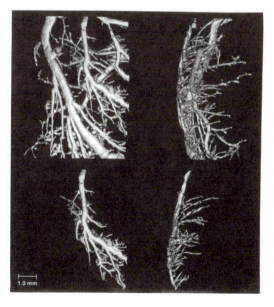

Figure 5. Detail of voxel–gradient display of image data such as used to make Figure 4. Note isolation of one vessel in lower panels. The voxel size is 21 μm.

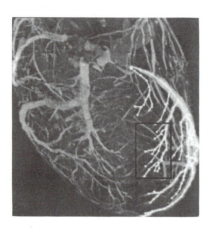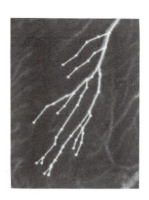

Figure 6. Automatically selected arteries in a brightest voxel display of the 3D image of a rat heat.

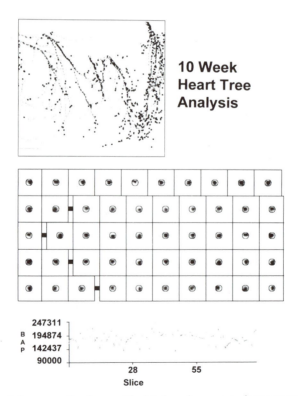

Figure 7. Computed cross–sectional area of the interbranch segments decreases exponentially with increasing branching order.

This tree must now be "traced" by the computer program [19], thereby providing the coordinates for the analysis program to do the actual measurements along the vessel branches. Figure 7 illustrates such a "trace" and the associated cross–sectional areas measured along a selected segment of the branch. From such analyses we obtain a table with vessel segment's order of branching, its length, cross–sectional area and branching angles.

RESULTS

Figure 8 shows how the branch cross sectional area changes with progressive branching. This is clearly an exponential relationship of the type described by analysis of manually analyzed specimens.

Figure 9 shows that if the smallest vessels (at the limit of spatial resolution) are aligned in all hearts (i.e., called order 14 in this data set) then all CSA–to–order relationships become indistinguishable. Figure 10 shows that the cubed relationship holds very well for all the three hearts studied.

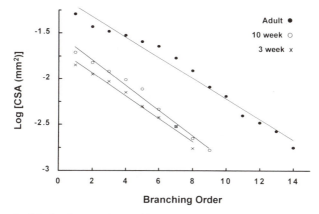

Figure 8. Aggregate data for three rat hearts. Note that as the rat age increases, the vessels are larger.

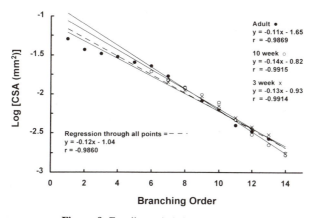

Figure 9. Equally scaled data from Figure 8.

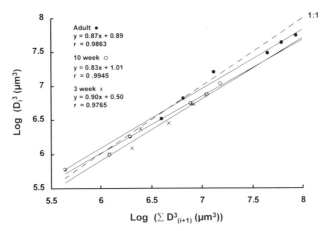

Figure 10. Diameter cubed relationship is maintained with maturation, an observation consistent with 'Murray' optimization.

DISCUSSION

Our results are consistent with the Murray optimization and with the hypothesis that nitric oxide−based mechanism controls vessel cross−sectional area. In addition, because we study intact vascular trees, we can explore the question as to whether the optimization holds for all segments or merely holds for an entire branch. The possible importance of the observation that this continuity of hierarchical branching segments is maintained throughout the vascular tree is suggested by the recent work of Zamir [16].

The method does have some limitations. Thus, the state of vasodilation of all vessel segments is not well controlled and the pressure of the microfil infusion may be locally altered because of unequal polymerization of the biopolymer. Ideally, we would want to observe this information in the living heart, which while possible technically, cannot be achieved with the current scanner.

CONCLUSIONS

Optimization of the coronary arterial tree, as well as nitric oxide−based mechanism for achieving this optimization, appear to be supported by our data.

Acknowledgments

The authors thank Ms. Denise Reyes for generating many of the computer displays used in this analysis, Ms. Julie Patterson for making the figures used in this manuscript and Ms. Delories Darling for typing the manuscript.

DISCUSSION

Dr. R. Beyar: Congratulation on a fascinating work. It seems like there is no limit on technology. When is the micro Cine−CT coming?

Dr. E.L. Ritman: It depends on how many dollars or shekels you have. With conventional X–ray sources, where you bombard a piece of metal with electrons, I do not think we can produce X–rays fast enough. Realize that no matter what size you are looking at, what scale, you need a certain number of photons per voxel to get a certain signal to noise. Say you have 1 micrometer cubed voxel, you need just as many voxels as a 1 mm^3 voxel in order to get the same signal to noise. You can imagine, here is a 1000x1000x1000 voxel image and you add up the photons, the X–ray dose rapidly becomes excessive. It is probably possible to do it with a synchrotron X–ray source. A synchroton is a device that allows you to make very bright, highly monochromatic, X–rays. With special X–ray optics, which could be used to generate several different angles of view simultaneously, rapid tomographic scanning may be possible. It may still not be possible to do Cine–CT, but you might be able to capture a "stop–action" scan of a living animal.

Dr. L. Axel: You rotate your specimen: how many steps do you do and how long does it take to acquire and reconstruct?

Dr. E.L. Ritman: The time depends on the resolution you want. There are rules that govern how many angles of view you need. People have worked out relationships between the size of the voxel and the number of angles of view and your detector size, etc. We normally do about 20 μm on a side cubic voxels, just for a start to see what is there. That requires about 750 angles of view around 360°, performed with a highly precise and accurate rotation state. The length of time depends on the size of the object diameter which determines how rapidly we build up the image. It takes at least 8 hr with the sort of hearts we have been looking at.

Dr. P. Hunter: This is extremely exciting. Perhaps you can answer the question that Dr. Beyar raised earlier about the relationship which we are trying to understand between the vessels and sheet structure or bundle structure. The capillaries are aligned with the fibers; how far up that system, in terms of larger and larger vessels, can you still see the alignment with the fiber direction?

Dr. E.L. Ritman: I have not looked at that specifically. Dr. Westerhof, some time ago, said that he was working on the papillary muscle and said that all the vessels run along parallel to the fibers. I looked at that in the rat hearts we have scanned and indeed, all of the vessels of all sizes run parallel to the fibers. Unfortunately, I have not looked at that issue in more detail. Some of the earlier cross–sections show the main vessels running around the epicardium and then the branches just dive straight to the wall. Vessels smaller than the ones that go transmurally are the ones that seem to be lined up with the muscle fiber bundles and they must be of the order of 50 micrometers or so in diameter.

Dr. S. Sideman: What is the significance of the angle of the branches?

Dr. E.L. Ritman: The angle of the branch, in Murray's hypothesis (which is a trade–off between the energy needed to make and maintain a tree vs operating it) is that if they almost align with the main vessel, they need less work to pump blood through them than if they are at right angles On the other hand, it takes the vessel longer to get around to the tissue beside the branching point when the branches are almost aligned with the parent vessel. Hence, the amount of vessel you have to build is increased. You can see from that presentation of the issue there is going to be a trade–off between the angle as to how quickly you get to all regions vs how much work you have to do to get there.

Dr. S. Sideman: Then there is no one angle of branching.

Dr. E.L. Ritman: No. You can have a certain, non optimal, angle in a particular branching, but then the next one probably corrects for that. Often they are not symmetrical bifurcations. As a rule, they are asymmetrical. It seems to work out on average, but that is one of the questions I want to address: is there optimization of branch angle on average or is this always done? Maybe there are several optimization mechanisms at work in parallel that on the average express this relationship. On the other hand, one mechanism may stray one way for some reason and then the other mechanism goes the other way to make up for it. I do not know how it works but that is what we would like to explore.

Dr. D. Adam: You alluded to the option of going down below 10 μm. What do you see as the maximal resolution that you may obtain with the new micro–CT that you have designed?

Dr. E.L. Ritman: We have not made that measurement because it is quite tough to make. The true measurement of the resolution, that is how precisely can you separate two objects, is not necessarily the issue. The point about blood vessels is often how small a vessel can you meaningfully see and measure, which may be accomplished without truly resolving a lone vessel. We have reconstructed down to 3 micrometer on a side cubic voxels and that was in order to do what we though we need to do to resolve the 10 micrometer microspheres. Three micrometer sounds pretty small, but that is only half of a capillary and that is barely enough for adequate visualization of individual capillaries. I cannot tell you whether we can achieve meaningful resolution to go beyond that. We have not tried that yet.

Dr. D. Adam: Do you do any processing on the images in order to obtain the high resolution that you have reached?

Dr. E.L. Ritman: You can do lots of processing but it is only going to be as good as the optical system. We spend a lot of effort on the optical system. The trick is to find out what is the largest voxel you can get away with to basically match the optical resolution. These are all questions I do not yet know the answer to yet.

Dr. J.B. Bassingthwaighte: One of the things that I would like to do with the kind of data that you are getting would be to measure segment lengths, element lengths, banding angles, etc., and be able to reconstruct the network on a statistical basis. How do you go about taking the data from where you are, to getting a battery of numbers out of it that might be put into Kassab's connectivity matrix, positional matrix, etc.?

Dr. E.L. Ritman: You have put your finger on a real problem. Say you have 10 levels of branching. After 10 levels you have 1000 little branches, you add them all up, so that is 2000 branches, and we actually got up to 14 levels of branching. Just the number of segments really challenges the computer you work with. To answer your question specifically, we know what has to be done but we are not close to be ready for that. We are still dealing with how do you name things as you go down the stream, so that you can, in a reasonably intelligent way, address the data.

Dr. J.B. Bassingthwaighte: Is it useful, in your view, to use Kassab's diameter–defined Strahler ordering system to try to capture this kind of information or is there a better way of doing it?

Dr. E.L. Ritman: We go for the Strahler scheme. There are many other methods which are good for particular purposes but I do not know which one would be best. Ideally you collect the data and name it in such a way that you can go with any ordering scheme you wish to use for a particular purpose. I would not want to restrict myself to one, but in having to pick one we went with the Strahler system.

Dr. N. Westerhof: It take it that your heart is in diastole?

Dr. E.L. Ritman: This is a dead heart.

Dr. N. Westerhof: But in principle, you could stop it in systole?

Dr. E.L. Ritman: Yes you could, but I would say most of these are in diastole because of the drugs we give. But we do have some discussions going with people to work out exactly what is the best way to stop a heart in what you might call systole.

REFERENCES

1.   van Bavel E, Spaan JAE. Branching patterns in the porcine coronary arterial tree. Estimation of flow heterogeneity. *Circ Res* 1972;71:1200–1212.

2.   Wieringa PA, Spaan JAE, Stassen HG, Laird JD. Heterogeneous flow distribution in a three–dimensional network simulation of the myocardial microcirculation – a hypothesis. *Microcirculation* 1982;2:195–216.

3.   Murray CD. The physiological principle of minimum work applied to the angle of branching of arteries. *J Gen Physiol* 1926;9:835–841.

4.   Murray CD. The physiological principle of minimum work. I. The vascular system and the cost of blood volume. *Proc Natl Acad Sci* 1926;12:207–214.

5.   Zamir M, Phipps BL, Langille BL, Wonnacott TH. Branching characteristics of coronary arteries in rats. *Can J Physiol Pharmacol* 1984;62:1453–1459.

6.   Roy AG, Woldenberg MJ. A generalization of the optimal models of arterial branching. *Bull Math Biol* 1982;44:349–360.

7.   Zamir M. Local geometry of arterial branching. Bull Math Biol. 1982;44:597–607.

8.   Rodbard S. Vascular caliber. *Cardiol* 1975;60:4–49.

9.   Mayrovitz HN, Roy J. Microvascular blood flow: evidence indicating a cubic dependence on arteriolar diameter. *Am J Physiol* 1983;245:H1031–H1038.

10.   Zamir M. The role of shear forces in arterial branching. *J Gen Physiol* 1976;67:213–222.

11.   Griffith TM, Edwards DH. Basal EDRF activity helps to keep the geometrical configuration of arterial bifurcations close to the Murray optimum. *J Theor Biol* 1990;146:545–573.

12.   Griffith TM, Edwards DH, Davies RLL, Harrison TJ, Evans KT. EDRF coordinates the behaviour of vascular resistance vessels. *Nature* 1987;329:442–445.

13.   Koller A, Kaley G. Endothelial regulation of wall shear stress and flow in skeletalmuscle microcirculation. *Am J Physiol* 1991;260:H862–H868.

14.   Griffith TM, Edwards DH, Davies RLL, Harrison TJ, Evans KT. Endothelium–derived relaxing factor (EDRF) and resistance vessels in an intact vascular bed: a microangiographic study of the rabbit isolated ear. *Br J Pharmacol* 1988;93:654–662.

15.   Davant B, Levin M. Popel AS. Effect of dispersion of vessel diameters and lengths in Stochastic Networks 1. Modeling of microcirculatory flow. *Microvascular Res* 1986;31:203–222.

16.   Zamir M. Measured structure and simulated dynamics of human coronary arteries. *Annals Biomed Eng* 1991;24:S-37 (Abst. 222).

17.   Flannery BP, Deckman HW, Roberge WG, D'Amico KL. Three–dimensional X–ray microtomography. *Science* 1987;237:1439–1444.

18.   Robb RA, Heffernan PB, Camp JJ, Hanson DP. A workstation for interactive display and quantitative analysis of 3–D and 4–D biomedical images. *Proc Tenth Annual Symp on Comput Appl in Med Care IEEE Cat* 1986;CH2341–6:240–256.

19.   Higgins WE, Spyra WJT, Ritman EL. Automatic extraction of the arterial tree from 3–D angiograms. *IEEE Eng Med Biol Soc 11th Annual Int Conf* 1989;CH2770–6/89/0563–0564.

CHAPTER 15

VASCULAR IMAGING BY ULTRASOUND: 3D RECONSTRUCTION OF FLOW VELOCITY FIELDS FOR ENDOTHELIAL SHEAR STRESS CALCULATION

Dan R. Adam and Pablo Burstein[1]

ABSTRACT

A new method for quantitative reconstruction of a three dimensional (3D) velocity field from ultrasound color doppler mapping (USCDM) images is used here to calculate the shear stress distribution on the endothelial layer of an artery. Measurements of a few spatially unrestricted USCDM transverse cross sectional images of the artery, and of several echo–ultrasound B–mode images of the same area, are required for reconstructing the geometry of the vessel's endothelial surface. The calculation is based on assuming a physical model of flow, and solving the Continuity and the Navier–Stokes equations numerically for a steady flow of an incompressible Newtonian fluid at constant temperature within a non–flexible tube. The correct choice of the penalty parameter in the finite element method (FEM) algorithm provides proper convergence of the reconstruction. The endothelial shear stress is calculated from the gradient of the velocity field at each point of the vessel's inner surface.

INTRODUCTION

Arterial disease processes are strongly related to the hemodynamics within the arteries [1]. Numerous observations correlate arterial pathologies, mainly arteriosclerosis, to certain locations in the arterial tree, and to certain flow patterns. An increasing number of reports have recently described mechanisms which partly explain the relationship

---

[1]Heart System Research Center, The Julius Silver Institute, Department of Biomedical Engineering, Technion–IIT, Haifa, Israel

Analytical and Quantitative Cardiology
Edited by Sideman and Beyar, Plenum Press, New York, 1997

between flow patterns and the vessel's pathological processes. The transduction pathways of shear stress into the endothelial cells are not fully known, but probably involve structural modification of membrane proteins, which may change/modulate local concentrations of ions, metabolites etc., or intracellular organelles. These induce short–term and long–term responses of the endothelial cells affect remodeling of the vessel. It has been shown, both *in vitro* [2] and *in vivo* [3], that acute or chronic increase of shear stress due to higher blood flow significantly enhance several genes, e.g. increase of the level of NO synthase3 mRNA and protein expression.

The transient response of the endothelial cells to a sudden increase in shear stress is affected by an influx of Ca^{2+} and K^+, protein phosphorylation and, among others, NO and prostacyclin are produced to relax the vessel's smooth muscle (and reduce the resistance to flow).

A somewhat different approach demonstrated *in vivo* [4] that augmented pulsatile perfusion increases coronary flow, in part by triggering NO release and adenosine. This data support the hypothesis that augmentation of pulsatile perfusion at the same mean pressure stimulates flow by the release of endothelium–mediated vasorelaxant factors such as NO. It was also found that the increase in flow in conscious animals during exercise triggered shear stress induced release of NO [5].

The probable mechanism which transducts the external forces acting on the endothelial cells to the intracellular processes was partially unveiled by the report that changes in the shear flow stimulate the coronary endothelial cells and modulate intracellular events, e.g. activation of G –proteins (specific GTP binding proteins) within 1 sec of flow onset [6]. This report proves that a mechanochemical signal transduction occurs in endothelial cells early as a response to the initiation of external fluid shear.

Sustained increase in shear stress modulates expression of thrombomodulin, adhesion molecules, and modifies production of these and other endothelial factors. Recently, *in vivo* measurements in a chronic high blood flow model demonstrated sustained increase in aortic endothelial NO synthase expression [7]. The significant *in vivo* increase of NOS3 mRNA and protein expression has been measured together with an enhancement of Ca^{2+} dependent NOS activity and cGMP content. Thus, sustained increase in shear stress modifies the position and morphology of the cells, and the expression of genes, e.g. PDGF, endothelin–1, thrombomodulin, and adhesion molecules. Functional and structural changes associated with these shear stress related changes of gene expression include atherosclerosis [8], chronic exercise adaptation, arteriovenous fistula and more [9].

The accumulated evidence on the relationship between fluid shear and endothelial processes and pathologies, and the transduction mechanisms which transfer the information into the cells, reemphasizes the importance of studying the flow patterns in the arteries. There is ample evidence to associate atherosclerotic processes with areas of very slow flow (e.g. near bifurcations) in the vicinity of regions of high flow velocities and high shear stresses. The study of arterial flow patterns may thus provide an insight into arterial pathogenesis.

Flow or flow velocity measurements are performed by a number of non–invasive imaging modalities: MRI, fast CT (cine–CT), UltraSound (US) [10–14]. Comparison of MRI and fast CT measurements [15] of flow phantoms and ultrasound [16] demonstrate good results. These methods, which measure the radiation from all directions in order to reconstruct the image, allow to sample the full 3D distribution of velocity, even when calculating and displaying a 2D cross–sectional image. The acquisition, though, is not done within a single heart beat, and therefore requires ECG gating and multiple–beat acquisition. Also, the spatial resolution of MRI flow velocity measurement is too low, and the acquisition, gated to the ECG, is averaged over many cycles [10–12]. The averaging procedure requires time and produces only average flow velocity data. Also the cost is extremely prohibitive. Validation of the flow velocity measurement has been reported [15, 16], but its implementation for routine blood velocity measurements seems still remote.

The measurement of flow velocity by Doppler US has some severe limitations: the measurement is intrinsically limited to the line of insonation. The measurement of flow velocity is possible. Once some limiting assumptions are made (e.g. developed flow in a cylindrical tube), and the image plane coincides with the vascular central longitudinal cross–section. Otherwise, as in the realistic acquisitions made in a clinical setup, the images obtained may produce erroneous values. Errors may also be introduced when the flow direction is not accounted for in the data analysis.

Doppler echo ultrasound mapping has the advantages of being non–invasive, nearly real–time and relatively inexpensive. There have been some attempts to reconstruct and quantify 3D flow profiles by using temporal and spatial sequential sets of 2D images, and any additional information available. Unfortunately, the acquisition of image sequences parallel to each other (or in a known, measured angle) of Doppler measurements is very difficult in practice, it introduces additional measurement errors, and its validation is complex. Here, again, in order to minimize the measurement error, the image plane must coincide with the vascular central longitudinal cross–section. The flow direction must be taken into account when calculating the flow velocity, unless the measurement is done with the beam parallel to the flow. Presently, mapping of the flow velocity patterns can be done only qualitatively.

Data produced by US Color Doppler Mapping (USCDM) images are 2D images of a 1D beam–aligned velocity component. Correct quantification of 1D velocity vector is difficult due to errors introduced by mean frequency estimation, quantization, statistical measurement noise, aliasing, etc. Once an effort is made to quantify the measurement of the 3D velocity field, additional errors are introduced (e.g. inaccurate spatial information of each pixel measured, and availability of sparse data, as only few samples are taken in the 3D space and only one velocity component is measured at each sample). Most of the efforts to reconstruct the 3D velocity vectors are based on "multiple lines of sight" methods, which use either one transducer at different locations, three transducers, or two transducers and transverse–Doppler [2]. The main drawback of these techniques is that each voxel must be accurately insonated by all the transducers, requiring a voxel by voxel procedure, and perfect alignment.

This study presents a new method for processing USCDM images which can provide the 3D velocity field within a tube–shaped artery and the related shear stress distribution imposed on it wall. The method depends on obtaining data by currently available equipment, which implies hand–held scanning transducers. There is, therefore, no restriction on the choice of transducer position and orientation at each measuring site, though its position and orientation are required, and must be recorded during the USCDM session. The methodology is presented here by using data taken from a model, thus enabling comparison of the reconstruction of the 3D flow velocity field and its related wall shear stress to exact known "measurements".

METHODS

The attempt to develop the method and prove its usefulness and accuracy is carried out in two stages:

1. Flow field simulation and data generation.
2. Flow field reconstruction from the simulated data.

Flow Field Simulation

The data was generated from a theoretical flow model of a cylindrical tube, which included a moderate "stenosis". The exact 3D geometric data of the wall as well as the 3D flow velocity vectorial field in each location within the tube is thus known. The cylindrical tube of radius r = 4 mm, and length l = 80 mm represents the common carotid artery (CCA). The narrowing of the lumen is of a hyperbolic shape, 20 mm in length. The stenotic region is located 30 mm from the inlet of the tube, with a maximal narrowing of 2 mm. The flow velocity vectorial field within this tube was produced by the FIDAP 7.0 program, assuming that

- The fluid is an incompressible, homogeneous, Newtonian fluid at a constant temperature.
- "Blood" characteristics: μ = 0.035 poise, ρ = 1.055 g/cm^3, Re = 600 at ~25 cm/sec.
- The flow is laminar and in steady state.
- The arterial wall is not flexible.
- The no slip condition applies.

Flow through the tube was calculated with the 3D vectorial values given at the nodes specified. Once the flow is known, two transverse planes were selected and two USCDM images, representing the inlet and outlet, are simulated by projecting the velocity vectors at each plane (obtained from the previous step) onto a predefined US beam direction. Finally, a normally distributed random noise ψ^2, is added to this velocity component, in a variety of signal to noise ratios.

Flow Field Reconstruction

The process of flow field reconstruction is composed of two stages: geometry reconstruction and proper flow field reconstruction.

Geometry reconstruction: A small number of B–mode obtained transversal cross-sectional boundaries are assumed to be exactly known (eight equally oriented and evenly distributed sections). These assumed known boundaries are generated by the same geometric equations used in the flow field simulation. In practice, these boundaries are tracked from real B–mode images, using an automatic (given the respective USCDM images) procedure, based on active contours, which produces a 'minimal energy' boundary. Their position in space is given by the concurrent measurement of the spatial location and orientation of the hand–held US probe. Spline interpolation is applied to these known transverse cross–sectional boundaries in order to reconstruct the remainder of the tube.

Proper flow field reconstruction: The 3D velocity field is reconstructed by numerically solving the Navier–Stokes and the Continuity equations:

$$\rho_0 \vec{u} \cdot \nabla \vec{u} = -\nabla p + \rho_0 \vec{f} + \mu \nabla^2 \vec{u} \tag{1}$$

$$\nabla \cdot \vec{u} = 0 \tag{2}$$

A penalty parameter approach (PPA) is adopted, by which:

$$\nabla \cdot \vec{u} = -\varepsilon p \tag{3}$$

where ε is the penalty parameter (a small number representing the fluid incompressibility). Disregarding external forces, we obtain:

$$\rho_0 \vec{u} \cdot \nabla \vec{u} = \frac{1}{\varepsilon} \nabla (\nabla \cdot \vec{u}) + \mu \nabla^2 \vec{u} \qquad (4)$$

The no–slip condition $\vec{u} = 0$ provides (Dirichlet) boundary conditions at the vessel wall. The two outermost USCDM, the first and last in the sequence of cross sections, provide the inlet and outlet velocity distributions, respectively. In order to simplify the solution, axial flow at the inlet and outlet planes is assumed, and its value is calculated as follows:

$$\vec{u} = \frac{f_D c}{2 f_0 \cos\theta} \hat{z} \qquad (5)$$

where f_0 and f_D are the transmitted and Doppler shifted frequencies, respectively, c is the US wave propagation speed, and θ is the angle between the velocity and the US beam.

Finally, the tube volume is discretized, and the problem is solved by the finite element method. A proper solution is obtained for such an ε which allows convergence to a feasible physical solution of the reconstructed field.

Shear stress calculation: Given the velocity vectors as a function of space, the shear stress is obtained by the following set of general equations (in tensorial notation):

$$\tau_i = \sigma_{ij} n_j \qquad (6)$$

$$\sigma_{ij} = -p \delta_{ij} + \mu (u_{i,j} + u_{j,i}) \qquad (7)$$

where τ_i, σ_{ij} and n_j are the shear stress vector, the stress tensor, and the unit normal vector at the boundary, respectively. δ_{ij} is Kronecker's delta.

For a 3D Cartesian coordinate system:

$$\sigma_{xx} = -p + 2\mu \frac{\partial u_x}{\partial x} \quad ; \quad \sigma_{yy} = -p + 2\mu \frac{\partial u_y}{\partial y} \quad ; \quad \sigma_{zz} = -p + 2\mu \frac{\partial u_z}{\partial z} \qquad (8)$$

$$\sigma_{xy} = \mu \left(\frac{\partial u_x}{\partial y} + \frac{\partial u_y}{\partial x} \right) \quad ; \quad \sigma_{yz} = \mu \left(\frac{\partial u_y}{\partial z} + \frac{\partial u_z}{\partial y} \right) \quad ; \quad \sigma_{xz} = \mu \left(\frac{\partial u_x}{\partial z} + \frac{\partial u_z}{\partial x} \right) \qquad (9)$$

RESULTS

Preliminary results for the three different noise levels, ψ^2, for the previously defined geometric conditions, show that ε in the range of 10e–4 to 10e–3 gives near–to–optimal reconstruction of the flow field, related to the minimization of the mean squared error (MSE) η:

$$\eta = \frac{1}{N} \sum_{i=1}^{N} \left\| \vec{u}_i - \hat{u}_i \right\|^2 \qquad (10)$$

where N is the number of simulated velocity vectors, $\bar{u}_i$ and $\hat{u}_i$ and are the original and the restored i–th vectors, respectively. The choice of ε in this range has almost no influence on the solution (low sensitivity). The error, η, was calculated for these conditions: for ε = 10e–4, and for noise levels ψ^2: 0, 6.25, and 25, the following MSE η were obtained, respectively: 0.9472, 5.5807, and 20.5291.

It is seen that, under the given simulation conditions, when noise levels are modified within the normal levels of measurement noise, there is no appreciable variation in η due to geometric uncertainty. $\psi^2 = 0$ represents an exception since, apart from numeric noise, there is no noise source other than geometric uncertainty. The distribution of shear stresses is as expected, since the conditions tested were steady state laminar flow. It is encouraging to learn that even under high, but acceptable levels of measurement noise, there is enough information in the flow velocity data measured at two cross–sections to calculate the distribution of stresses in a stenotic artery, even when the stenosis is severe.

DISCUSSION

The reconstructed geometry of the vessel is inaccurate, being based on the eight to 10 ultrasonically measured cross–sections where the vessel's boundaries are (assumed to be) exactly known. The geometric shape of the ·vessel 3D wall is generated by spline interpolation between these known boundaries, and therefore some errors are introduced. The reconstruction of the 3D flow velocity vectorial field in the lumen of this vessel, includes errors due to the reconstruction of the wall geometry, due to the USCDM flow velocity measurements at the two cross–sections, due to the calculation of the flow velocity vectors at these two planes, and due to the reconstruction of the 3D flow velocity field itself.

Under conditions of random measurement noise and the geometric uncertainty of the location of the arterial walls, the flow velocity field can be reconstructed, usually requiring large values of ε. This means that blood is considered as a slightly compressible fluid (which it is not), in order to compensate for the above mentioned errors. Good reconstruction is obtained with ε in the range of 10e–4 to 10e–3, with no need for time consuming optimal parameter search. Due to the PPA used, only two velocity boundary conditions (USCDM planes) need to be acquired, far enough from the suspected stenosis, in order to provide boundary conditions for the FEM algorithm. Additionally, about eight B–mode cross sections provided a satisfactory geometric reconstruction; the geometric reconstruction error could be made smaller by increasing the number of these planes.

The measurements required of the user are relatively small: two USCDM images of the vessel transverse cross–sections, and approximately eight B–mode cross–sections for the wall border determination; all these measurements must be done, with concurrent acquisition of the spatial location and orientation of the US hand–held probe.

CONCLUSIONS

The availability of a method for reconstruction of the 3D vectorial field of flow velocities within the lumen of a section of an artery, allows to calculate the distribution of flow velocities in each cross–section. It also provides a way to calculate the distribution of shear stress, as imposed on arterial wall, i.e., on the endothelial layer. Since there is no practical way to measure the shear stress in one particular location of the wall, or the distribution of stresses along the artery or the circumferential distribution, it is difficult to verify the results reported here. Because of these difficulties, the availability of these results is important. The method is limited to laminar, developed flow, with no bifurcation or a very severe stenosis. But even under these limitations, the technique is applicable for measurements during late diastole, in peripheral arteries (e.g. CCA, descending aorta, femoral arteries etc.). It may also be useful in providing lower bound estimates, since the higher flow velocities during systole will produce overall higher stresses (though at some specific locations flow velocity and shear stress may be very low due to flow separation). The reports [4–8], which associate shear stress with endothelial intracellular processes, usually relate to average values of shear stresses, usually calculated from the average flow velocity. The technique presented here estimates, even if in a limited way, the distribution of the shear stresses upon the intima. It provides a tool for studying the effects of localized shear stresses or the possible effects of stepwise distribution of shear stress where nearby sections of endothelial tissue are exposed to significantly different values of stresses.

Acknowledgment

This study was supported by the Technion's VPR fund for Promotion of Research.

DISCUSSION

Dr. R. Beyar: Is the new procedure you presented limited to axisymmetric geometry of the artery? Do you need to assume such a condition for the flow calculations, or can you accommodate any 3D shape?

Dr. D.R. Adam: No, we are not limited at all. As long as sufficient B–mode US cross–sections are obtained for proper reconstruction of the arterial walls, its 3D geometry can be reconstructed and the flow pattern can be calculated.

Dr. R. Beyar: Very often the situation in severe stenosis is that flow separation occurs with jets. Can the procedure allow for separation to occur?

Dr. D.R. Adam: Flow separation is allowed as long as the flow regime does not turn turbulent.

Dr. L. Axel: You seem to dismiss MR because of cost considerations, but one basic difference between MR and ultrasound is that ultrasound is intrinsically limited to measurement along the line of the sound, whereas MR allows you to sample the full 3D distribution of velocity, even with a planar image, though not within a single beat.

Dr. D.R. Adam: Yes, it is of course true that US is intrinsically limited to measuring velocity along the line of sound. But if one imagines the design of a more complex US system, one may think of multiple transducers, insonating each volume element from several known orientations and then the 3D flow velocity vector can be obtained.

Dr. E. Ritman: One can estimate the shear stress at the endothelium using the flow and diameter of the vessel if one makes some assumptions about viscosity, laminar flow etc. You have some more realistic data, I presume. How does that commonly used expression of shear, in terms of flow and diameter, relate to what you might call a better estimate?

Dr. D.R. Adam: Our assumption are very much the same and the estimation is, therefore, of the same accuracy. The procedure presented here, though, allows for different geometries (e.g. non–

symmetric, change of size, etc.) and complex flow profiles. It is therefore a method which can be used with realistic data of various shapes of arteries, and not just a tube.

Dr. H. Azhari: Did you account for the pulsatility of the wall, or did you assume a rigid geometry? Also, in order to solve the finite element you have to assume something about the flow. Did you assume potential flow or something else?

Dr. D.R. Adam: In order to assure a laminar regime, we find ourselves limited to the diastolic period, where diameter changes are small enough to consider flow in a stiff pipe. In principle, the method can accommodate pulsatility of the wall, but the calculations and computation time will be long. Concerning the second part of your question: we do not assume potential flow, but a viscous one (according to blood characteristics).

Dr. N. Westerhof: There may also be movement of the coronary vessels in the axial direction. Would that not complicate the matter?

Dr. D.R. Adam: One possible solution is to also acquire a longitudinal cross–section in which the axial movement can be recorded and measured. The measured and calculated flow velocities can then be adjusted accordingly. This solution will require, again, the assumption of repeatability of the recorded data (quasi–stationarity) over the different heart beats.

Dr. R. Beyar: The role of the shear stress is probably very important. These analytical tools can probably allow you to predict, if you can get enough data, a realistic value to the response of the structure to the stresses. There may be a big role of the cyclic shear stress rather than the quasistatic stress in the endothelial cell. The dynamic shear stress component, which is probably very large, has to be accounted for in the future.

Dr. D.R. Adam: I started this project at the NIH in 1992. AT that time I was asked to find clinical or pathophysiological justification to study the shear stress near the arterial wall. That was 5 years ago, but now the need has been established. We have presented here a method which can be applied during diastole. The method can be extended to periods in which there is rapid change of flow velocity. However, the method fails once turbulence occurs.

Dr. U. Dinnar: Shear stress is defined as the difference in velocity over a very short distant. This is hard to get in this example because the short distance is on the same scale as the error that you have. It looks to me that to get a realistic point–by–point shear stress is very complicated.

Dr. R. Beyar: When one tries to measure near the wall, one is confronted by a huge resolution problem. Dr. Adam's procedure is based on measuring the full flow profile in two cross–sections, and then using a finite element model; the shear stress comes out as an estimate. Whether it is correct or not is another question.

REFERENCES

1.   Nerem RM, Levesque MJ. Fluid mechanics in atherosclerosis. In: *Handbook of Bioengineering* (Skalak R, Chien S, editors), McGraw Hill: NY, 1987, pp. 21.1 21.22.
2.   Fox MD, Gardiner M. Three–dimensional doppler velocimetry of flow jets. *IEEE Trans Biomed Eng* 1988;35:834–841.
3.   Schrank E, Phillips DJ, Morits WE, Strandness DE Jr. A triangulation method for the quantitative measurement of arterial blood velocity magnitude and directions in humams. *Ultrasound in Med Biol* 1990;16(5):499–509.
4.   Recchia FA, Senzaki H, Saeki A, Byrne BJ, Kass DA. Pulse pressure–related changes in coronary flow *in vivo* are modulated by nitric oxide and adenosine. *Circ Res* 1996; 79:849–856.

5. Bernstein RD, Ochoa FY, Xu X, Forfia P, Shen W, Thompson CI, Hintze TH. Function and production of nitric oxide in the coronary circulation of the conscious dog during exercise. *Circ Res* 1996;79:840–848.

6. Gudi SRP, Clark CG, Frangos JA. Fluid flow rapidly activates g proteins in human endothelial cells. *Circ Res* 1996;79:834–839.

7. Nadaud S, Philippe M, Arnal JF, Michel JB, Soubrier F. Sustained increase in aortic endothelial nitric oxide synthase expression *in vivo* in a model of chronic high blood flow. *Circ Res* 1996;79:857–863.

8. Vonderleyen HE, Gibbons GH, Morishita R, Lewis NP, Zhang L, Nakajima M, Kaneda Y, Cooke JP, Dzau VJ. Gene therapy inhibiting neointimal vascular lesion: *in vivo* transfer of endothelial cell nitric oxide synthase gene. *Proc Natl Acad Sci USA* 1995;92:1137–1141.

9. Zarins CK, Zatina MA, Giddens DR, Ku DN, Glagov S. Shear stress regulation of artery lumen diameter in experimental atherogenesis. *J Vasc Surg* 1987;5(3):413–420.

10. Van Dijk P: Direct cardiac NMR imaging of heart wall and blood flow velocity. *J Comput Assist Tomogr* 1984;8:429–436.

11. Bryant DJ, Payne JA, Firmin DN, Longmore DB. Measurement of flow with NMR imaging using a gradient pulse and phase difference technique. J Comput Assist Tomogr 1984; 8: 588–593.

12. Mohiaddin RH, Amanuma MA, Kilner PJ, Pennel DJ, Manzara C, Longmore DB. MR phase–shift velocity mapping of mitral and pulmonary venous flow. *J Comput Assist Tomogr* 1991;15:237–243.

13. Wang T, Wu X, Chung N, Ritman EL. Myocardial blood flow estimated by synchronous, multislice, high–speed computed tomography. *IEEE Trans Med Imaging* 1989;8:70–77.

14. Bailliart O, Bonnin P, Capderou A, Savin E, Kedra AW, Martineaud JP. Simultaneous ultrasonic measurement of carotic blood–flow and intracerebral hemodynamics in man. *Arch Int de Physiol de Biochem et de Biophysic* 1993;101(2):149–154.

15. Van Rossum A, Sprenger KH, Peels FC, et al. *In vivo* validation of quantitative flow imaging in arteries and veins using magnetic resonance phase shift techniques. Society of Magnetic Resonance in Medicine, Berkly CA, 9th Annual Sci Meeting, Amsterdam, 1989; 205.

16. Kilner PJ, Firmin DN, Rees RSO, et al. Magnetic resonance jet velocity mapping for assessment of valve and great vessel stenosis. *Radiology* 1991;178: 229–235.

CHAPTER 16

COMPENSATORY ENLARGEMENT, REMODELING, AND RESTENOSIS

Gad Keren[1]

ABSTRACT

Coronary atherosclerosis is associated with vessel remodeling and dilatation. Quantitative analysis of arterial morphometry documents that as the cross sectional area of the plaque increases within a diseased vessel segment, the outer wall of the artery expands in an attempt to compensate for the accumulation of plaque. This focal compensatory enlargement maintains cross sectional area at stenotic sites of arteries, and the angiographic appearance of the vessel may be normal, despite marked accumulation of atherosclerotic plaque. Compensatory enlargement may develop as a response to increased shear stress caused by atherosclerotic plaque in conjunction with endothelial dependent factors, or alternatively, due to medial attenuation with loss of underlying structural support. The mechanism of arterial remodeling plays an important role in the development of arterial restenosis late after balloon dilatation or other interventional modalities. Stents prevent the remodeling process and restenosis with stents is the result of a relatively uniform neointimal tissue proliferation throughout the stent. Endovascular stents induce tissue proliferation both within the endoluminal stent surface and in the tissue layers surrounding the metallic Palmaz–Schatz stent struts. The therapeutic goals to prevent restenosis have to be oriented towards prevention of acute recoil, reduction of intimal, medial and adventitial prolific response and the phenomenon of inadequate arterial remodeling.

INTRODUCTION

Coronary atherosclerosis is associated with vessel remodeling and dilatation and thus the angiographic appearance of the vessel may be normal despite marked accumulation of

---

[1]Department of Cardiology, Tel Aviv Medical Center, Tel Aviv University, Tel Aviv, Israel

atherosclerotic plaque. Quantitative analysis of arterial morphometry documents that as the cross sectional area of the plaque increases within a diseased vessel segment the outer wall of the artery expands in an attempt to compensate for the accumulation of plaque. This focal compensatory enlargement has been described as a mechanism to maintain luminal cross–sectional area in human femoral, carotid and coronary arteries. A significant correlation was found between vessel area and plaque area in the original presentation of this concept by Glagov and coworkers [1]. In their study, 136 left main coronary segments underwent careful histopathologic examination for lumen area, total vessel area and lesion area. Total vessel area correlated significantly with lesion area and lumen area was maintained up to 40% vessel stenosis, as determined from the ratio of lesion area divided by internal elastic lamina area. When the ratio was higher than 40% the lumen decreased and significant lumen narrowing developed. The important conclusion was that compensatory enlargement maintain lumen size up to 40% stenosis but fail to do so for larger ratio [1]. This idea was later corroborated by intravascular ultrasound (IVUS) and epicardial echocardiography in coronary arteries [2–4], in femoral arteries [5], carotid arteries and more recently in saphenous veins used as arterial conduits in bypass operation [6]. Accordingly, clinically and angiographically significant coronary artery disease develops when a focal failure of compensatory dilatation occurs in response to atherosclerotic plaque deposition.

Compensatory enlargement may develop as a response to increased shear stress caused by atherosclerotic plaque in conjunction with endothelial dependent factors. Alternatively, it may be due to medial attenuation with loss of underlying structural support. The accumulation of atherosclerotic plaque is associated with significant inflammatory response, cytokine and growth factor secretion.

Losordo et al. [5] used IVUS in 62 paired adjacent normal and diseased sites in the superficial femoral arteries of 20 patients undergoing peripheral vascular interventions. They have shown a decrease in lumen cross sectional area from 21 mm^2 at normal sites to 16 mm^2 at adjacent diseased sites. This decrease in lumen area was associated with an increase in plaque area and vessel area from 32 mm^2 to 37 mm^2. A regression analysis disclosed a significant correlation between cross sectional area of the plaque and total arterial area at the lesion site without affecting adjacent normal segments of the vessel. Wong et al. [2], performed a segment by segment analysis of intracoronary ultrasound images in 15 patients and showed that maximal plaque area was not significantly different between those having more than 50% narrowing by quantitative angiography and those who did not show any significant disease indicating compensatory enlargement of the vessel due to plaque accumulation in some of the patients.

Nishioka et al. [4] studied the mechanism of compensatory enlargement in human coronary arteries using IVUS in 30 patients with coronary artery disease. They have defined compensatory enlargement to be present when the lesion site total vessel cross sectional area was larger than the proximal normal segment, inadequate compensatory enlargement when the lesion vessel cross sectional area was smaller than the distal reference site and intermediate remodeling when the vessel cross sectional area at the lesion site was intermediate between the two reference sites. Compensatory enlargement was observed in 19 (54%) of 35 lesions, inadequate enlargement in 26% and intermediate remodeling in 20% of lesions. In the compensatory enlargement group the vessel wall area increased markedly (182%) and exceeded the lumen area reduction and was partially (82%) compensated by the vessel cross sectional area increase. In the inadequate compensatory enlargement group, the cross sectional area reduction contributed to 39% of the lumen area reduction at the lesion site, whereas wall area increase explained 61% of the lumen area reduction at the lesion site. The inadequate compensatory enlargement resulting in relative vessel constriction at the lesion site appears to be an important contributing factor along with plaque proliferation to vascular stenosis.

Mendelsson and coworkers [6] evaluated the response of saphenous vein bypass grafts to progressive atherosclerosis. They suggested that the reaction to flow and shear forces in veins may be similar to arteries but veins may lack the endothelial mediated function required for remodeling. Twenty four discrete lesions and reference sites in 21 saphenous vein grafts were studied. Lesion vessel area was larger than the reference area in 23 of 24 vessels and there was a significant correlation between plaque and vessel area. Similar to the reports for native coronary arteries, the ability to increase plaque burden is impeded in vein grafts and more than 30 to 40% of the vessel area is occupied by plaque, undergoing compensatory enlargement similar to muscular arteries.

RESTENOSIS MECHANISMS: LATE OUTCOME AFTER INTERVENTIONS

Restenosis remains the major limitation of transcatheter coronary revascularization. The original hypothesis of the mechanisms underlying restenosis includes:

1. Acute lumen loss due to elastic recoil.
2. Neointimal growth mainly as a result of smooth muscle cell proliferation.
3. Extracellular matrix formation and deposition in the subintima and at the area of neointimal proliferation.

However, this paradigm has failed in view of two observations: First, all the pharmacotherapeutic agents used in clinical trials to prevent restenosis have failed, even when the therapeutic agents were found highly efficacious in animal models of restenosis. Moreover, recent animal models, substantiated by angiographic and IVUS studies suggest that arterial remodeling, is the major factor underlying restenosis and should be taken into consideration when planning treatment strategies for prevention of restenosis.

Kakuta et al. [7] have used percutaneous transluminal angioplasty (PTCA) in the iliac artery of the atherosclerotic rabbits to cause arterial stenosis. Histologic evaluation of the vessels immediately and at 4 weeks revealed that stenotic vessels had smaller arterial area compared to non–stenotic vessels, while there was no significant difference in the plaque and media area. The authors conclude that iliac arteries compensate for neointimal formation after angioplasty by vessel enlargement. The extent of this enlargement is the main determinant of chronic lumen size. A similar study was performed by Post and Borst [8] who evaluated the effect of barotrauma and thermal trauma to arteries of rabbits and microswines. Their conclusions were that restenosis after this trauma is mainly due to intimal hyperplasia and arterial remodeling. In a later study, Andersen and Falk [9] have again clearly shown that arterial remodeling is more important than neointimal formation in determining late lumen loss. Adventitial proliferation and thickening were extensive indicating that the adventitia is significantly involved in the process of restenosis. This hypothesis was further corroborated by Shi and Zalewski [10] who used BrDu labeling and immunohistochemistry to study the sequence of cell activation in a Porcine PTCA injury model. They have shown that adventitial fibroblasts migrate to the neointima and differentiate to myofibroblasts. These myofibroblasts are involved in tissue contraction and may represent a mechanism for geometric remodeling which sometimes unfavorably results in vessel constriction.

Neointimal formation is the vessel's response to deep injury that may be either physical or biological. The response involves all the layers of the vessels, mainly smooth muscle cells, adventitial fibroblasts with significant matrix formation.

Many clinical, angiographic, and more recently IVUS variables were evaluated as possible predictors for restenosis. Review of the subject demonstrates that different conclusions can be drawn from the various studies. In an early study of 100 patients undergoing PTCA, Honye [11] suggested that restenosis occurs more frequently in lesions with relatively soft atheroma and insufficient plaque fracture. Only significant fracture of the plaque is associated with prevention of restenosis.

Tenaglia and coworkers [12], performed PTCA, directional coronary atherectomy (DCA) or laser therapy in 68 patients assisted by an initial IVUS imaging. Six month angiographic follow-up, and 1 year clinical follow-up showed that dissections detected in 42% of patients were associated with adverse clinical outcome, including cardiac death, myocardial infarction, coronary bypass surgery and mainly restenosis.

Feld et al. [13] determined the value of IVUS compared to angioscopy in predicting outcome of interventional procedures such as PTCA, DCA, laser angioplasty and stent implantation. They performed interventional procedures in 60 patients followed by either IVUS, angioscopy, or both. Follow-up at 1 year was clinical and coronary angiography was undertaken wherever needed. Predictive of adverse outcome were clinical presentation, thrombolytic therapy, angioscopic plaque rupture prior to procedure, and the detection of thrombus pre and post procedure. The conclusion was that angioscopy rather than IVUS or angiography was predictive of adverse outcome in patients with complex lesions after interventions.

In the PICTURE trial [14], 200 patients were enrolled to try and evaluate whether post PTCA IVUS imaging can predict 6 months restenosis. Variables studied were the appearance of dissection, tears, plaque types, plaque area, total vessel area, lumen area and other ratios. Interestingly, none of the post PTCA IVUS variables were predictive of angiographic restenosis at 6 months. Jain et al. [15] have investigated IVUS derived parameters that can predict restenosis in 33 patients and lesions, after balloon angioplasty (n=25), and DCA (n=8). After 6 months follow-up in 30 patients, they found major dissections in 78% of patients with angiographic restenosis compared to 10% of patients without restenosis, whereas plaque fracture was more abundant in patients without restenosis. Plaque burden calculated as plaque area/external elastic lamina (EEL) area was significantly more severe in patients with angiographic restenosis compared to patients without restenosis. The authors concluded that the absence of plaque fracture, existence of a major dissection and greater plaque burden identify patients in whom restenosis is more likely to occur after catheter based interventions. The rate of arterial recoil was similar for both groups.

Mintz et al. [16] performed IVUS imaging in 360 non-stented native coronary artery lesions for whom angiographic follow-up was obtained within a few months. The angiographic predictors of restenosis were the use of rotational atherectomy, lesions longer than 10 mm, vessel tortuosity, total occlusion lesions and preintervention TIMI flow less than 3. Lumen cross sectional area, minimal lumen diameter, and eccentricity index obtained from IVUS imaging prior to intervention correlated with the occurrence of restenosis. The highest correlation was found for percent cross sectional narrowing calculated as plaque plus media cross sectional area divided by external elastic membrane cross sectional area. Similarly, these variables obtained in the post intervention IVUS imaging phase correlated significantly with restenosis.

Blasini et al. [17] showed, by IVUS after PTCA and at 6 months follow-up, that most of the late lumen loss is due to arterial remodeling. In an extensive study Mintz et al. [18], performed IVUS imaging, in 212 lesions, treated with PTCA, DCA, rotational atherectomy and laser angioplasty. They have found that in patients who developed restenosis, the reduction in lumen size was attributed to a reduction in total vessel area (EEL area). This phenomenon was not encountered in the non-restenotic lesions. Over time lumen size decreased by an average of 4.1 mm^2 in patients who developed restenosis compared to 1.2 mm^2 in those who did not develop restenosis. These changes were attributed mainly to a 3.1 mm^2 drop in the total vessel size in the restenosis group compared to 0.8 mm^2 in the non–restenosis group. The conclusion of the authors was that, restenosis is determined after interventions mainly by the extent and direction of remodeling of the vessel.

The current hypothesis of the mechanism underlying restenosis can be summarized as follows: Immediately after the barotrauma, or any other deep injury to the vessel wall, a thrombotic phase ensues with an inflammatory response, cytokines and growth factors secretion. These changes are followed by two long term processes of cellular proliferation associated with matrix deposition and arterial remodeling.

The changing concept of the underlying pathophysiology of restenosis calls for a change in treatment strategy with significantly more emphasis given to prevention of remodeling mainly with the use of stents.

CORONARY STENTS

Coronary stenting was initially used as a safe and effective bail–out procedure to prevent impending vessel closure after balloon dilatation and in patients with recurrent restenosis. However, deployment of these metallic devices has recently been shown to reduce the frequency of restenosis in de novo lesions in selected groups of patients compared to balloon angioplasty. Until the introduction of effective antithrombotic therapy, stent placement was associated with 1–3% thrombotic complications.

IVUS seemed a perfect imaging modality to assess stent deployment characteristics and long term results since metal, similar to calcium, is highly echogenic. Indeed, stent struts or coils are well visualized by IVUS and imaging by IVUS is significantly improved compared to fluoroscopy and angiography in most stents. The IVUS measurements of the stent and reference lumen dimensions and cross sectional area were found highly reproducible with low inter and intraobserver variability. This imaging modality was used extensively over the last few years in an effort to improve our understanding of stent deployment characteristics and define IVUS guidelines for implantation. Full stent expansion to the appropriate size, complete apposition and symmetry both axially and longitudinally have been found to be important criteria that may help to avoid events of acute and sub–acute stent thrombosis. Moreover, arterial remodeling is reduced by stent deployment though tissue growth is augmented. The initial IVUS stent studies were performed after Palmaz–Schatz stent implantation. Acutely stents were usually concentric with an inner layer of highly reflective struts, that obscure a middle hypoechoic layer composed of media and compressed atheroma and an outer echogenic adventitia. The lumen of the stented vessels was usually clear of flaps or thrombi. The stent struts were sometimes expanded in an asymmetric fashion. Chronic changes included a thin layer of neointimal hyperplasia in a significant number of patients.

The initial IVUS observations were later expanded with careful comprehensive and longitudinal studies performed to assess the determinants of acute success and late restenosis after stent implantation. Nakamura et al. [19], compared IVUS imaging with coronary angiography in 63 patients who underwent Palmaz Schatz stent insertion for native coronary artery stenosis. The angiographic and IVUS data were used to decide whether stent placement results were satisfactory and further balloon dilatation was performed whenever necessary. The authors concluded that IVUS evaluation after stent insertion demonstrates a significant degree of underestimation compared with coronary angiography. Using IVUS, more than 80% of patients underwent further dilatation despite the initial appearance of an optimal angiographic result. The result of the study supported the view that IVUS guided careful stent deployment with adherence to criteria of size, symmetry and apposition may reduce the need for anticoagulation. In a later study from the same center, Goldberg and coworkers [20], guided stent deployment with the use of angiography and IVUS to obtain optimal results in 40 patients. The angiographic percent diameter stenosis was 74% at baseline and increased to an average of 8% after apparent successful angiographic result and to −6% negative residual stenosis after IVUS guided correction. These changes were associated with marked increase in lumen cross sectional area obtained by IVUS and improvement in eccentricity index from 0.84 to 0.89 at the final post IVUS dilatation. The study further demonstrated that stents are not expanded uniformly along the long axis, and IVUS guided higher pressure and larger balloon inflation results in intra–stent cross sectional area that will translate to a significant increase in flow through the vessel. This may, on the long run, result in lower incidence of thrombotic events and restenosis.

Recent studies suggest that arterial remodeling after balloon angioplasty may have a more significant role compared to neointimal proliferation in causing restenosis. The process of remodeling involves changes that occur in the adventitia and media and may be halted by the deployment of stents. Two factors may contribute to stent restenosis. First, stents trigger the development of neointima and second is the possible chronic recoil and reduction in stent size. Hoffman [21] performed serial IVUS studies in 142 stents to determine the relative contribution of both these factors in causing restenosis. The acute angiographic and ultrasound results were excellent and the JJIS stents were quite uniform in size longitudinally except for the narrowest portion at the articulation site where most of the prolapsed tissue was detected. On later follow–up studies, lumen size decreased markedly, with only minor change in stent size. In stent intimal proliferation was significant throughout the stent lumen and accumulated more at the central articulation site. Late lumen loss correlated strongly with tissue growth and weakly with stent recoil and remodeling. The authors concluded that stents prevent the remodeling process and restenosis of stents is the result of relatively uniform neointimal tissue proliferation throughout the stent. A second study [22] showed that endovascular stents induce tissue proliferation both within the endoluminal stent surface and in the tissue layers surrounding the metallic Palmaz–Schatz stent struts. Similar to previous findings, tissue proliferation was greater in restenotic than in non–restenotic stents. Tissue proliferation surrounding the stent was accompanied by adaptive remodeling and increase in external elastic membrane cross sectional area [22].

CONCLUSIONS

Compensatory enlargement and arterial remodeling are dynamic processes that occur in the vessel wall as a reaction to biological, biochemical or physical injury with plaque deposition and neointimal proliferation. When the response is compensatory and total vessel area increases, vessel lumen may be maintained without stenosis. However, restenosis develops when the dilatation is insufficient.

The therapeutic targets to prevent restenosis can be summarized as follows:
a)   Acute recoil after coronary intervention can be prevented by stent implantation.
b)   Chronic remodeling can be modified by stents, though research is currently performed to define optimal deployment and adjunct pharmacotherapy.

c)   Prevention of tissue growth, whether originating from the media or adventitia, can be prevented by future developments in pharmacotherapy or site specific radiation therapy.

DISCUSSION

Dr. E. Ritman: What bothers me is the adventitial proliferation. How do you explain that? One possible mechanism is that the vaso vasora are damaged and that we are in fact looking at some interesting effects in the adventitia because of that. Or do you think there is actually something diffusing out from the endothelium?

Dr. G. Keren: We have been biased to think that it is the media that is involved in this process, and actually the adventitia is very much involved. I do not believe that the endothelium is the main issue, and that something from the endothelium infiltrates through the media into the adventitia and affects there. It has to be a local factor, and you can see how localized it is in the area of injury. I do not have an explanation as to whether there is some cytokine secretion there and why there is such a proliferation there. Nothing can at this point be studied from IVUS regarding adventitial involvement because you can not see the adventitia with IVUS. There is such an attenuation of the signal that you do not know what is going on down in the adventitia, and where the adventitia ends. So answers from human studies with IVUS can not be helpful. Going back to the basic research, there are many questions and few answers.

Dr. H. Strauss: Even though the smooth muscle cells may not be proliferating, they still may be able to liberate cell signalling molecules that could influence other cells in the environment. The other factor, of course, is neurotrophic stimulation. Has anybody examined the effects of denervation to see whether it can modulate this process?

Dr. G. Keren: I am not familiar with this kind of data.

Dr. M.S. Gotsman: Technology has outstripped our biological knowledge. We are putting very big balloons into very small arteries and we are simply creating a lot of damage. We used to pray and hope it would get better. Now we are putting in stents and they are staying open. However, we have damaged the arterial wall so much that what we have is a very acute inflammatory response and a very acute healing response. All the mechanisms of wound healing are in fact working here. Ultrasound is showing us what we are doing, but we do not know the actual mechanisms at work.

Dr. J. Saffitz: An important point to keep in mind is that virtually all the animal models of human vascular disease are imperfect. The hypercholesterolemic rabbit, for example, is characterized by an intimal lesion that is extremely rich in lipid and has very little fibrous and smooth muscle cell components. Many of the other injuries occur in essentially normal vessels where the response to injury is going to be different than what you have in a patient in whom you are dilating a lesion that is already probably decades old and has many degenerative features that do not occur in the animal models. It is difficult to conclude about smooth muscle cell proliferation by looking at what happens in animal models and trying to jump to the human situation.

There is something else I have always wondered about. I have heard it mentioned that soft plaque components can be compressed. But I do not understand how that can possibly happen.

Dr. G. Keren: It happens. There is proof that it redistributes. What happens is that the total area of the vessel dilates. If you look at the width on the long axis, you think it is compressed, but actually it is redistributed; there is no loss of mass.

Dr. A. McColloch: Do you think that stretch associated with the procedure, or subsequent to it, could be the signal for the adventitial accumulation? Wilson and Ives [*Wilson E, Sudhir K, Ives HE. Mechanical strain of rat vascular smooth muscle cells is sensed by specific extracellular matrix/integrin interactions. J Clin Invest 1995;96(5):2364–2372*] have shown that stretching induces vascular smooth muscle cell proliferation. In various fibroblasts, stretch increases extracellular matrix gene expression and protein synthesis.

Dr. G. Keren: I believe it is the stretch more than other signals. The BRDU studies show that it occurs quite early.

Dr. U. Dinnar: Do you have an estimate as to how long it takes before the phenomena stabilizes, or stops?

Dr. G. Keren: I do not know. I am trying to figure it out. I think it takes a few months to stabilize.

Dr. M.S. Gotsman: There are three reactive phases in the arterial wall after an interventional procedure. The first phase consists of simple retraction which follows dilatation, and this occurs almost immediately as the artery is an elastic structure. The clinical counterpart corresponds to one week of clinical improvement of angina pectoris, and then the symptomatology returns as the constricting artery returns to its previous diameter. We have shown in our angiographic studies, presented at these meetings some years ago, that the restenotic lesions were identical to the original lesions when observed angiographically. Secondly, there is adventitial, medial and intimal proliferation which occurs and is usually complete within three months. With stents, this can take up to a year so that the proliferative process lasts a long time. The third is positive remodeling in which the arterial lumen expands when flow increases.

Dr. G. Keren: I do not know that it stabilizes. I assume it takes a few months until it reaches a certain steady point. But if the neointima starts to grow, I am talking about stents, I believe it goes on. It is an ongoing process. In some cases it is like a little tumor.

Dr. U. Dinnar: Suppose you find a method to stop intimal growth. How long would you have to continue this procedure?

Dr. H. Strauss: Now I am confused. I thought that some of these studies such as the recently reported Reopro study have suggested that if the agent is given for a brief period, then you can prevent long–term sequelae by somehow interrupting the cell signalling molecules from being liberated from, or binding to, their receptor sites. These data suggest that you may not necessarily have to intervene pharmacologically through the entire time course of the evolution of this lesion.

Dr. G. Keren: The radiation studies that suggest that there is some effect on restenosis by radiation, are acute. You sort of break the cycle in the beginning but I do not think it answers the question as to how long it takes to stabilize.

Dr. J. Saffitz: If you look pathologically, histologically, you can get a somewhat different picture. It is difficult to interpret exactly what is going on histologically with ultrasound. Many of the cyto-kines are not so strongly mitogenic as much as they induce migration. So you may find that smooth muscle cells from the media are proliferating, but they do not proliferate until they migrate into the intima and then they fall under the influence of mitogens. This may be missed in these studies. You can not conclude that smooth muscle cells are not proliferating, because they clearly are.

Dr. M. Morad: There have been some recent atrial remodeling studies on the cellular level suggesting that some activity of the ion channels in such atrial cells have been altered. Is there any study on that level, on remodelled intimal cells?

Dr. G. Keren: I am not familiar with this.

REFERENCES

1. Glagov S, Weisenberg E, Zairns CK, Stankunavicius R, Colletis GJ. Compensatory enlargement of human atherosclerotic coronary arteries. *N Engl J Med* 1987;316:1371–1375.
2. Wong CB, Porter TR, Xie F, Deligonul U. Segmental analysis of coronary arteries with equivalent plaque burden by intravascular ultrasound in patients with and without angiographically significant coronary artery disease. *Am J Cardiol* 1995;76:598–601.
3. Weissman NJ, Mendelsohn FO, Palacios IF, Weyman AE. Development of coronary compensatory enlargement in vivo: sequential assessments with intravascular ultrasound. *Am Heart J* 1995;130:1283–1285.
4. Nishioka T, Luo N, Eigler L, Berglund H, Kim C–J, Siegel RJ. Contribution of inadequate compensatory enlargement to development of human coronary artery stenosis: an in vivo intravascular ultrasound study. *J Am Coll Cardiol* 1996;27:1571–1576.
5. Losordo DW, Rosenfield K, Kaufman J, Pieczsk A, Isner JM. Focal compensatory enlargement of human arteries in response to progressive atherosclerosis in vivo documentation using intravascular ultrasound. *Circulation* 1994;89:2570–2577.
6. Mendelsohn FO, Foster GP, Palacios IF, Weyman AE, Weissman NJ. *In vivo* assessment by intravascular ultrasound of enlargement in saphenous vein bypass grafts. *Am J Cardiology* 1995;76:1066–1069.
7. Kakuta T, Currier JW, Haudenshield CC, Ryan TJ, Faxon DP. Differences in compensatory vessel enlargement, not intimal formation, account for restenosis after angioplasty in the hypercholesterolemic rabbit model. *Circulation* 1994;89:2809–2815.
8. Post MJ, Borst C, Kuntz RE. The relative importance of arterial remodeling compared with intimal hyperplasia in lumen narrowing after balloon angioplasty in the hypercholesterolemic rabbit. *Circulation* 1994;89:2816–2821.
9. Andersen HR, Maeng M, Thorwest M, Falk E. Remodeling rather than neointimal formation explains luminal narrowing after deep vessel wall injury. *Circulation* 1996;93:1716–1724.
10. Shi Y, O'Brien JE, Fard A, Mannion JD, Wang D, Zalewski A. Adventitial myofibroblasts contribute to neointimal formation in injured porcine coronary arteries. *Circulation* 1996;94:1655–1664.
11. Honye J, Mahon DJ, Jain A, White CI, Ramee SR, Wallis JB, Al Zarka A, Tobis JM. Morphological effects of coronary balloon angioplasty in vivo assessed by intravascular ultrasound imaging. *Circulation* 1992;85:1012–1025.
12. Tenagliia AN, Buller CE, Kisslo KN, Phillips HR, Stack RS. Intracoronary ultrasound predictors of adverse outcomes after coronary artery interventions. *J Am Coll cardiol* 1992;20:1385–1390.
13. Feld S, Ganim M, Carell ES, Kjellgren O, KirkeeideRL, Vaughan WK, kelly R, McGhie AI, Kramer N, Loyd D, Andersson HV, Schroth G, Smalling RW. Comparison of angioscopy, intravascular ultrasound imaging and quantitative coronary angiography in predicting clinical outcome after coronary intervention in high risk patients. *J Am Coll Cardiol* 1996;28:97–105.
14. Peters RJ, The PICTURE study group. Prediction of the risk of angiographic restenosis by intracoronary ultrasound imaging after coronary balloon angioplasty. *J Am Coll Cardiol* 1995:February, 35A (Abstract 701–3).
15. Jain SP, Jain A, Collins TJ, Ramee SR, White CJ. Predictors of restenosis; a morphometric quantitative evaluation by intravascular ultrasound. *Am Heart J* 1994;128:664–673.
16. Mintz GS, Popma JJ, Pichard AD, Kent KM, Satler LF, Chuang C, Griffin J, Leon MB. Intravascular ultrasound predictors of restenosis after transcatheter coronary revascularization. *J Am Coll Cardiol* 1996;27:1678–1687.
17. Blasini R, Mudra H, Klauss V, Regar E, Schomig A. Remodeling of coronary arteries after balloon angioplasty: in vivo documentation in patients using consecutive intravascular ultrasound. *J Am Coll Cardiol* 1995;February:139A (Abstract 731–3).
18. Mintz GS, Popma JJ, Pichard AD, Kent KM, Satler LF, Wong C, Hong MK, Kovach JA, Leon MB. Arterial remodeling after coronary angioplasty: a serial intravascular ultrasound study. *Circulation* 1996;94:35–43.
19. Nakamura S, Colombo A, Gaglione A, Almagor Y, Goldberg SL, Maiello L, Finci L, Tobis JM. Intracoronary ultrasound observations during stent implantation. *Circulation* 1994;89:2026–2034.

20.   Goldberg SL, Colombo A, Nakamura S, Almagor Y, Maiello L, Tobis JM. Benefit of intracoronary
      ultrasound in the deployment of Palmaz Schatz stents. *J Am Coll Cardiol* 1994;24:996–1003.
21.   Hoffman R, Mintz GS, Dussaillant GR, Popma JJ, Pichard AD, Satler LF, Kent KM, Griffin J, Leon
      MB. Patterns and mechanisms of in–stent restenosis: a serial intravascular ultrasound study.
      Circulation 1996;94:1247–1254.
22.   Hoffman R, Mintz GS, Popma JF, Satler LF, Pichard AD, Kent KM, Walsh C, Mackell P, Leon MB.
      Chronic arterial responses to stent implantation: a serial intravascular ultrasound analysis of Palmaz
      Schatz stents in native coronary arteries. *J Am Coll Cardiol* 1996;28:1134–1139.

CHAPTER 17

ATHEROSCLEROSIS STUDIES BY INTRACORONARY ULTRASOUND

Mervyn S. Gotsman, Morris Mosseri, Yoseph Rozenman, Dan Admon,
Chaim Lotan, and Hisham Nassar[1]

ABSTRACT

Intravascular ultrasound (IVUS) is a new technique of tomographic visualization of the coronary arteries: its lumen, wall and pathology. Three dimensional (3D) reconstruction shows the tubular structure of the arterial wall and its pathology. IVUS has many advantages over coronary angiography: it has better resolution and shows many hidden lesions. IVUS has helped uncover the underlying mechanisms of percutaneous transluminal coronary angioplasty (PTCA), restenosis, the use and value of other interventional techniques such as directional coronary atherectomy (DCA), rotational atherectomy and stent implantation, and has great value in planning complex interventional procedures. The new American Heart Association (AHA) classification of coronary atherosclerosis pathology can be demonstrated by IVUS. IVUS is sensitive for studies of atheroma regression and progression and shows the coronary artery lesions after cardiac transplantation.

INTRODUCTION

Atherosclerosis is the primary cause of death and morbidity in the Western World. Coronary atherosclerosis causes severe angina pectoris, myocardial infarction and sudden death. Mortality has fallen in the last 25 years, but older patients remain alive and there has been an explosion in the prevalence of the disease within this increasingly aged population [1]. New insights into pathogenesis and pathology have improved our understanding of the underlying disease process while percutaneous interventional cardiology offers a simple and

---

[1]The Cardiology Department, Hadassah University Hospital, Jerusalem, Israel

Analytical and Quantitative Cardiology
Edited by Sideman and Beyar, Plenum Press, New York, 1997

effective approach to long–term definitive management. These procedures require precise anatomical localization and measurement of the obstructive lesions: coronary angiography is at present the "working gold standard" of diagnosis [2, 3]. Ultrasound transducers have been miniaturized, so that a fairly simple disposable transducer (mechanical or phased–array) can be directed down the coronary artery to provide a precise tomographic image of the vessel lumen, its wall and identify the nature of the underlying pathology [4]. Three dimensional computer reconstruction can provide a complete picture of the overall anatomy.

This presentation deals with the quantitative and qualitative demonstration and identification, by IVUS, of coronary atherosclerosis before and after various interventions. The impact of this knowledge on interventional procedures and its value in assessing the results of the different interventions will be discussed.

The AHA Classification of Atheroma

The AHA has adopted the new pathological classification of Stary [5, 6].

Type I occurs in young children and consists of the accumulation of foam cells in the subintima. Circulating low–density lipoprotein (LDL) particles migrate into the subintima, attach to the subendothelial matrix and are oxidized. Monocytic chemotactic protein attracts monocytes; they migrate into the subintima and change into tissue macrophages. Their scavenger receptors ingest the modified and oxidized LDL. The cells swell and form foam cells. Lesions start at arterial bifurcations.

Type II lesions are visible *fatty streaks* on the inner surfaces of the arteries. The lesions contain strata of confluent macrophage foam cells together with smooth muscle cells which migrate and ingest lipid droplets.

Type III is *pre atheroma* with minimal intimal thickening, multiple foam cells and extracellular lipid droplets and particles. The extracellular lipid disrupts the coherence of adjacent intimal smooth muscle cells and form small circumscribed foci.

Type IV lesions, *true atheroma*, consist of a dense accumulation of extracellular lipid which form an intimal lake. There is co–localization of the extracellular lipid as a clear lipid core with a superficial cap. The lesions may rupture and are potentially dangerous.

Type V lesions, *fibro atheroma*, consist of a central core, but the cap has become thicker and contains more collagen.

Type VI lesions demonstrate unstable, *complicated plaque* [7]. Elevated serum LDL levels promote active monocyte–macrophage traffic: cells are located primarily at the plaque shoulder. Lymphocytes and activated mast cells also aggregate in the shoulder, secrete powerful proteolytic enzymes such as metalloproteinases and collagenase and dissolve the intercellular matrix. Plaque disruption occurs in the unstable plaque which has a soft, large core with a thin, vulnerable cap. The plaque has intrinsic vulnerability and is subject to fatigue. There are extrinsic triggers of plaque disruption such as circumferential tensile, compressive, bending, longitudinal friction, and hemodynamic stresses and these are related to other triggering factors. These small, potentially active vulnerable plaques, are unstable, and the ruptured plaque initiates intramural and intraluminal thrombosis. We seek to identify these progenitors of rupture.

Type VII is a mineralized *calcified lesion*. Calcification starts on the medial side of the intima.

Type VIII is the *fibrotic lesion* which consists predominantly of collagen. Type VII and VIII lesions are stable, but islands of Type IV and VI pathology may coexist in the same artery.

METHODOLOGY

The IVUS Imaging System

The cardiovascular imaging system transducer (CVIS, Sunningdale, USA) incorporates a piezo electric transducer and a rotating mirror [4]. The transducer directs an ultrasound beam at the mirror which is rotated at high speed by a drive cable, and the beam continuously scans a 360° cross–section of the artery. The flexible design allows the catheter to be advanced to the most tortuous distal coronary arteries and the composite drive cable produces one–to–one torque, transmitting undistorted rotation of the mirror. The coronary artery is cannulated with an appropriate guiding catheter and a 0.014" guidewire passed down the artery. The CVIS 2.9 Fr ultrasound catheter is threaded over the wire into the artery past the lesion. The proximal end of the drive cable is mounted on a constant speed mechanical pullback device and the piezo electric crystal is withdrawn at constant speed while recording the ultrasound image on a video tape recorder. The tip is monitored by radiological screening. The controlled withdrawal creates a series of tomographic slices of the arterial lumen, its wall and associated pathology at known distances from the introducer system and provides information about the precise site of its tip in the artery. A computer software system permits 3D reconstruction of the tomographic slices [8, 9].

Ultrasound Images of the Normal Arterial Wall

The ultrasound image can show the three layers of the arterial wall: intima, media and adventitia. The luminal–intimal interface appears as a sharp ultrasound opaque image: the media is lighter (less opaque) with similar characteristics to the lumen, so that if the lumen is normal and thin, the medial intimal interface may be difficult to identify. The adventitia is less echo dense and appears as a lighter image. In most patients, three clear layers are visible but in some the intima is not clearly apparent and the media and adventitia fade into one another so that only two layers are seen clearly [10, 11] (Fig. 1).

Plaque Pathology

Most patients have mixed atheroma with a combination of the different pathologies and each can be identified on the ultrasound tomographic slice. The pathology of the

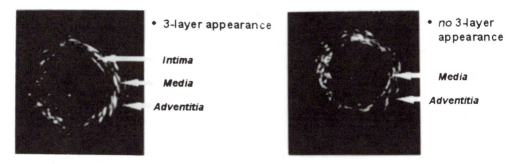

Figure 1. a) The normal artery showing the three–layered appearance. **b)** The normal artery showing the two–layered appearance.

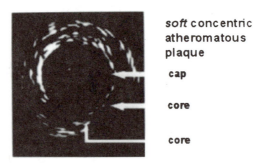

Figure 2. Soft atheromatous plaque showing the translucent atheromatous core.

plaque is usually well noted. Soft atheroma (Types III–VI) appears as an ultrasound lucentarea between the intima and media, but occasionally it fades into the media so that precise demarcation may be difficult (Fig. 2). Cap thickening can also be demonstrated. Fibrous plaques (Type VIII) are more ultrasound opaque and resemble the adventitia. Calcified lesions are easy to identify, since they reflect the ultrasound beam and cause an intense radio opaque image [12, 13]. The ultrasound is usually not transmitted to the outer layers of the artery and creates a translucent space (lucent shadow) behind the calcified lesion (Fig. 3).

Endoluminal thrombi are difficult to distinguish from flowing luminal blood [14]. Arterial wall dissections after angioplasty and ruptured plaques can be identified. Mechanical devices such as stents are intensely ultrasound opaque and are clearly seen, even though they are radio lucent at coronary angiography [15].

Quantitative Measurements

Quantitative coronary angiography (QCA) is the current measurement standard for assessing the degree of obstruction of coronary arteries and the response to interventional procedures [2]. By comparison, quantitative IVUS is much more accurate because of the

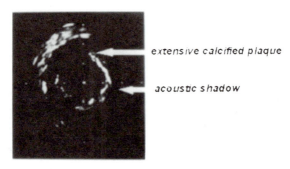

Figure 3. The calcified plaque showing the echo–dense calcified plaque (from 1:00–5:00 o'clock or 150° of plaque in the intima).

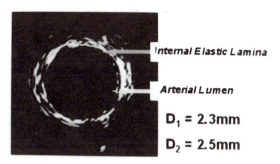

Internal Elastic Lamina

Arterial Lumen

$D_1 = 2.3\text{mm}$

$D_2 = 2.5\text{mm}$

Figure 4. Measurement of arterial diameters.

greater resolution of the system and the tomographic images can be more accurately measured if the tissue interfaces are clear [11, 15, 16].

It is possible to measure the luminal diameter in each polar coordinate and the diameter of the medial–adventitial interfaces (Fig. 4). The tomographic slice is 2D and it is easy to convert the boundaries and diameters into areas. These measure the free luminal area, the medial bounded area, the lesion or plaque area, and the percentage area of obstruction (Fig. 5). When sequential images are reconstructed and measured, values are defined for each image and measuring lesion length and the 3D reconstruction permits precise measurement of the volume of the atheromatous lesion [9]. The 3D reconstruction produces a tubular image of the pathology and shows the extent and volume of the atheromatous mass, and its components. Quantification of calcification is expressed by measuring the arc, depth and length of each calcified plaque.

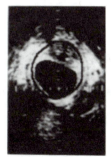

Free Luminal Area	14.7 mm²
Media-bounded Area	29.2 mm²
Lesion Area	14.7 mm²
Percent obstruction	50%
Mean Luminal Diameter	4.3mm
Maximal Diameter	5.0mm
Minimal Diameter	4.0mm

Figure 5. Quantitative measurement of the coronary artery and its luminal and mural pathology. (Taken from Atlas of Intravascular Ultrasound, Ed. John McB. Hodgson, Assoc. Ed. Helen M. Sheehan, Raven Press, New York, Fig. 3, pg. 31, with permission.)

PATHOLOGICAL PHENOMENA

Remodeling of the Coronary Vessels

Intracoronary ultrasound has a great advantage: it demonstrates the area and length of the lumen and also the thickness and nature of the arterial wall. The latter is not observed by angiography. This delineation shows remodeling of the wall (Fig. 6). Glagov [17] has shown that initial accumulation of atheroma in pathological specimens is associated with maintenance of normal luminal cross–sectional area: the arterial wall thickens and the lumen expands so that the luminal cross–sectional area remains normal despite a significant atheromatous burden. This is seen well with IVUS so that a normal luminal cross–sectional area with increased wall thickness is a first sign of atheroma: at a later stage the atheromatous plaque protrudes into the lumen [18, 19].

IVUS has shown [20] that vessel wall recoil occurs after apparently successful coronary artery dilatation with a balloon, and the vessel returns to its normal diameter. Restoration of normal arterial flow with a normal arterial lumen after angioplasty can cause further dilatation of narrowed segments, a phenomenon known as *positive remodeling* [21].

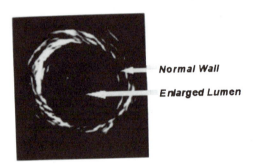

Figure 6. The enlarged, dilated remodeled ectatic coronary artery (diameter: 5 mm).

Diffuse Disease and Asymmetry

The degree of coronary atherosclerosis on angiography is assessed by arterial narrowing associated with a normal contiguous normal segment. Cardiac surgeons have noted that in many patients with angiographically small arteries, the vessels have a heavy atheromatous burden [22]. Patients with a sleeve of atheroma appear to have a small artery but do not have important localized narrowing despite significant anginal symptoms. This paradox has been elucidated by IVUS: the artery is really very narrow with a long sleeve of atheroma but without significant intraluminal protrusions. This produces a narrow artery with important long obstructive lesions (Fig. 7). Measurement of reference segments for assessing the degree stenosis can be fallacious and hence the use of the angiographic concept: "minimal lumen diameter". Eccentric lesions, particularly if the angiographic beam is not at right angles to the lesion, can be confusing since in some views the artery appearsto be significantly narrowed but the arterial diameter may be normal in the right angle view (Fig. 8). Lesions are also hidden at bifurcations, and when two arterial shadows are superimposed. A dissected wall or ruptured intima has a hazy angiographic subintima

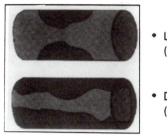

- Localised Lesion
  (the plaque)

- Diffuse Disease
  (the sleeve)

Figure 7. Localized and diffuse disease in the coronary artery. The localized lesion is well defined by angiography while diffuse disease appears as a narrow artery without significant localized obstructions.

and contrast which permeates between the cracks gives a false impression of a normal arterial lumen size [3].

Atheroma Progression and Regression

Studies of atheroma progression have been restricted to physiological examinations using Thallium SPECT imaging [23, 24] or quantitative angiography [25]. The changes in angiographic lesions have been very small and have shown a lack of progression, rather than regression, in patients treated with the new therapeutic strategies (Ileal bypass, severe dietary therapy or Statin drugs). IVUS is a more sensitive method of detecting and measuring the total atheromatous mass and ongoing studies are addressing themselves to regression in treated patients.

Cardiac Transplant Atherosclerosis

This is a unique form of generalized diffuse coronary atherosclerosis, due in part to humoral and cellular rejection processes. IVUS has shown incipient or important atheroma in transplanted donor hearts immediately after transplantation, regression of atheroma after implantation in some patients, and the inexorable process of diffuse

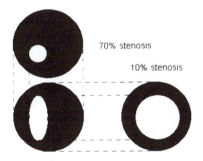

70% stenosis

10% stenosis

Figure 8. The illusion of eccentric plaque. The eccentric lesion (bottom left) appears to have a 70% stenosis when viewed from the front but only 10%, when viewed from the side.

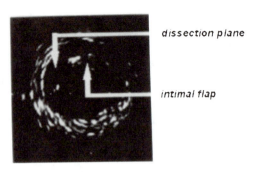

Figure 9. Coronary arterial dissection after PTCA.

atheromatous progression in others. This is often undetected by simple angiography which shows only a long thin tapering coronary artery with a sleeve of atheroma. The underlying pathology is a diffuse atheromatous process that can only be detected by a tomographic procedure which shows the true wall thickness [24, 26, 27].

INTERVENTIONAL PROCEDURES

Post PTCA Restenosis

IVUS plays an important role in identifying the severity, extent and pathological nature of the atheromatous process [28, 29]. Pathological studies have shown three mechanisms of arterial dilatation after PTCA: 1) Simple dilatation of the elastic arterial wall; 2) remodeling of the atheroma; and 3) intimal cracking and dilatation of the torn arterial wall.

The final angiogram after angioplasty, usually does not distinguish between these processes, nor does it identify fragmented intima unless there is a clear hazy outline or dissection with residual contrast medium outside the arterial lumen (Fig. 9). A dissected plaque superimposed on a luminal shadow is invisible. IVUS shows these three pathologies clearly (Fig. 10).

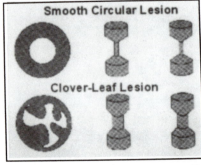

Figure 10. The illusion of the clover leaf lesion. The lumen appears to be falsely enlarged.

IVUS has been invaluable in demonstrating the true nature of restenosis [21, 22, 28–30]. In two–thirds of arteries with restenosis there is recoil of the stretched segment. This usually occurs within 2–3 weeks of the dilatation and is associated with a return of symptoms. One–third is a consequence of intimal–medial repair with migration and phenotypic modulation of adventitial myofibroblasts or medial muscle myocytes and thelaying down of new proteoglycans and collagen. There is also positive remodeling where increased blood flow in the dilated artery causes further arterial dilatation. Each of these mechanisms can be identified by IVUS which provides a clear tomographic image of the arterial wall rather than a naked lumenogram.

Complex Procedures

Patients with soft or fibrous plaques respond well to simple PTCA. Calcified lesions, particularly of the intima or with a wide angle of calcification or long lesions, do not respond well to PTCA or directional atherectomy. PTCA fractures the arterial wall between the calcified sheets and leaves multiple luminal fronds which are an excellent nidus for thrombosis, the release of platelet derived and other growth factors, and intense medial–intimal hyperplasia. In some patients, the calcified segment does not respond to dilatation and only the normal elastic wall expands. Subsequently this retracts. Calcified lesions are treated best by initial rotational atherectomy, so that the hard intimal calcified layer is removed [31]. This is followed by low pressure balloon dilatation with or without subsequent stent implantation.

Calcified lesions are unsuitable for atherectomy since the atherectomy device can not cut the calcified lesions [32, 33]. If the arterial wall recoils, or the intima fragments with sessile fronds, then stent implantation is mandatory. IVUS is also excellent for demonstrating the nature of coronary artery vein graft pathology [34, 35].

Intracoronary Stenting

The development of intracoronary stenting in the last six years has revolutionized coronary interventional procedures [15, 36]. The stent has proven invaluable in severe intimal dissection or intimal collapse after an interventional procedure: the stents compress the arterial wall and anchors the ruptured tissues. If the arterial wall recoils, this can be scaffolded by a stent and 60% of restenosis will be prevented. Unfortunately, stent implantation induces a more aggressive repair process and more intimal–medial proliferation. IVUS is particularly helpful in understanding the mechanism of stent placement and expansion since the stent is intensely ultrasound reflective. The classical seminal studies of Colombo [15] and Leon and associates [37] have shown that in many patients, the Palmaz–Schatz stent was partially deployed with incomplete expansion. This was due to the use of smaller balloons under low pressure with differential expansion in a variable compliant arterial wall [38]. IVUS has shown that if the stent is significantly smaller than the natural arterial lumen, a low–flow potential space exists between the stent and the arterial wall, particularly if expansion is asymmetrical. These factors favor stasis and turbulence with thrombosis and subsequent stent occlusion 1–2 weeks after implantation [39]. Subsequent studies have shown that high balloon pressure (18–20 atmospheres) can produce excellent stent expansion with close wall apposition, but balloons that are too large damage the adventia and the vessel responds with intense repair and restenosis. It is now clear that balloon dilatation with a perfect sized balloon matched to the arterial diameter of the normal reference segment using high pressure inflation creates good stent wall apposition [40, 41] (Fig. 11). Recurrent balloon dilatation using higher and higher iteration

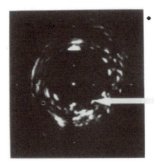

• *Concentric. circular. symmetric* expansion and *application* of stent struts

Stent struts

Figure 11. Good stent apposition. Stent struts are well applied to the arterial intima with a circular configuration.

of pressure produce good stent apposition [42, 43]. Stents are radio lucent so that only IVUS can show the true nature of stent application, expansion, eccentricity, the nature of the disease in the reference segment and the mechanisms of restenosis (Fig. 12). It has also shown that newer reticulated stents may not need high balloon pressures for inflation since they have a different design to the slotted tube Palmaz–Schatz stent.

DISCUSSION

Imaging procedures have been designed to reconstruct planar IVUS tomographic images in 3D space. The IVUS examination is performed and recorded while pulling back the probe automatically at a constant speed (usually 0.5 – 1.0 mm/sec). A computer software system reconstructs the vessel by arranging the segmental short axis images. The computer image can then be rotated or swiveled to look at the vessel from different angles, cut into new slices and provide measurements. The methods have been validated and are correlated with histological sections and manual planimetry of planar IVUS [8, 9].

The technique has several limitations. The vessels are reconstructed assuming a cylindrical shape and tortuosity is ignored. The planar image slices are assumed to be

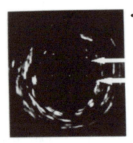

• repair with cellular proliferation

Ingrowth

Stent struts

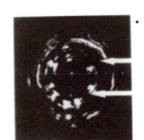

• mostly *outgrowth*

Outgrowth

Stent struts

Figure 12. Instent restenosis: **a)** In–growth inside the stent struts. **b)** Fibrocellular proliferation around the stent with stent constriction.

perpendicular to the long axis of the artery, but in tortuous vessels this is not correct. Currently, there is no way to detect the position of the probe in space in relation to the heart (myocardium and pericardium), and the operator must rely on the emergent side branches. The IVUS probe may also rotate along its long axis during pull back and this distorts the true arterial axis. Three dimensional reconstruction assumes that the imaging catheter is centered within the lumen of the artery. If this is not true, the luminal cross-sectional area and volume may be overestimated.

Atherosclerosis is heterogeneous and may have different components according to the Stary classification. Computerized algorithms cannot always recognize and distinguish the vessel layers from one another. Threshold settings, may modify tissue identification and exclude the lumen. Automatic edge detection can be unreliable and manual editing of the tissue–lumen interface may be needed.

Imaging vessels with a lumen diameter less than that of the imaging catheter will always underestimate the narrowing severity. Systolic and diastolic movements of the heart and arteries introduce circumferential and axial deformation in the 3D reconstruction. This has been overcome, partially, by cardiac "gating" to the electrocardiogram, but this requires very slow (minutes) pull–back time through the artery.

CONCLUSIONS

IVUS gives a true tomographic image of the arterial lumen and its wall. While angiography depicts the lumen, it also has several limitations, including lack of definition of the underlying pathology, inability to see the vessel wall, inability to recognize diffuse sleeves of atheroma, inaccuracy of assessing hazy wall outlines, and lack of 3D tomo-graphic imaging. Complex lesions, bifurcations and eccentric lesions are often poorly demonstrated. IVUS overcomes these limitations and has opened a new window of visual-izing the pathological anatomy, nature, extent, precise localization and quantitative measurement of coronary atherosclerosis. The technique has relatively high resolution, though invasive and expensive as each patient needs a new disposable catheter tipped transducer [44]. IVUS has a bright future in the assessment of coronary artery pathology, its progression and regression and directing and assessing the outcome of different interventional procedures.

DISCUSSION

Dr. E. Ritman: Some people are now using X-ray CT to look for coronary calcification as an early index of coronary artery disease. In your experience, have you always seen calcification with atheroma?

Dr. M.S. Gotsman: The pictures from angiography, spiral CT, and IVUS are slightly different. The spiral CT is superb in the out-patient to identify coronary artery calcification. Nonetheless, I am not sure that we know the precise correlation between the spiral CT and IVUS pictures. There is a very poor correlation with angiographic calcification and IVUS calcification. Angiographic calcification also does not tell us whether this is in the media or the adventia. Nor does it tell us the extensive distribution nor its dispersion.

Dr. G. Keren: There is no calcium in every plaque when you look with IVUS. Even in an extensive atherosclerotic vessel, you may find some calcium in 60–70% of the vessels that you look at. Calcium is quite rarely seen in vein graft.

Dr. E. Ritman: Do you ever see calcium without atheroma?

Dr. M. Gotsman: I have not seen calcium without atheroma, but this does not mean that it does not exist. We have tried to determine whether: a) the plaque is soft, fibrous or calcified; b) the extent and distribution of the calcification in the plaque. When you dilate the artery, it cracks circumferentially between the layers of calcified plaque because of the differential compliance of the artery. We have been examining balloon dilatation with a model in which we know the precise pressure and volume inside the balloon. We have compared this with IVUS and its calcification before and after balloon dilatation.

Dr. N. Westerhof: After increasing flow you see a consistent increase in diameter in some patients. Do you have any idea what the mechanism is?

Dr. M.S. Gotsman: I simply think it is the increased flow. But the biological mechanism, I do not know.

Dr. N. Westerhof: It could be that the endothelium plays a role, but is that likely in those patients?

Dr. M.S. Gotsman: Probably not. If we look at endothelial dysfunction underneath the atheromatous block, we know that production of nitric oxide is impaired.

Dr. L. Axel: The problem with Imatron–related fast CT methods is that you can have plaque without calcification and you can have calcification without hemodynamically significant plaque. Statistically, the more calcium you have, the more likely you are to have disease, but the disease does not match up one–for–one with the severe plaque. It is only a statistical correlation rather than real matching.

Dr. E. Ritman: People use CT to see if you have calcification as a marker of atheroma. Hence, if you do not have coronary calcification people tend to feel more comfortable, but it sounds like that is false comfort.

Dr. L. Axel: You can have an MI without calcification.

Dr. E. Ritman: That is another problem, though. You can have just endothelial damage without atheroma and that will clot up your artery and you will have problems.

Dr. G. Keren: When you perform IVUS, you usually do it in one vessel. When you do spiral CT you look at all the vessels. So the chances of finding some calcification is actually greater when you use the spiral CT. There is no correlation between the severity of disease and calcification. The most severe lesion would not be the calcified lesion, but rather the contrary.

Dr. U. Dinnar: You have related to severity of disease by the minimal cross section. Should there not be a number associated with the minimal cross section and the length? What about the length?

Dr. M.S. Gotsman: I am certain that we can calculate the length of the atheromatous lesion. This can be done by QCA or IVUS. The real problem is that we do not know the normal diameter of an artery and whether it is lined by a sleeve of atheroma. We should know the normal diameter and standard deviation of the artery in different populations. IVUS allows us to calculate the volume of atheromatous mass.

Dr. E. Ritman: Lance Gould [*Circ Res 43: 242–253, 1978*] has published such a formula. It has been used to compute the impact of the actual geometry (i.e., absolute lumen diameter) rather than the relative geometry (i.e., percent diameter narrowing).

Dr. S. Sideman: I would like to relate to the art of using stents. I understand there are 30 or 40 different kinds of stents and I assume that it is not very easy to determine at this stage which is better. What about stents made of polymers, which can have the advantage of providing self-effecting drug release. Is it promising enough to become a commercial product or is it just talk?

Dr. R. Beyar: There have been many attempts in the past 10 years to try and have a biodegradable stent because most people did not like the idea of leaving metal in the coronary arteries for life. However, all the studies to date with degradable stents have failed, sometimes because of mechanical properties: they would break during degradation. But the major problem has been that they provoked an intense inflammatory response which led to reocclusion of the vessel.

Another approach currently under investigation is to cover stents with biopolymer as a method of drug delivery and release, playing with controlled drug release, hoping that a combination of the right polymer and the right drug will prevent the proliferative response. However, the right materials have not been found yet. Another venue is covering stents with a drug like heparin, covalently linked to the metal. I do not know what will yield the best results.

Dr. J. Downey: How useful are animal models in developing stents?

Dr. R. Beyar: Usually you want to make sure that the device you are using is safe, before you go to patients, so the animal model is very important to test the entire process of stenting safety. Obviously the animal model will never match the clinical model; that is always problematic. The proliferative response of a normal artery, whether it is a dog or a pig, and even an atherosclerotic artery, may be different from what happens in a human patient. Obviously everybody, including the FDA, want to have the final conclusion about stents from well controlled clinical studies, after meeting the initial safety criteria in animals. I am confident that one can learn a lot from animal models in terms of the proliferative response.

Dr. J. Downey: But now we are down to much more sophisticated criteria. Can we use these second generation criteria, do we know what to look for in the animal models to direct these studies to more than just safety?

Dr. R. Beyar: People are still looking at the six month response to stenting. If you see an exaggerated response, and you have a data base of the response to previous stents. You can use that for comparison. However, one must realize that the proliferative response is also a function of the deployment process. If you overexpand the artery, you can get with the same stent a markedly larger proliferative response. So you have to do the study very carefully, compare it to previous studies, and be able to show that the proliferative response is comparable to other stents. This is what has been done.

Dr. E. Ritman: You made an interesting observation. You show that the endothelial cells do not line up with recovery. Does that happen due to just the damage of the endothelium in the first place and do we know where these cells come from? Are they local cells that just proliferate or do they come from somewhere else?

Dr. R. Beyar: I have talked with a few people who are doing endothelial work. We have seen it consistently in all our preparations. The endothelial cells suddenly become oval rather than elongated. What is the mechanism? I do not know. There have been previous studies showing how the intimal formation covers the stents. Actually, it covers the stents from the endothelial cells around it. The speed of re–endothelialization may be a parameter which affects the biological process to some extent. But whether this round shape of the endothelium is seen in atherosclerotic tissue or just because of flow disturbance, I do not know. Dr. Resnick has shown (Chapter 13) that in the region of bifurcation you get round cells, but stents are not in a flow field of a bifurcation. After 6 months you do not have this irregularity of the stent anymore. You have a smooth surface through the stent. Longitudinally, with a fully open stent, the flow field should still result in a linear arrangement of the endothelial cell. I do not think that we know how the endothelial cells arrange themselves to align with the flow. Therefore, the round cells after stenting is a puzzle.

Dr. J. Saffitz: Isner [*Human Gene Therapy 1996;7(8):989–1011*] from Boston has done research in this area. He would say, I think, that this abnormal endothelium is also functionally abnormal. It does not make nitric oxide in response to normal stimuli. He has also found that if you use a vascular endothelial growth factor, you can not only increase the speed with which the endothelium recovers the wound, as well as the speed with which it assumes normal shape and function.

You mention the issue of regression from 6–12 months in the restenosis lesions. More than three quarters of the mass of the neointima is made of matrix. One thought is that perhaps you are getting maturation of the matrix, where the collagen fibers are cross–linking and the actual volume of matrix is shrinking, much in the way that a scar that replaces a myocardial infarction will eventually shrink. I wonder what is known about this regression phenomenon and whether matrix maturation might have any role.

Dr. R. Beyar: There might be maturation of the matrix and soothing out of the inflammatory response. Many factors can play in this response. I do not think that this has been appropriately studied yet.

Dr. M. Morad: I like the coated stents. They are fascinating. It is interesting that heparin–coated stents are an improvement. One property of heparin not fully appreciated is that it is a good calcium channel blocker. I wonder if somebody has coated stents with EGTA? That may also stop proliferation. It may be worth a shot.

Dr. R. Beyar: If you could show that, it would be a major achievement.

Dr. P. Hunter: On the issue of the shape of the endothelial cells, I believe there had been studies that show that the normal elongated pattern of endothelial cells in the direction of the flow is partly related to shear but is also related to the cells aligning orthogonal to the direction of stretch under normal stretching conditions.

Dr. R. Beyar: It might be that taking off the pulsatility from the stented segment has a role, but again, this hypothesis has to be proven.

Dr. P. Hunter: There is experimental evidence that has been published [*Dartsch PC, Betz E. Response of cultured endothelial cells to mechanical stimulation. Basic Res Cardiol 1989;84:268– 281*] that addresses that very issue.

Dr. R. Beyar: That is interesting. Thank you.

REFERENCES

1. Rouleau JL, Talajic M, Sussex B, Potvin L, Warnica With, Davies RF, Gardner M, Stewart D, Plante S, Dupuis R, Lauzon C, Ferguson J, Mikes E, Balnozan Very, Savard P. Myocardial infarction patients in the 1990s – Their risk factors, stratification and survival in Canada: The Canadian assessment of myocardial infarction (CAMI) Study. *J Am Coll Cardiol* 1996;27:1119–1127.

2. Rensing BJ, Hermans WRM, Deckers JW, de Feyter PJ, Tijssen JGP, Serruys PW. Lumen narrowing after percutaneous transluminal coronary balloon angioplasty follows a near gaussian distribution: a quantitative angiographic study in 1, 445 successfully dilated lesions. *J Am Coll Cardiol* 1992;19:939–945.

3. Topol EJ, Nissen SE. Our preoccupation with coronary luminology: The dissociation between clinical and angiographic findings in ischemic heart disease. *Circulation* 1995;92:2333–2342.

4. Hodgson John McB, Sheehan Helen M. *Atlas of Intravascular Ultrasound,* Raven Press, New York, 1994.

5. Stary HC:Evolution of atherosclerotic plaques in the coronary arteries of young adults. *Arteriosclerosis* 1983;3:471a.

6. A report from the Committee on Vascular Lesions of the Council on Arteriosclerosis, American Heart Association. A Definition of advanced types of atherosclerotic lesions and a histological classification of atherosclerosis. *Circulation* 1995;92:1355–1374.

7. Fuster V, Stein B, Ambrose JA, Badimon L, Badimon JJ, Chesebro JH. Atherosclerotic plaque rupture and thrombosis: Evolving concepts. *Circulation* 1990;82:II47–II59.

8. Roelandt J, di Mario C, Pandian N, Wehguang L, Keane D, Slager CJ. Three–dimensional reconstruction of intracoronary ultrasound images. Rationale, approaches, problems and directions. *Circulation* 1994;90:1044–1055.

9. Rosenfield K, Losordo DW, Ramaswamy K, Pastore JO, Langeuin RE, Razui S, Kobowsky BD, Isner JM. Three–dimensional reconstruction of human coronary and peripheral arteries from images recorded during two–dimensional intravascular ultrasound examination. *Circulation* 1991;84:1938–56.

10. Nissen SE, De Franco AC, Tuzcu EM, Moliterno DJ. Coronary intravascular ultrasound diagnostic and interventional applications. *Coron Artery Dis* 1995;6:355–67.

11. Nissen S, Gurley J, Grines C, Booth DC, McClure R, Berk M, Fischer C, DeMaria AN. Intravascular ultrasound assessment of lumen size and wall morphology in normal subjects and patients with coronary artery disease. *Circulation* 1991;84:1087–1099.

12. Mintz GS, Popma JJ, Pichard AD, Kent KM, Satler LF, Chuang YC, Ditrano CJ, Leon MB. Patterns of calcification in coronary artery disease. A statistical analysis of intravascular ultrasound and coronary angiography in 1155 lesions. *Circulation* 1995;91:1959–65.

13. Mintz GS, Douek P, Pichard A, Kent KM, Satler LF, Popma JJ, Leon MB. Target lesion calcification in coronary artery disease: An intravascular ultrasound study. *J Am Coll Cardiol* 1992;20:1149–1155.

14. Frimerman A, Miller H, Hallman M, Laniado S, Keren G. Intravascular ultrasound characterization of thrombi of different composition. *Am J Cardiol* 1994;73:1053–1057.

15. Colombo A, Hall P, Nakamura S, Almagor Y, Maiello L, Martini G, Gaglione A, Goldberg SL, Tobis JM. Intracoronary stenting without anticoagulation accomplished with intravascular ultrasound guidance. *Circulation* 1995;91:1676–88.

16. Nissen SE, Gurley JC. Application of intravascular ultrasound for detection and quantitation of coronary atherosclerosis. *Intracoronary J Card Imaging* 1991;6:165–77.

17. Glagov S, Weisenberg E, Zarins CK, Stankunavicius K, Kolettis GJ. Compensatory enlargement of human atherosclerotic coronary arteries. *N Engl J Med* 1987;316:1371–1375.

18. Hermiller J, Tenaglia A, Kisslo K, Phillips HR, Bashore TM, Stack RS, Davidson CJ. *In vivo* validation of compensatory enlargement of atherosclerotic coronary arteries. *Am J Cardiol* 1993;71:665–668.

19. McPherson D, Sirna S, Hiratzka L, Thorpe L, Armstrong ML, Marcus ML, Kember RE. Coronary arterial remodeling studied by high–frequency epicardial echocardiography: An early compensatory mechanism in patients with obstructive coronary atherosclerosis. *J Am Coll Cardiol* 1991;17:79–86.

20. Potkin BN, Keren G, Mintz GS, Douek PC, Richard AD, Salter LF, Kent KM, Leon MB. Arterial responses to balloon coronary angioplasty: An intravascular ultrasound study. *J Am Coll Cardiol* 1992;20:942–951.

21. Mintz G, Pichard A, Kent K, Satler L, Popma J, Leon M. Intravascular ultrasound comparison of restenotic and de novo coronary artery narrowings. *Am J Cardiol* 1994;74:1278–1280.

22. Mintz GS, Painter JA, Pichard AD, Kent KM, Satler LF, Popma JJ, Chuang YC, Bucher TA, Sokolowicz LE, Leon MB. Atherosclerosis in angiographically "normal" coronary artery reference segments: An intravascular ultrasound study with clinical correlations. *J Am Coll Cardiol* 1995;25:1479–1485.

23. Gould KL. Identifying and measuring severity of coronary artery stenosis: Quantitative coronary arteriography and positron emission tomography. *Circulation* 1989;78:237–245.

24. Cohn JM, Wilensky RL, O'Donnell JA, Bourdillon PDV, Dillon JC, Feigenbaum H. Exercise echocardiography, angiography, and intracoronary ultrasound after cardiac transplantation. *Am J Cardiol* 1996;77:1216–1219.

25. Brown BG. Workshop VI – Regression of atherosclerosis: What does it mean? *Am J Med 90* 1991;(Suppl 2A):53S–55S.

26. Rickenbacher PR, Pinto FJ, Chenzbraun A, Botas J, Lewis NP, Alderman EL, Valantine HA, Hunt SA, Schroeder JS, Popp RL, Yeung AC. Incidence and severity of transplant coronary artery disease

early and up to 15 years after transplantation as detected by intravascular ultrasound. *J Am Coll Cardiol* 1995;25:171–7.

27. Ventura HO, Ramee SR, Jain A, White CJ, Collins TJ, Mesa JE, Murgo JP. Coronary artery imaging with intravascular ultrasound in patients following cardiac transplantations. *Transplantation* 1992;53:216–9.

28. DiMario C, Gil R, Camenzind E, Ozaki Y, von Birgelen C, Umans Very, de Jaegere P, de Feyter PJ, Roelandt JR, Seruys PW. Quantitative assessment with intracoronary ultrasound of the mechanisms of restenosis after percutaneous transluminal coronary angioplasty and directional coronary atherectomy. *Am J Cardiol* 1995;75:772–7.

29. Jain SP, Jain A, Collins TJ, Ramee SR, White CJ. Predictors of restenosis: a morphometric and quantitative evaluation by intravascular ultrasound. *Am Heart J* 1994;128:664–673.

30. Mintz G, Pichard A, Kovach J, Kent KM, Satler LF, Javier SP, Popma JJ, Leon MB. Impact of preintervention intravascular ultrasound imaging on transcatheter treatment strategies in coronary artery disease. *Am J Cardiol* 1994;73:423–430.

31. MacIsaac AI, Bass TA, Buchbinder M, Cowley MJ, Leon MB, Warth DC, Whitlow Pl. High speed rotational atherectomy: outcome in calcified and noncalcified coronary artery lesions. *J Am Coll Cardiol* 1995;26:731–736.

32. Umans VA, Baptista J, di Mario C, von Birgelen C, Quaedvlieg P, de Feyter PJ, Serruys PW. Angiographic, ultrasonic, and angioscopic assessment of the coronary artery wall and lumen area configuration after directional atherectomy: the mechanism revisited. *Am Heart J* 1995;130:217–227.

33. Matar FA, Mintz GS, Pinnow E, Javier SP, Popma JJ, Kent KM, Satler LF, Pichard AD, Leon MB. Multivariate predictors of intravascular ultrasound end points after directional coronary atherectomy. *J Am Coll Cardiol* 1995;25:318–24.

34. Jain S, Roubin G, Nanda N, Dean L, Agrawal S, Pinheiro L. Intravascular ultrasound imaging of saphenous vein graft stenosis. *Am J Cardiol* 1992;69:133–136.

35. Painter JA, Mintz GS, Wong SC, Popma JJ, Pichard AD, Kent KM, Satler LF, Hong MK, Leon MG. Intravascular ultrasound assessment of biliary stent implantation in saphenous vein grafts. *Am J Cardiol* 1995;75:731–734.

36. Serruys PW, Strauss BH, van Beusekom HM, van der Giessen WJ. Stenting of coronary arteries: Has a modern Pandora's box been opened? *J Am Coll Cardiol* 1991;17:143B–154B.

37. Dussaillant Great, Mintz GS, Pichard AD, Kent KM, Satler LF, Popma JJ, Wong SC, Leon MB. Small stent size and intimal hyperplasia contribute to restenosis: A volumetric intravascular ultrasound analysis. *J Am Coll Cardiol* 1995;26:720–724.

38. Mudra H, Klauss V, Blasini R, Kroetz M, Rieber J, Regar E, Theisen K. Ultrasound guidance of Palmaz–Schatz intracoronary stenting with a combined intravascular ultrasound balloon catheter. *Circulation* 1994;90:1252–1261.

39. Gershlick AH, Aggarwal RK. Stent thrombosis revisited. *Euro Heart J* 1996;17:1623–1628.

40. Kiemeneij F, Laarman GJ, Slagboom T. Percutaneous transradial coronary Palmaz–Schatz stent implantation, guided by intravascular ultrasound. *Cathet Cardiovasc Diagn* 1995;34:133–136.

41. Gorge G, Haude M, Ge J, Voegele E, Gerber T, Rupprecht HJ, Meyer J, Erbel R. Intravascular ultrasound after low and high inflation pressure coronary artery stent implantation. *J Am Coll Cardiol* 1995;26:725–730.

42. Macaya C, Serruys PW, Ruygrok P, Suryapranata H, Mast G, Klugmann S, Urban P, den Heijer P, Koch K, Simon R, Morice MC, Crean P, Bonnier H, Wijns With, Danchin N, Bourdonnec C, Morel MA, for the Benestent Study Group: Continued benefit of coronary stenting versus balloon angioplasty: one–year clinical follow–up of Benestent Trial. *J Am Coll Cardiol* 1996;27:255–261.

43. Di Mario C, Keane D, Serruys PW. Sizing of stents: Quantitative coronary angiography or intravascular ultrasound? In: *Endoluminal Stenting*, Editor: Sigwart U, With.B. Saunders Company Ltd, London, 1996:272–279.

44. Talley JD, Mauldin PD, Becker ER, Stikovac M, Leesar MA. Cost and therapeutic modification of intracoronary ultrasound–assisted coronary angioplasty. *Am J Cardiol* 1996;77:1278–1282.

V. Myocardial Structure and Function

CHAPTER 18

TISSUE REMODELING WITH MICRO–STRUCTURALLY BASED MATERIAL LAWS

Peter Hunter[1] and Theo Arts[2]

ABSTRACT

Cardiomyocytes and the extracellular collagen matrix which holds them together respond to changes in their mechanical environment by adapting their orientation, size and composition. We examine local mechanical feedback mechanisms affecting the fiber orientation, sheet orientation and passive fiber direction stiffness, using an axisymmetric finite element model of the left ventricle (LV), with material constitutive laws based on the fibrous–sheet microstructure of myocardium.

INTRODUCTION

Anatomically accurate models of the normally functioning dog heart have been developed to analyze the large deformation mechanics of ventricular diastole and systole [1, 2], the sequence of myocardial activation [3], the coupling between these two processes [4, 5] and, to a lesser extent, coronary blood flow and oxygen transport [6]. These models incorporate accurate descriptions of ventricular geometry and the fibrous–sheet structure of myocardial tissue, based on detailed measurements of geometry and fiber directions [7] and the organization and material properties of the extracellular collagen matrix [8–10]. One application of these models is in the improved diagnosis of diseased hearts and the more rational design of therapeutic methods.

Most current continuum models assume the material properties of the tissue are static. In reality, however, there is an astonishing level of continuous material adaptation

---

[1]Department of Engineering Science, University of Auckland, New Zealand; and [2]Department of Biophysics, University of Maastricht, The Netherlands

by the cells to their mechanical and biochemical environment, even for healthy tissue operating under normal physiological conditions [11, 12]. There is loss of contractile filaments and an increase in connective tissue within hours of reducing the load of the myocytes [13]. With increased load the myocytes thicken by laying down more filaments (predominantly in parallel during pressure overload hypertrophy and in series and parallel during volume overload hypertrophy [14]), and there is a corresponding adaptation of the extracellular collagen matrix [15, 16]. A clear example of the role of stretch and/or tension in maintaining the structural integrity of the myocardial cell is the observation that unloaded papillary muscles (with their chordae tendineae cut) show rapid and profound cellular degeneration [17]. Even the orientation of the myocytes continuously adapts to the current distributions of stress and/or strain [18].

Cardiac structure, composition and function are thus regulated dynamically by the myocyte loading environment. However, the mechanisms by which a mechanical stimulus initiates a growth response are unclear. Some possibilities are: stretch (or stress) induced secretion of myocyte–derived autocrine growth factors (e.g. angiotensin II) [19, 20] or endothelial cell–derived paracrine growth factors (e.g. endothelin–1) [21]; stretch sensitive myocyte membrane channels [22]; stretch sensitive fibroblasts (which, as well as respond–ing to growth stimuli by producing more collagen, communicate with the myocytes both structurally, via adhesion proteins and the transmembrane integrins, and electrotonically) [23, 24]; and mechanically induced cell wounding [12]. Some of these pathways result in changes in the expression of genes coding for contractile proteins (and many other cell components) within hours of the mechanical load changes [25–28].

In this chapter we extend an earlier analysis of fiber angle adaptation with a cylindrical model [29, 30] by performing a large deformation analysis with a 3D prolate spheroidal finite element model in which the fibrous/sheet structure of myocardium and its material properties based on this structure are both spatially varying. In particular, we examine local mechanical feedback mechanisms affecting the orientation of fibers and sheets and the passive fiber direction stiffness. The cell metabolic activity is assumed to be at normal levels so as to avoid, at this stage, the considerable additional complexity of the changing metabolic environment that occurs in anoxia and ischaemia.

MICRO–STRUCTURALLY BASED CONSTITUTIVE LAWS

Studies of the microstructure of myocardial tissue [8] have shown that the myocardium consists of layers of interconnected sheets of tissue separated by "cleavage planes". Each sheet is 3 to 4 cells thick (about 100 μm) and loosely coupled together by the perimysial collagen network – predominantly types I and III collagen. The muscle fibers, which lie in the plane of a sheet, are bound together by the endomysial collagen network more strongly in the plane of the sheet than transverse to it. Three microstructural axes are evident: one along the fiber direction, the *fiber axis*; one orthogonal to the fiber axis but also in the plane of the sheet, the *sheet axis*; and a third, orthogonal to these two, directed across the cleavage planes, the *sheet normal*.

The passive elastic properties of cardiac muscle are determined largely by the extracellular matrix. In particular, the uniaxial mechanical properties of cardiac muscle in the fiber direction are dominated by large coiled perimysial fibers [31, 32], but with some contribution from the intracellular structural proteins titin [33, 34]. The uniaxial stress–strain properties are quite different in the three orthogonal directions, reflecting in part the organization of collagen relative to these three axes (Fig. 1). The most striking difference in material behavior along the three axes is the limiting strain for an elastic response. If the

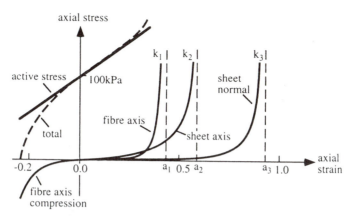

Figure 1. The uniaxial stress–strain relations along the fiber axis, sheet axis and sheet normal directions. The J-shaped curves for the passive material properties are defined by three parameters, one giving the elastic strain limit (a_j), one the curvature (not labelled) and one the scaling coefficient (k_j) which determines the contribution that each strain energy component makes to the total strain energy of the tissue. There are three similar relations for the behavior in shear (see Eq. (1)). The curve on the lower left is the passive compressive stress in the fiber direction at negative fiber strain and arises, via tissue incompressibility, from stretching of collagen fibers in the plane lateral to the muscle fiber axis. The active fiber tension and the total tension in the fiber direction (active + passive) are also shown.

tissue is stretched along the fiber direction the limiting axial·strain is typically about 0.34 (although this figure varies with position in the myocardium) and along the sheet axis the limiting strain is typically 0.68 [10]. In the direction of the sheet normal very little tension is developed below a strain of 0.5 but tension increases rapidly above this and cannot be stretched beyond about 1.0 without irreversible damage.

The passive stress–strain behavior of myocardium may be defined mathematically using the microstructurally based strain "pole–zero" energy function given in Eq. (1) [35]. Each term in this constitutive equation is of the form $W = kE^2(a-E)^{-\beta}$, where E is a component of the Green strain tensor (referenced to the fiber material coordinates), a is the elastic limit for that component (the "pole"), β controls the sharp rise in strain energy as a strain component reaches its elastic limit, and k is a coefficient weighing the contribution of the strain energy for that particular strain component to the total strain energy for the material. The empirically determined form of this expression, derived from biaxial tests on thin myocardial sheets [10, 36], captures the essential features described above: the behavior along one particular axis is almost independent of the degree of stretch along the other two axes and the axial stress is very low at low axial strain but rises rapidly as the strain reaches a well defined limiting value for that axis.

$$W = k_1 \frac{e_{11}^2}{(a_1 - e_{11})^{\beta_1}} + k_2 \frac{e_{22}^2}{(a_2 - e_{22})^{\beta_2}} + k_3 \frac{e_{33}^2}{(a_3 - e_{33})^{\beta_3}}$$
$$+ k_{12} \frac{e_{12}^2}{(a_{12} - e_{12})^{\beta_{12}}} + k_{23} \frac{e_{23}^2}{(a_{23} - e_{23})^{\beta_{23}}} + k_{31} \frac{e_{31}^2}{(a_{31} - e_{31})^{\beta_{31}}}$$

(1)

The six terms in the pole–zero law correspond to the six independent components of the Green strain tensor e_{ij}. Each component independently contributes to the total strain energy of the tissue. The behavior in compression along a material axis is largely dictated by lateral stretching arising from the constant volume (incompressibility) properties of the tissue. A biophysical model of the tissue microstructure can be used to determine dependencies among the material parameters [5].

REMODELING WITH AN AXISYMMETRIC MODEL OF THE HEART WALL

Our aim is to understand how the structure of the physiologically normal heart develops and how that structure changes in response to abnormal hemodynamic loading conditions. As a first step towards this goal we examine the mechanics of an axisymmetric finite element model which, although geometrically simple, nonetheless has many of the pertinent structural features of a real LV, such as the approximately prolate spheroidal shape, a spatially varying fibrous/sheet structure, large deformation, and nonlinear spatially varying material properties. Because of its relative simplicity the stress and strain distributions in the model can be computed rapidly and the understanding gained on this model will later be applied to the more anatomically accurate model of both left and right ventricles [7, 9].

The axisymmetric prolate spheroidal model is shown in Fig. 2. Parameters defining the geometry and fiber and sheet orientations are defined at four nodes. A description of the basis functions and finite deformation elasticity equations governing the mechanics are given in [37, 38]. The passive and active constitutive laws are described in [35]. The initial (undeformed) LV volume is 40 mm^3 and the wall volume is 100 mm^3. The stress and strain components in this single element model are converged only to within 20% but this was deemed acceptable for this initial study in which we are interested in gross trends only.

We choose here to investigate three aspects of myocardial structure: (i) the orientation of the muscle fibers, (ii) the orientation of the sheets, and (iii) the passive stiffness of the tissue in the fiber direction. We propose that these three components of the structure and composition of myocardium are determined by particular loading conditions associated with different phases of the cardiac cycle: pre–ejection systole, end–systole and end–diastole, respectively.

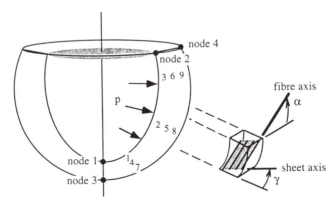

Figure 2. An axisymmetric prolate spheroidal model of the LV. One element is used with four nodes as shown. The fibrous–sheet structure of the myocardium is defined by the fiber angle α (the angle between the fiber axis and the circumferential direction) and the sheet angle γ (the angle between the sheet axis and the transmural direction). The points within the wall labelled 1..9 identify material points at which the stress and strain tensors are calculated from the large deformation finite element solution. p is the LV pressure.

Muscle Fiber Orientation

Loading conditions at the pre–ejection systolic phase of the cardiac cycle are chosen to examine fiber orientation because the forces acting on the fibers are much greater during systole than diastole and the stress fields at pre–ejection are not complicated by the large lateral forces associated with end–systole. Support for a stress feedback mechanism for fiber orientation comes from studies which show that pressure overload hypertrophy changes fiber orientation but volume overload hypertrophy does not [18, 39].

The model with homogenous material properties (see legend to Fig. 1) is inflated passively to an end–diastolic volume of 60 mm^3. The volume is then held constant during active contraction which raises ventricular pressure to about 15 kPa. All four nodal sheet angles are set to zero. The fiber angle at each of the two apex nodes (1 and 3) is zero, at the endocardial base node 2 the angle is –90° and at epicardial base node 4 it varies from 20° to 90°. For the purposes of this study we assume zero imbrication angle (i.e., the fibers lie in planes tangent to the wall). The stress and strain distributions are computed at each choice of node 4 fiber angle. The fiber stresses t_{11} in the basal subepicardium and two adjacent points (to illustrate the transmural and base–to–apex gradients) are shown in Fig. 3 as a function of the node 4 fiber angle. At low values of fiber angle the fiber stress t_{11} is high and there is a large transmural gradient of fiber stress. As the fiber angle increases both the fiber stress and the transmural gradient diminish until at about 70° the local fiber stress is minimum and at about 80° the gradients disappear. This agrees well with measured epicardial fiber angles in the free wall of the dog heart [7].

A possible feedback signal for controlling fiber angle on the epicardium would therefore seem to be the fiber axis stress (or spatial gradients of this stress). By finding an orientation which minimizes the local fiber stress the transmural and longitudinal gradients are also minimized. It is not yet clear, however, whether this feedback signal is sufficient to correctly determine endocardial fiber angles and further study is required to confirm the

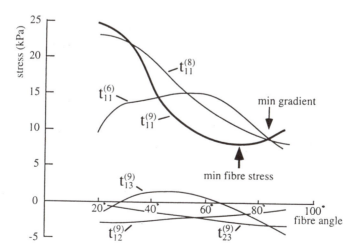

Figure 3. Pre–ejection systolic fiber stress (t_{11}) at material points 6, 8 and 9 labelled in Fig. 2, and shear stress (t_{12}, t_{13}, t_{23}) at point 9, plotted as a function of node 4 fiber angle. Note that point 9, from the basal subepicardium, is adjacent to node 4, while points 6 and 8 are further into and down the wall, respectively. The fiber angle at which fiber stress $t_{11}^{(9)}$ minimized (dark arrow) is close to the angle at which transmural and longitudinal fiber stress gradients are at a minimum (light arrow).

importance of fiber stress *per se* rather than, for example, the fiber shortening that results from this stress.

Sheet Angle

The study by LeGrice *et al.* [40] has shown that the direction of maximum shear at two subendocardial sites in the dog heart (one free wall and one in the septal wall) correlates well with the measured sheet orientation at those sites (44° and −67°, respectively) and that, because the cleavage planes between the sheets correspond to slippage planes, the high shear strain along these planes helps to maximize wall thickening at end–systole. In seeking a feedback mechanism for control of sheet angle it is logical to examine the dependence of shear and wall thickening on sheet angle.

The model (with zero epicardial sheet angles) was made to contract against a low ventricular pressure (4 kPa) to ensure a large ejection fraction. Figure 4 shows various components of subendocardial strain plotted against the endocardial sheet angle. The inter-sheet shear strain $\overset{v}{e}_{23}$ rises sharply in magnitude to a peak at a sheet angle of 55°. A similar behavior is seen for negative sheet angles. This agrees (fortuitously well, given the geometric simplicity of our axisymmetric model) with the mean absolute value (½(44°+67°)= 55.5°) found by LeGrice *et al.* [40] at subendocardial sites in the dog heart. The most significant finding is the sharpness of the shear strain peak. The other fiber coordinate shears $\overset{v}{e}_{12}$ and $\overset{v}{e}_{13}$ are an order of magnitude smaller and show no significant peaks. When the fiber coordinate strains are transformed to wall coordinates (ξ) the wall thickening strain e^{ξ}_{33} is maximum at 65°, only slightly above the optimal value of 55°, and the principal shear direction therefore coincides with the sheet orientation, as observed experimentally [40].

The large shear strain occurring in the subendocardium at end–systole would therefore appear to promote the development of layers or sheets of strongly bound myocytes which can readily slide over one another and contribute to the substantial wall thickening required to achieve a high ejection fraction.

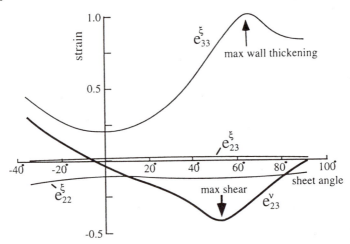

Figure 4. End–systolic shear strain with respect to fiber–sheet axes ($\overset{v}{e}_{23}$) and three components of the strain tensor expressed in wall coordinates (e^{ξ}_{ij}) plotted as a function of endocardial sheet angle. All strains are from a point in the subendocardium midway between apex and base (point 2 in Fig. 2). The wall thickening strain (e^{ξ}_{33}) is maximized at a sheet angle (upper arrow) slightly greater than the sheet angle which maximizes inter–sheet shear (lower arrow).

Passive Muscle Fiber Stiffness

A similar adaptation of the extracellular collagen matrix may be responsible for ensuring a uniform distribution of sarcomere length at end–diastole. Large coiled perimysial collagen fibers appear to be responsible for setting the limits of fiber extension. The parallel changes in sarcomere length and collagen fiber tortuosity have been quantified by Mackenna *et al.* [32] who show how the J–shape of the stress–strain curve arises from the bending stiffness of these "twisted ribbons". The pole position (a_1) of the fiber axis stress–strain curve shown in Fig. 1 is evidently set by the uncoiled length of these fibers, and the magnitude (k_1) and curvature (β_1) parameters are determined by the degree of fiber crosslinking (together with a small contribution from the intracellular structural proteins). In this final example we examine the effect of a feedback signal from fiber stretch on the axial stiffness parameter k_1.

The model is inflated to an end–diastolic pressure of 2 kPa and the distribution of fiber strain is calculated for various nodal values of k_1 (see Eq. (1)) and residual strain. The nodal fiber angles are 0°, −90°, 70°, 70° and sheet angles are 55°, 55°, 0°, 0° as determined from the previous two studies. The value of k_1 at node 1 is initially set to 10 to avoid an overly compliant apex in this geometrically simplified model. Transmural plots of fiber axis strain (which determines sarcomere length) are shown in Fig. 5 at the three locations indicated by the numbers 147, 258 and 369 (apical, midwall and basal, respectively) in Fig. 2. Figure 5a shows the fiber strains for material parameters k_1=10, 1, 1, 1 (kPa) at nodes 1, 2, 3, 4, respectively, with no residual strain included. The large basal subendo–cardial strain in Fig. 5a is substantially reduced by increasing endocardial stiffness (k_1=20, 10, 1, 1), as shown in Fig. 5b. Further reduction of the longitudinal gradients in fiber strain are achieved by further stiffening but no changes in nodal values of k_1 could remove the transmural gradients of fiber strain. However, applying a 10% gradient in residual strain, as suggested by residual strain measurements [41] (i.e., 10% longer sarcomeres at the epicardium than endocardium) does indeed substantially reduce the fiber strain gradient, as shown in Fig. 5c.

These results indicate that: (a) spatial variation in passive fiber axis stiffness (k_1 parameter), using a local feedback signal from fiber axis strain, can remove the longitudinal gradients in strain which would otherwise exist; (b) transmural gradients cannot be completely removed by stiffness changes (i.e., gradients in collagen density); but (c) transmural gradients can be removed by a 10% gradient in residual strain (as observed experimentally [41]).

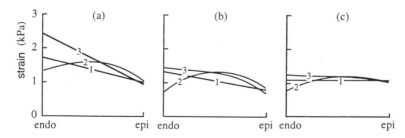

Figure 5. End–diastolic fiber strains shown as transmural plots near apex (1), midventricle (2) and base (3). **a)** Uniform fiber stiffness except at endocardial apex. **b)** Effect of stiffening up endocardial base is to reduce longitudinal fiber strain gradients in subendocardium. **c)** Effect of adding a 10% residual strain gradient is to reduce transmural fiber strain gradients.

CONCLUSION

Myocardial structure and composition are continuously regulated by the mechanical loading environment of the cells. An understanding of the mechanical factors determining the structure of the normal adult heart should help elucidate the various hypertrophic responses to abnormal hemodynamic loads. Using a prolate spheroidal finite element model of the LV we have examined the development of (a) fiber orientation by pre–ejection systolic fiber stress, (b) sheet orientation by end–systolic shear strain, and (c) passive fiber axis stiffness by fiber strain. In all three cases a local mechanical response was found to give an adequate feedback signal to control remodeling without the need for any control "reference points".

The geometrically simple model used in this study needs to be extended to the full anatomically accurate model of both left and right ventricles [7, 9] to test whether these feedback signals are sufficient to explain the known regional variations of fibrous/sheet structure [40] and extracellular collagen matrix density [42]. Other issues awaiting investigation are: the development of fiber imbrication angle [43], particularly near the LV apex; the factors affecting myocyte growth and resorption in the development of normal ventricular geometry; and the regional variation of ion channel densities, as highlighted by the recent discovery of M–cells in the mid–myocardium [44].

Acknowledgements

We are very grateful to the Netherlands Organization for Scientific Research (NWO) for supporting PJH during the three month period in Maastricht when this work was carried out.

DISCUSSION

Dr. R. Beyar: Is the sheet orientation in the model completely independent of the fiber orientation or are they linked together somehow?

Dr. P.J. Hunter: They are independent.

Dr. R. Beyar: I understand that the sheet is a plane of maximum shear?

Dr. P.J. Hunter: It turns out to be a plane of maximum shear, at least on the subendocardium. The same argument can not be used so strongly in the epicardium because the role of shear is much reduced in the epicardium. But in the endocardium it is.

Dr. R. Beyar: So it is indeed a plane of maximum shear. We have also seen that the sheet is also a plane which is the weakest in terms of stress–strain relationship. Is there any data on whether the sheet contains the penetrating blood vessel, or is its only role in enhancing thickening by participating in the shear process?

Dr. P.J. Hunter: What we know is that the capillaries lie within the sheets. We have studied the sheets using scanning e.m. (this is the work of Ian LeGrice and Bruce Smaill in the Physiology Department in Auckland), and under confocal microscopy. It is certain that the capillaries lay firmly embedded within the sheets along the direction of the myocytes on pretty much a one–to–one basis.

What happens with the larger vessels we do not know, but a student, Nic Smith, is working with Ian LeGrice in Auckland, to study the way the vessels develop in relation to the sheet architecture. We grow the coronary structure into the wall in a way that is consistent with the larger blood vessels lying in the cleavage planes between the sheets. We are making the assumption here, which is yet to be fully verified experimentally, that the blood vessels lie in the cleavage planes and end up as capillaries within the sheets, aligned with the myocytes. There are some very interesting issues between the mechanics and the blood vessels in relation to the sheet architecture.

Dr. D. Noble: I was intrigued by what you had to say earlier on in the discussion (Chapter 18) on M cells. Part of your comment was that there is more space between the sheets in the middle so there are more cleavages there.

Dr. P. Hunter: Longer gaps before the sheets branch and interconnect again.

Dr. D. Noble: You have already given one possible use of those, which is to fit in the circulation. That is nice. But do you have anything specific in mind in relation to the M cells and why there would be any function in having a different electrophysiology corresponding to that different structure?

Dr. P. Hunter: I am only speculating because we have not done the modeling studies to justify it, but I will go ahead anyway. I was once talking to Art Winfrey about the sheet structure and he pointed out to me that he had written a paper in the late 80s when he was looking at reentrant arrhythmias and vortices, showing that you needed some sort of insulating layers in the base apex direction in order to stabilize the heart. He proposed, long before we knew about the sheet structure of the heart, that there would need to be some series of insulating layers in exactly that orientation in the mid–myocardium to stabilize the normal rhythm of the heart. Basically, he said in that paper, "why doesn't the heart fibrillate far more often than it does?" He was very interested in finding that there was evidence of an insulating layer that could help provide that stabilizing effect. The M cell story from Antzelevitch [*Antzelevitch C, Sicouri S, Litovsky SH, Lukas A, Krishnan SC, Di Diego JM, Gintant GA, Liu DW. Heterogeneity within the ventricular wall. Electrophysiology and pharmacology of epicardial, endocardial and M cells. Circ Res 1991;69:1427–1449*] is also interesting. One of the properties of the M cells is that they are almost like Purkinje fibers in terms of the higher sodium channel densities and the higher upstroke speed. A simple speculation is that if you rapidly activate the subendocardium, you then want to have a mechanism for quickly conducting that activation to the epicardium and the way to do it, given that you have got these sheet structures, would be to have a faster conducting system in the mid–myocardial sheets.

Dr. D. Noble: I certainly think that we need something like this because one of the messages that is coming out of the simulations in which we and other groups around the world are incorporating the detailed cell models into big networks and into whole heart simulation using your anatomy modeling is that fibrillation is, if anything, too easy to induce. It seems to me that if that were all there were to it, we would not be around this table discussing it!

Dr. S. Sideman: Sometime ago we tried to identify arrhythmia and fibrillation by simulating the propagation of the electrical activation front. Mike Rosen of Columbia Universiy suggested that we can identify fibrillation in our analytical study by the simultaneous appearance of a number of local reentries and arrhythmias. Do you have any comment on that, from your model?

Dr. P. Hunter: Sasha Panfilov [*Panfilov AV, Keener JP. Reentry in an anatomical model of the heart. Chaos, Sol, Fract 1995;5:681–689*] is the one who has done the most on this question, still using modified FitzHugh–Nagumo models. He has looked at reentry and the breakdown of arrhythmias to fibrillation based on our geometry.

Dr. D. Noble: Once you incorporate biophysically detailed models into whole heart anatomy and you create a rapid tachycardia, it seems to break down with the greatest of ease into rotors that just wander around, and on the ECG at least that would produce something that looks like fibrillation.

REFERENCES

1. Hunter PJ, McCulloch AD, Nielsen PMF, Smaill BH. A finite element model of passive ventricular mechanics. In: Spilker RL and Simon BR, eds. *Computational Methods in Bioengineering*, ASME, BED, 1988;9:387–397.
2. Guccione JM, Costa KD, McCulloch AD. Finite element stress analysis of left ventricular mechanics in the beating dog heart. *J Biomech* 1995;28:1167–1177.
3. Panfilov A, Keener JP. Re–entry in an anatomical model of the heart. *Chaos, Solitons & Fractals* 1995;5:681–689.
4. Hunter PJ, Smaill BH, Nielsen PMF, LeGrice IJ. A mathematical model of cardiac anatomy. In: Panfilov S, Holden A, eds. *Computational Biology of the Heart*, John Wiley 1996;Chapt. 6 (In press).
5. Hunter PJ, Nash MP, Sands GB. Computational electro–mechanics of the heart. In Panfilov S, Holden A, eds. *Computational Biology of the Heart*, John Wiley 1996;Chapt. 12 (In press).
6. Mawson DA, Hunter PJ, Kenwright DN, Loiselle DS. Oxygen exchange in the isolated, arrested guinea–pig heart: theoretical and experimental observations. *Biophys J* 1994;66:789–800.
7. Nielsen PMF, LeGrice IJ, Smaill BH, Hunter PJ. A mathematical model of the geometry and fibrous structure of the heart. *Am J Physiol* 1991;29:H1365–H1378.
8. LeGrice IJ, Smaill BH, Chai LZ, Edgar SG, Gavin JB, Hunter PJ. Laminar structure of the heart: ventricular myocyte arrangement and connective tissue architecture in the dog. *Am J Physiol* 1995;269:H571–H582.
9. LeGrice IJ, Hunter PJ, Smaill BH. Laminar structure of the heart: Mathematical model. *Am J Physiol* 1997; (in Press).
10. Smaill BH, Hunter PJ. Structure and function of the diastolic heart: Material properties of passive myocardium. In: Glass L, Hunter PJ, McCulloch AD, eds. *Theory of Heart: Biomechanics, Biophysics and Nonlinear Dynamics of Cardiac Function*, Springer–Verlag 1991;Chapt. 1.
11. Terracio L, Tingstorm A, Peters WH, Borg TK. A potential role for mechanical stimulation in cardiac development. *Ann NY Acad Sci* 1990;588:48–60.
12. Clarke MSF, Caldwell RW, Chiao H, Miyake K, McNeil PL. Contraction–induced cell wounding and release of fibroblast growth factor in heart. *Circ Res* 1995;76:927–934.
13. Cooper G, Tomanek RJ. Load regulation of the structure, composition and function of mammalian myocardium. *Circ Res* 1982;50:788–798.
14. Campbell SE, Korecky B, Rakusan K. Remodelling of myocyte dimensions in hypertrophic and atrophic rat hearts. *Circ Res* 1991;68:984–996.
15. Doering CW, Jalil JE, Janicki JS, Pick R, Aghili S, Abrahams C, Weber KT. Collagen network remodelling and diastolic stiffness of the rat left ventricle with pressure overload hypertrophy. *Cardiovasc Res* 1988;22:686–695.
16. Harper J, Harper E, Covell JW. Collagen characterization in volume–overload– and pressure–overload–induced cardiac hypertrophy in minipigs. *Am J Physiol* 1993;265:H434–H438.
17. Tomanek RJ, Cooper G: Morphological changes in the mechanically unloaded myocardial cell. *Anat Rec* 1981;200:271–280.
18. Carew TE, Covell JW. Fiber orientation in hypertrophied canine left ventricle. *Am J Physiol* 1979;236:H487–H493.
19. Baker KM, Aceto JF. Angiotensin II stimulation of protein synthesis and cell growth in chick heart cells. *Am J Physiol* 1990;259:H610–H618.
20. Sadoshima JIM, Yuhui X, Slayter HS, Izumo S. Autocrine release of angiotensin II mediates stretch–induced hypertrophy of cardiac myocytes in vitro. *Cell* 1993;75:977–984.
21. Dartsch PC, Betz E. Response of cultured endothelial cells to mechanical stimulation. *Basic Res Cardiol* 1989;84:268–281.
22. Lab MJ. Mechanoelectric feedback (transduction) in heart: concepts and implications. *Cardiovasc Res* 1996;32:3–14.
23. Kohl P, Noble D. Mechanosensitive connective tissue: potential influence on heart rhythm. *Cardiovasc Res* 1996;32:62–68.

24.   De Maziere AMGL, van Ginneken ACG, Wilders R, Jongsma HJ, Bouman LN. Spatial and functional relationship between myocytes and fibroblasts in the rabbit sinoatrial node. *J Mol Cell Cardiol* 1992;24:567–578.

25.   Swynghedauw B. Remodeling of the heart in response to chronic mechanical overload. *Eur Heart J* 1989;10:935–943.

26.   Schneider MD, Roberts R, Parker TG. Modulation of cardiac genes by mechanical stress. The oncogene signalling hypothesis. *Mol Biol Med* 1991;8:167–183.

27.   Villarreal FJ, Dillmann WH. Cardiac hypertrophy–induced changes in mRNA levels for TGF-β_1, fibronectin, and collagen. *Am J Physiol* 1992;262:H1861–H1866.

28.   Van Bilsen M, Chien KR. Growth and hypertrophy of the heart: towards an understanding of cardiac specific and inducible gene expression. *Cardiovasc Res* 1993;27:1140–1149.

29.   Arts T, Prinzen FW, Snoeckx LHEH, Rijcken JM, Reneman RS. Adaptation of cardiac structure by mechanical feedback in the environment if the cell: A model study. *Biophys J* 1994;66:953–961.

30.   Arts T, Prinzen FW, Snoeckx LHEH, Reneman RS. A model approach to the adaptation of cardiac structure by mechanical feedback in the environment of the cell. In: Sideman S, Beyar R, eds. *Molecular and subcellular cardiology: Effects of structure and function*, Plenum Press 1995;22:217–228.

31.   Robinson TF, Cohen–Gould L, Factor SM, Eghbali M, Blumenfeld OO. Structure and function of connective tissue in cardiac muscle. Collagen types I and III in endomysial struts and pericellular fibers. *SEM* 1988;2:1005–1015.

32.   MacKenna DA, Omens JH, Covell JW. Left ventricular perimysial collagen fibers uncoil rather than stretch during diastolic filling. *Basic Res Cardiol* 1996;91:111–122.

33.   Linke WA, Popov VI, Pollack GH. Passive and active tension in single cardiac myofibrils. *Biophys J* 1994;67:782–792.

34.   Trombitas K, Jin J–P, Granzier H. The mechanically active domain of titin in cardiac muscle. *Circ Res* 1995;77:856–861.

35.   Hunter PJ. Myocardial constitutive laws for continuum mechanics models of the heart. In: Sideman S, Beyar R, eds. *Molecular and subcellular cardiology: Effects of structure and function*, Plenum Press 1995;30:303–318.

36.   Nielsen PMF, Hunter PJ, Smaill BH. Biaxial testing of membrane biomaterials: Testing equipment and procedures. *J Biomech Eng* 1991;13:295–300.

37.   Costa KD, Hunter PJ, Rogers JM, Guccione JM, Waldman LK, McCulloch AD. A three–dimensional finite element method for large elastic deformations of ventricular myocardium: Part I – Cylindrical and spherical polar coordinates. *J Biomech Eng* 1996;118:452–463.

38.   Costa KD, Hunter PJ, Wayne JS, Waldman LK, Guccione JM, McCulloch AD. A three–dimensional finite element method for large elastic deformations of ventricular myocardium: Part II – Prolate spherical coordinates. *J Biomech Eng* 1996;118:464–472.

39.   Anversa P, Ricci R, Olivetti G. Quantitative structural analysis of the myocardium during physiologic growth and induced cardiac hypertrophy: A review. *J Am Coll Cardiol* 1986;7:1140–1149.

40.   LeGrice IJ, Takayama Y, Covell JW. Transverse shear along myocardial cleavage planes provides a mechanism for normal systolic wall thickening. *Circ Res* 1995;77:182–193.

41.   Omens JH, Fung YC. Residual strain in rat left ventricle. *Circ Res* 1990;66:37–45.

42.   Omens JH, Milkes DE, Covell JW. Effects of pressure overload on the passive mechanics of the rat left ventricle. *Annals Biomed Eng* 1995;23:152–163.

43.   Bovendeerd PHM, Arts T, Huyghe JM, Van Campen DH, Reneman RS. Dependence of left ventricular wall mechanics on myocardial fiber orientation: a model study. *J Biomech* 1992;25:1129–1140.

44.   Antzelevitch C, Sicouri S, Litovsky SH, Lukas A, Krishnan SC, Di Diego JM, Gintant GA, Liu DW. Heterogeneity within the ventricular wall. Electrophysiology and pharmacology of epicardial, endocardial and M cells. *Circ Res* 1991;69:1427–1449.

CHAPTER 19

MULTIAXIAL MYOCARDIAL MECHANICS AND EXTRACELLULAR MATRIX REMODELING: MECHANOCHEMICAL REGULATION OF CARDIAC FIBROBLAST FUNCTION

Ann A. Lee and Andrew D. McCulloch[1]

ABSTRACT

Substantial evidence suggests that not only does the structure of the cardiac extracellular matrix affect the mechanical properties of myocardium, but that mechanical loading affects the synthesis of the extracellular matrix. However, loading conditions *in vivo* are nonhomogeneous and multiaxial. An experimental approach that combines mechanics and cell biology is used to examine the mechanisms of extracellular matrix remodeling in the heart. The results indicate that differential biological responses in adult cardiac fibroblasts can be correlated with specific physical signals, such as the magnitude and two dimensional (2D) pattern of strain. Some effects of flow–function relations are discussed.

INTRODUCTION

Over the past decade, experimental studies of regional mechanics in the intact ventricular wall have shown that myocardial deformations in the normal and diseased heart are highly nonhomogeneous and multiaxial [1–3]. Many of these studies suggest an important role of the cardiac extracellular matrix (ECM)—the hierarchical network of collagen and other interstitial proteins that interconnect and reinforce ventricular

[1]Department of Bioengineering and Institute for Biomedical Engineering University of California San Diego, La Jolla, California, USA

Analytical and Quantitative Cardiology
Edited by Sideman and Beyar, Plenum Press, New York, 1997

myocytes—in determining myocardial strain distributions. For example, Waldman and colleagues [4] showed that although the principal axis of maximum shortening is aligned with the myofiber axis at the subepicardium during systole, it is almost perpendicular to the fiber axis on the endocardium. Thus, collagen extracellular connections provide strong transmural coupling between adjacent layers of the ventricular myocardium. This "tethering" phenomenon is also observed during subendocardial ischemia. Many investigators have observed profound epicardial segment dysfunction during partial coronary artery stenosis despite little or no loss of subepicardial perfusion [5]. Our studies of three dimensional (3D) myocardial deformations have also revealed large transverse shear strains, especially in the longitudinal–radial plane [2, 6], that are largely unexplained but known to be significantly altered during acute ischemia [7]. Recently, it has been shown that the perimysial collagen matrix organizes myocytes into laminar cleavage planes, or sheets [8], oriented so that they tend to accommodate the majority of transverse shearing by interlaminar sliding during systole [6].

The ECM is probably even more important in regulating diastolic ventricular mechanics. Altered diastolic stiffness is associated with a variety of pathologies that are accompanied by fibrosis (such as myocardial infarction and ventricular pressure overload) or matrix degradation (such as acute myocardial ischemia and stunning [9]). It has also been suggested that the ECM might be important during rapid filling by releasing elastic energy stored during systole [10]. Also, the fibrous anisotropy of resting ventricular myocardium [11] may be explained at least in part by the predominant alignment of the large coiled perimysial collagen fibers parallel to the myofiber axis [12].

Not only does ECM structure affect multiaxial myocardial mechanics, but there is accumulating evidence that myocardial strains can regulate matrix synthesis and remodeling. In pressure–overload hypertrophy or wound healing after myocardial infarction, remodeling of the ECM under changing conditions of hemodynamic forces and biochemical stimuli can contribute significantly to cardiac mechanical dysfunction [13, 14].

Since cardiac fibroblasts have been identified as the cell types primarily responsible for the production of cardiac ECM components, including fibronectin (FN) and fibrillar collagens, we have been investigating the mechanochemical regulation of these cells to understand the mechanisms of cardiac ECM remodeling. Here, we describe our studies on the specific roles of multiaxial strains and angiotensin II (Ang II) in the cellular regulation of FN, fibrillar collagen, and transforming growth factor-β_1 (TGF-β_1). The *in vitro* testing systems developed for these studies is also being used to identify candidate mechanotransducers in adult cardiac fibroblasts. ECM transmits information from the extracellular environment to cells by influencing cell shape and function, especially during cardiac development and disease [15]. This chapter provides a brief introduction to the known regulatory factors of the cardiac ECM and the experimental approaches which have been developed to study the role of mechanical forces in cell growth and function.

FACTORS AFFECTING REGULATION

Remodeling of the Extracellular Matrix

The diverse components of the cardiac ECM include collagens, proteoglycans, noncollagenous glycoproteins, growth factors, and extracellular proteases [15]. Major ECM components of interest are the fibrillar collagen types I and III, the main structural proteins of the connective tissue network, and FN, a glycoprotein that is important for the attachment of cells to the interstitial network and that influences cell growth, migration, and wound repair [16, 17]. In fibrosis accompanying pressure–overload hypertrophy, the over–accumulation of fibrillar collagens has been shown to adversely increase myocardial stiffness [14]. Relative increases in FN expression have also been observed in several models of cardiac hypertrophy [18, 19]. Since the composition and distribution of FN and the fibrillar collagens are significantly altered during scarring after myocardial infarction, these ECM proteins are also thought to be influenced by both chemical and mechanical factors present during tissue wound healing [20].

Cardiac fibroblasts, which number nearly two–thirds of the cells in the heart, have been identified as the cell types primarily responsible for the production of cardiac ECM components, including FN and the fibrillar collagens [21, 22]. Since there are a multitude of components in the cardiac ECM, *in vitro* models have been extremely important in the identification and testing of specific regulatory factors and their roles in cardiac ECM remodeling [15]. The following major factors in the regulation of growth and function of cardiac fibroblasts have been identified: (i) *renal–cardiovascular hormones*, such as Ang II, aldosterone, and endothelin; (ii) *regulatory peptides*, such as TGF–β_1, platelet–derived growth factor (PDGF), and basic fibroblast growth factor (bFGF); (iii) *mechanical stretch and adhesion*; and (iv) *cytokines*, such as interleukin–1 (IL–1).

In particular, Ang II has been established as a major regulator of growth and ECM synthesis both in neonatal and adult cardiac fibroblasts and has been an important factor in the determination of numerous signal transduction pathways in these cells [23]. Recent studies on the role of Ang II in stretch–induced cardiac myocyte hypertrophy suggest that Ang II may also be associated with stretch–activated mechanisms in other cardiac cell types [15, 24]. There has also been growing interest in regulatory peptides such as TGF–β_1 and PDGF as they may play significant roles in regeneration and repair processes in the heart. Exogenous TGF–β_1 has been shown to directly regulate cardiac ECM components such as fibrillar collagens and extracellular proteases [25, 26]. The establishment of TGF–β_1 as a major autocrine/paracrine growth factor in cell types such as vascular smooth muscle cells [27] and proximal tubular cells [28] has raised the possibility that this growth factor plays similar autocrine/paracrine roles in cardiac fibroblasts, which are the principal cellular origin of myocardial TGF–β_1 [29].

In addition to *in vivo* evidence of the influence of mechanical forces on ECM remodeling, several *in vitro* studies in neonatal cardiac fibroblasts have shown that uniaxial stretch can activate nuclear events [30] and stimulate collagen type III gene and protein expression [31]. However, it is not clear whether adult cardiac fibroblasts respond similarly to stretch since neonatal cardiac fibroblasts have exhibited functionally different characteristics of growth and differentiation compared with the adult phenotype [15, 32]. The potential mechanisms of mechanotransduction in the adult cells are also not well–characterized although collagen gel contraction studies suggest the likely involvement of integrins [33]. Since adult cardiac fibroblasts are responsible for a variety of structural and functional changes in cardiac tissue remodeling, it will be important to elucidate the roles of mechanical and chemical factors in the regulation of these cells.

Mechanical Forces in Growth and Differentiation

The ability of mechanical factors to influence the growth and remodeling of biological tissues has long been an important issue for developmental morphologists and cell biologists. Questions about the basic principles of tissue organization and the genera–tion of biological pattern were at the forefront of the emerging modern field of biology [34, 35]. In his book *On Growth and Form*, published in 1917, D'Arcy Thompson observed "...the very important physiological truth that a condition of strain, the result of a stress, is a direct stimulus to growth itself. This indeed is no less than one of the cardinal facts of theoretical biology" [36]. However, interest in the mechanical approach in biology was subordinated by growing emphasis on biochemical, molecular, and genetic analyses [34].

The establishment of cell culture techniques during the 1950's and 1960's stimulated rapid progress in the field of cell biology in the following two decades by enabling the identification of novel chemical growth factors and the understanding of their mechanisms of action through transmembrane receptors and intracellular signaling pathways [37]. Along with the advances in growth factor regulation of cell function, major progress has been made over the last 20 years in the chemical characterization of the biopolymers that comprise the cytoskeleton—the microfilaments, microtubules, and intermediate filaments [38]. While the dynamic roles of these architectural elements during changes in cell shape, division, and motility are not well understood, studies on embryological development have indicated that the cytoskeleton may be a primary determinant of tissue remodeling. For example, during gastrulation, major cell shape changes that drive tissue bending and invagination have been attributed to mechanical interactions within the cytoskeleton [39]. Observations that gastrulation can also be redirected by applying external mechanical force or by disrupting load–bearing intermediate filaments suggest the possibility of specificity of cellular responses to mechanical stimuli.

However, the basic principles of regulation of cell and tissue structure and function by internal and external mechanical forces still remain undefined. One area of investigation is cell regulation by shape change, e.g. by spreading, which is an important determinant of growth and differentiation and is thought to be influenced by alterations in the cytoskeletal force balance [40]. Recent reports have also proposed that, while growth factors stimulate cell proliferation, the development of tissue patterns may be determined primarily by local growth differentials established by local mechanical changes [34]. Thus, the questions originally raised by early developmental biologists have generated renewed interest in examining the mechanical regulation of cellular function in numerous tissues, including blood vessels and myocardium [37, 41–43]. A comprehensive understanding of the role of mechanical forces in cells will provide a framework with which to interpret the interactions between physical and chemical regulatory factors, such as growth factors, and associated signaling pathways.

Mechanisms for sensing and responding to mechanical stimuli have been observed in diverse biological systems, including microbes, plants, and animals. For example, stretch–sensitive ion channels have been found in *E. coli*, yeast, insects, amphibians, birds, reptiles, and mammals [44]. In mammals, tissues such as bone and muscle have long been observed to grow or resorb in adaptation to altered mechanical loads [45]. Organ systems including the heart, lung, skeleton and blood vessels all undergo significant remodeling under changing mechanical environments [41, 45, 46].

The development of *in vitro* models for growth factor studies have contributed to recent improvements in our understanding of the role of mechanical forces in cellular function [37]. The most popular paradigm for the mechanical regulation of cells proposes that mechanical stimulus, such as fluid shear stress, mechanical stretch, or hydrostatic pressure, is transmitted or transduced across the cell membrane to stimulate signaling pathways which may elicit a multitude of cellular responses (Fig. 1A) [44].

Strong evidence indicates that in most anchorage–dependent cells, mechanotrans-duction mechanisms are a combination of force transmission through cytoskeletal elements and biochemical signal transduction at mechanotransducer sites. Figure 1B shows potential sites of mechanical transmission and transduction in cells, including: (i) stretch–sensitive ion channels; (ii) integrins and focal adhesions (sites of ECM–integrin–cytoskeleton contact); (iii) G–protein–coupled receptors; (iv) cell–cell attachments, via cadherins; and

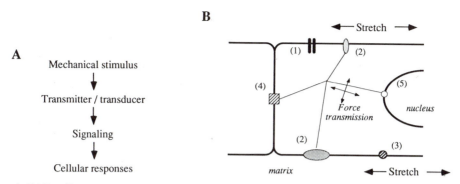

Figure 1. (A) Paradigm for mechanical regulation in cells. **(B)** Potential sites of mechanical transmission and transduction in cells: (1) stretch–sensitive ion channels; (2) integrins and focal adhesions; (3) G–protein–coupled receptors; (4) cell–cell attachments; (5) nuclear membrane sites. Cytoskeletal elements may transfer forces to potential intracellular mechanotransducers. Modified from Davies and Tripathi [44].

(v) the nuclear membrane with possible attachments to cytoskeletal elements [44, 47]. Second messengers which have been induced by mechanical stimulation include cAMP [24, 48], inositol phosphates (IP) [49], intracellular Ca^{2+} [50, 51], protein kinase C (PKC) [52], and the mitogen–activated protein (MAP) kinases [30]. *In vitro* studies have shown that mechanical forces can induce a wide array of cellular responses including the stimulation of transcription factors, immediate early response genes, mRNA regulation, protein synthesis, autocrine/paracrine mediators, cytoskeletal reorganization, and cell proliferation, adhesion, and migration (see [37, 42, 53] for reviews). The discovery of a shear stress responsive element (SSRE) in the promoter of the PDGF–B gene and other genes from fluid flow studies suggests that cells may contain unique shear–stress or stretch–regulated transcription factors and corresponding DNA binding sites [54].

Thus, with the aid of analytical tools from cell and molecular biology, knowledge of the effects of mechanical stimulation in cells has advanced rapidly in recent years. However, the fundamental questions "What are the basic principles of tissue construction?" and "How is biological pattern generated?" can still not be answered [34]. As embryologists have noted, the generation of tissue pattern during development requires the establishment of local differentials in cell shape and mechanical stresses which are temporally and spatially dynamic [36, 39]. For example, local mechanical force transmission has been postulated to directly affect certain cellular mechanisms such as chemical polymerization or nuclear matrix rearrangement which may physically regulate gene expression [34]. Therefore, to fully understand mechanochemical regulation of cells and tissues, it will be essential to develop quantitative relationships between external mechanical stimuli and cellular responses. Meaningful interpretation of experiments studying the effects of mechanical forces on cellular function will depend on the ability to quantify both mechanical and biochemical parameters *in vitro*.

METHODS

While studies of the effects of fluid shear stress in endothelial cells have often been quantitative (see [42] for review), most experimental models used to study mechanical stretch and cellular function do not define or quantify the multiaxial deformation of cells stretched on an elastic substrate [37, 55]. In those studies, a single measure is most often used to describe the 2D substrate deformation and this quantity is subsequently correlated with measurements of cell function. The specificity of cellular responses to stretch will be difficult to determine from these studies because the substrate deformation is often nonuniform and multiaxial and the state of cellular deformation may vary due to cell polarity, cytoskeletal structure, or adhesion properties. The uniaxial and biaxial devices which have been used extensively in cell stretch studies often produce nonhomogeneous strain fields, e.g. 0–30% in radial strain [56, 57], and only one study to date has reported 2D strains in stretched cells [2]. A suitable experimental strain system should meet the following engineering design criteria, verified by calibration tests: (1) provide reproducible strain selection for controlling substrate deformation; and (2) allow for *in situ* visualization of cells for the specific and quantitative correlation of cellular strain and functional responses. A uniform field of strain may also be desirable to reduce variations that arise from cell plating orientations and cellular responses to strain gradients. In some cases it may also be desirable to control the spreading and orientation of cells *in vitro*, either by polymerizing the matrix that coats the elastic substrate or by fabricating elastic membranes with a grooved surface [58].

Studies of Mechanochemical Regulation in Cardiac Fibroblasts

Current thought in cell biology asserts that generation of tissue pattern is critically dependent on temporal and spatial cellular responses to specific physical and biochemical regulatory signals [34, 39]. Therefore, a key question in the study of the mechanochemical regulation of cellular function is: Do cells respond to specific physical parameters of mechanical stretch? As Ingber stated in his review of the mechanical regulation of the cytoskeleton [34]: "If this mechanochemical vision of cell and tissue development is accurate, then future experiments must be designed in which mechanical as well as soluble factors can be varied in a controlled manner."

Our overall aim was to conduct a quantitative investigation of the role of specific physical parameters of biaxial strain in the differential regulation of FN, fibrillar collagen, and TGF-β_1 in adult cardiac fibroblasts. In developing an experimental approach to achieve this aim, the following questions were also asked: Can we establish a cell culture model to identify relevant functional markers that may be regulated by mechanical stretch? Can we control and measure 2D strains in cultured cells? And can we use this quantitative experimental strain system to identify candidate mechanisms of mechanotransduction *in vitro*? The following studies addressed these questions, which are fundamental to the experimental study of the mechanochemical regulation of adult cardiac fibroblast function.

Our specific goal was to establish a cell culture model to identify potential stretch–sensitive markers, such as ECM proteins and TGF-β_1, which have been observed to change during cardiac ECM remodeling. Since Ang II has been established as a major regulator of cardiac ECM components and a potential mediator in stretch–induced hypertrophy, this chemical factor was selected as an agonist to identify the growth factor TGF-β_1 as a potential autocrine/paracrine mechanism which may be regulated by mechanical stretch in adult cardiac fibroblasts.

Next, we developed a quantitative experimental system to control and measure 2D uniform equibiaxial strains in cultured cells. Cellular deformation was quantified *in situ* in this system by imaging and finite strain analysis. The suitability of the equibiaxial stretch device for the study of numerous cell types and the potential applications of single–well and multiwell versions of the device to cellular and molecular studies of mechanotransduction was evaluated. We developed a device that applies homogeneous equibiaxial strains of 0–10% to a cell culture substrate and quantitatively verified transmission of substrate deformation to cultured cardiac cells. Clamped elastic membranes in both single–well and multiwell versions of the device were uniformly stretched by indentation with a plastic ring, resulting in strain that was directly proportional to the pitch:radius ratio.

The selection of cardiac ECM markers in the adult rat cardiac fibroblast model and the development of a quantitative experimental system for mechanical stretch allowed us to address the final goal: to examine the role of specific mechanical parameters, such as cell area and strain magnitudes, in the regulation of FN, fibrillar collagen, and TGF–β_1 in adult cardiac fibroblasts. These used a combination of uniaxial and equibiaxial testing to evaluate the influence of cell shape changes and other determinants of differential ECM expression in these cells.

RESULTS

Angiotensin II Stimulates TGF–β_1 in Adult Cardiac Fibroblasts

The ability of Ang II to regulate the gene expression, biological activity, and protein production of TGF–β_1 in cultured adult rat cardiac fibroblasts was recently examined [59]. Treatment of fibroblast cultures with 10^{-9} M Ang II induced a two–fold increase in TGF–β_1 mRNA levels within 4 h that was sustained through 24 h. TGF–β_1–like activity measured using a bioassay was significantly increased in Ang II–treated cultures compared with. Specificity for TGF–β_1–like activity was confirmed through its neutralization with a TGF–β_1 specific antibody (100 µg/mL). Total concentration of TGF–β_1 (latent plus active forms) in conditioned media from treated cardiac fibroblasts was also significantly greater than control. These findings suggest that factors regulating cardiac hypertrophy and myocardial fibrosis, such as Ang II or mechanical stretch, may stimulate the involvement of autocrine/paracrine mechanisms, including the production and release of TGF–β_1 by cardiac fibroblasts.

Testing the Equibiaxial Strain System for Cultured Cells

The ability of our new cell strain system to apply repeatable, homogeneous equibiaxial stretch to elastic substrata was tested, and we determined how reliably these strains are transmitted to cultured cardiac fibroblasts [60]. 2D deformations were measured by tracking fluorescent microspheres attached to the substrate and to cultured adult rat cardiac fibroblasts. For nominal stretches up to 18%, strains along circumferential and radial axes were equal in magnitude and homogeneously distributed with negligible shear. For 5% stretch, circumferential and radial strains in the substrate were 0.046±0.005 and 0.048±0.004 (NS), respectively, and shear strain (0.001±0.003) was not significantly different from zero. The reproducible application and quantification of homogeneous equibiaxial strain in cultured cells provides a quantitative approach for correlating mechanical stimuli to cellular transduction mechanisms.

Differential Responses to Biaxial Strain

A combination of uniaxial and equibiaxial strain testing was used in adult rat cardiac fibroblasts to examine specific physical regulators of ECM gene and protein expression and TGF–β_1 [61, 62]. Levels of mRNA for FN and collagen type III in cells stretched uniaxially by 10% increased three–fold when compared with control but decreased significantly at 20% extension. Uniaxial stretch also stimulated significant increases both in FN protein production and TGF–β_1 activity. Mean cell surface strains for 10% substrate stretch were 0.107±0.018 and 0.042±0.013, with negligible shear (0.011±0.020), demonstrating that "uniaxial stretch" is really a specific state of biaxial cell strain. Cell area changes applied by 10% and 20% nominal extension in the uniaxial system were equivalent to 3% and 6% strains, respectively, in the equibiaxial system. Similar to uniaxial stretch, mRNA levels for ECM proteins increased for changes in cell area applied by 3% equibiaxial strain and decreased under 6% strain. TGF–β_1 activity in fibroblast conditioned media showed no changes at 3% equibiaxial strain but increased with increasing magnitudes of 6% and 10% strain.

Consequently, we have concluded that: (1) Cell area changes may be a significant determinant of differential responses in mRNA levels for cardiac ECM proteins; and (2) stretch–induced TGF–β_1 activity may be dependent on strain magnitudes in either tensile or compressive testing. In contrast to previous studies which correlated single strain values with cellular responses to stretch, these results suggest that in adult cardiac fibroblasts, different magnitudes and patterns of 2D strain may be important in determining the differential responses of cells to mechanical stimulation.

DISCUSSION

The mechanical environment in the heart is nonuniform, multidimensional, and dynamic. During cardiac hypertrophy or scarring after myocardial infarction, tissue remodeling generates different compositions and structural patterns in the ECM network, which often contribute to cardiac dysfunction. Since soluble growth factors alone cannot account for the formation of tissue pattern [34], we investigated whether the regulation of selected ECM components in adult cardiac fibroblasts may correlate with specific kinematic parameters of biaxial strain. In these studies, we established an *in vitro* model and identified an autocrine/paracrine TGF–β_1 mechanism, developed a quantitative approach to biaxial testing of cultured cells, and showed that the differential regulation of cardiac ECM components may be influenced in part by specific physical parameters, such as cell area strain or maximum strain magnitude. Furthermore, our studies indicated that focal adhesions and G–protein–coupled receptors are two candidate mechanotransducers that may be involved in the specificity of mechanical signaling in these cells.

The identification of an autocrine/paracrine TGF–β_1 mechanism regulated by both mechanical stretch and Ang II has important implications in cardiac tissue remodeling. In cardiac myocytes, TGF–β_1 can regulate contractile activity and induce gene expression essential for myocyte hypertrophy [63]. In cardiac fibroblasts, TGF–β_1 is considered a primary regulator of fibrillar collagen and FN synthesis during growth and disease [23]. As recent studies have indicated the increasing importance of the paracrine effects of cardiac fibroblasts in the myocardium, the presence of a functional autocrine/paracrine mechanism of TGF–β_1 in these cells may have significant effects on cellular growth and remodeling for all cardiac cell types during hypertrophy or scarring [23, 32]. Furthermore, TGF–β_1 may be a potential mediator in the development of interventional therapies, including gene therapy, for controlling fibrosis and scarring. Hence, the understanding of TGF–β_1 regulation by local chemical and mechanical factors will be essential in the determination of its role in cardiac tissue remodeling.

The experimental strain system developed in this research was essential for correlating uniform measures of 2D cell strains to functional responses. In particular, the ability to select substrate strains in a reproducible manner and to measure cellular strain and function *in situ* allowed for the design and development of meaningful experiments for studying the specificity of mechanical signaling in cells. The observation that cells may elicit specific responses to different magnitudes and patterns of 2D strain supports the current belief in cell biology that physical regulators such as cell shape are critical for the local growth differentials during tissue formation [40]. In particular, physical changes in nuclear shape have been considered a potential determinant of DNA synthesis and the control of gene expression [64, 65]. Our observation of the marked correlation between ECM mRNA levels and cell area strains in cardiac fibroblasts indicates that it may be interesting to examine further the possibility that nuclear shape changes may influence gene expression. In contrast, the apparent dose dependent response of autocrine TGF–β_1 to maximum tensile or compressive strain magnitudes in these cells suggests that different cellular responses, such as protein synthesis, may be sensitive to alternative physical parameters of strain.

The demonstration that cardiac fibroblasts may be differentially regulated by specific states of biaxial strain indicates that current methods of uniaxial and biaxial testing may not be sufficient to elucidate the effects of stretch on cell function. For example, a recent study using a nonhomogeneous biaxial stretch device concluded that cardiac fibroblasts may not respond to stretch unless cultured in high concentrations of serum [66]. Our results demonstrating the distinct biphasic response of ECM mRNAs to different biaxial loading suggest that the use of nonhomogeneous experimental systems (e.g. with 0 – 30% radial strains) may in fact potentially mask any differential effects of stretch in cultured cells. While our studies are suggestive of the potential role of cell area strain and maximum strain magnitudes in the determination of cellular function, it will be necessary to pursue further a comprehensive characterization of the effects of biaxial strain parameters on cell responses. In particular, the effects of compression and shear will need to be fully quantified.

Finally, while 2D cell culture testing will be useful to quantify specific effects of mechanical and chemical factors in cellular function, it has been suggested that cells may need 3D scaffolding with a design and level of information content which can direct a tissue–building response [67]. In particular, cells engaged in tissue building may depend on three kinds of stimuli: chemical factors, applied forces, and structural stimuli. For future studies, it will be necessary to extend the quantitative experimental approaches developed for 2D testing to the 3D characterization of mechanical forces in cell function. Potential experimental approaches toward the development of a comprehensive understanding of cellular function during tissue remodeling include the use of cell culture matrices and 3D strain analysis, which may be useful in the long–term goal of creating functional biological tissues.

CONCLUSION

Combining mechanics with cell and molecular biology, an interdisciplinary experimental approach has been outlined to examine the cellular mechanisms of ECM remodeling in the heart. The results indicate that differential biological responses in adult cardiac fibroblasts can be correlated with specific local physical signals, such as the magnitude and 2D mode of mechanical strain. These studies suggest that remodeling of the cardiac ECM in response to altered regional myocardial loading may be mediated by specific cellular mechanotransduction mechanisms.

Acknowledgments

The authors are grateful to our collaborators, Drs. Francisco Villarreal, James Covell, Wolfgang Dillmann, Deidre MacKenna and Tammo Delhaas. The assistance of John Clemmens is also gratefully acknowledged. This research was supported by NIH grant HL41603 and NSF grant BES9157961.

The authors are grateful to our collaborators, Drs. Francisco Villarreal, James Covell, Wolfgang Dillmann, Deidre MacKenna and Tammo Delhaas. The assistance of John Clemmens is also gratefully acknowledged. This research was supported by NIH grant HL41603 and NSF grant BES9157961.

DISCUSSION

Dr. H. Azhari: Have you looked at the principal strains in your studies of flow–function relations in ischemic myocardium? As you probably know, the maximal deformation does not necessarily occur in the direction of the fibers. In fact, it has been known that it is actually perpendicular to the direction of the fibers near the endocardium. Maybe that would come up with a more sensitive relationship between flow and function?

Dr. A.D. McCulloch: The principal systolic strain does show the expected trend which, as you say, is that maximum shortening is not the same as fiber shortening and, in fact, it is closer to the crossfiber direction in the subendocardium. You are correct that, being large, the subendocardial principal strain is a more sensitive indicator of regional flow than fiber strain. However, there is an interaction effect of transmural location on the relationship between principal strain and perfusion. From the point of view of finding a flow–function relationship that is independent of location, the fiber strain is a better candidate.

Dr. S. Sideman: The functional border zone is different for left anterior descending coronary artery occlusion vs left circumflex occlusion. Could you elaborate on that?

Dr. A.D. McCulloch: A similar result was reported by Kim Gallagher and colleagues in an abstract at the American Heart Association meeting several years ago [Circ 1987;76(suppl. IV):373] where they measured wall thickening and found evidence of a difference in the width of the functional border zone between those two beds. The widths we measured, although different, were not significantly different. A combination of the greater hyperfunction in the nonischemic region for circumflex occlusion and the narrower zone gave rise to a significantly sharper gradient in function across the boundary. My interpretation of this is a mechanical one, namely that the difference is in the orientation of the perfusion boundaries relative to the muscle fiber direction.

Dr. S. Sideman: When we put a pacer in different places on the surface of the heart, we get different responses. Would that be in some way connected with this phenomena?

Dr. A.D. McCulloch: Ventricular pacing is definitely another situation where there is evidence of this sort of interaction, in that case between early and late activated regions. These types of interactions occur not only during ischemia, but during asynchronous activation as well. I think that similar mechanisms may apply.

Dr. L. Axel: Using MR, we, as well as researchers at Johns Hopkins, have looked at the relationship of the principal strains to the fiber angle and found that although there is a lot of cross–fiber shortening in the subendocardium, when you resolve the component along the fiber direction, it is quite uniform. Also, in the setting of a recent infarct, we have done acute ischemia experiments. Again, we see the transition zone between the area of dysfunction and the somewhat hyperfunction in the remote areas, with a continuous distribution angle of principal strain between the circumferentially located strain in the region of the infarction (basically stretching), and the radial contraction in the more remote areas, with a fairly smooth transition between them.

Dr. A.D. McCulloch: Although the functional border zone has not been defined for myocardial infarction and for later phases, an equivalent phenomenon does exist. In fact, there was a poster by Rochitte et al from Zerhouni's group at the 1996 Heart Association meeting, showing similar relationships in the human by magnetic resonance tagging.

Dr. R. Beyar: In a paper in Circulation [*Gibbons CA et al. Circulation 1995;92:130–141*] from work at Calgary we show that torsional twist measured by apical rotation is markedly reduced by LAD occlusion. Considering the interaction effect, the depth effect vs the flow effect, do you think that this interaction effect may be related to the twist which effects the different layers of the endocardium and the epicardium in a different way and which is abolished during ischemia?

Dr. A.D. McCulloch: The interaction or lack of interaction in the fiber direction is undoubtedly due in part to the torsion that occurs at baseline, because torsion, as you and others have shown, is responsible for minimizing the transmural gradient of fiber function at baseline, which is important for the relative lack of an interaction effect in the fiber direction. We found that the small systolic shear strain which was positive at baseline, corresponding to right–handed systolic torsion, went pretty much to zero during ischemia. The biggest difference in shearing was in one of the components of the transverse shear, which changed sign and was dramatically altered during ischemia.

Dr. J. Downey: One of the problems with this kind of work is that one has to now exactly where the flow border is. What is your pixel size? What size cubes did you chop the heart into?

Dr. A.D. McCulloch: That is an important issue. We determined the flow border indirectly. Our blocks were about 1 cm on the side and we did not attempt to separate them anatomically, as previous investigators have done, to identify that sharp transition in flow at the boundary. So the flow profiles that we got were smooth and that is an artifact of our sampling. This is why we then computed a boundary from the flow profile and expressed the results with respect to distance from the boundary. However, to see whether that was valid, we compared the boundary computed from the flow distributions that we identified by perfusing monasteryl blue at the end of the study into the ischemic region. There was good agreement to within a resolution of our measurements, of 1 mm or so, between the dye–demarcated boundary and the computed boundary from the flow distribution.

Dr. J. Downey: Your model seems to assume that the flow boundary goes perpendicular into tissue from the epicardial surface. As you know, if you slice these things the borders go every which way so that what may be very ischemic epicardially, may have quite well perfused tissue under it. How do you correct for that?

Dr. A.D. McCulloch: We have not corrected for it directly other than by sectioning the tissue and looking at the differences in the dye boundary. In individual regions and individual hearts there can be transmural variations. But on average, the location of the boundary on the endocardium was essentially the same as the epicardium. This is unlikely to be the case, particularly during nontransmural ischemia.

Dr. J. Downey: What is the current thinking on adjacent fiber tethering?

Dr. A.D. McCulloch: The hypothesis that I would like to propose from this work is that the tethering, or interaction between ischemic and nonischemic myocardium is strongest when fibers are parallel to the perfusion boundary and becomes weaker as the orientations of the fibers and the perfusion boundary diverge. This is similar to the parallel fiber hypothesis proposed by Wyatt *et al.* [*Am J Cardiol* 1976;37:366–372].

REFERENCES

1. Omens JH, May KD, McCulloch AD. Transmural distribution of three–dimensional strain in the isolated arrested canine left ventricle. *Am J Physiol* 1991;261:H918–H928.
2. Waldman LK, Fung YC, Covell JW. Transmural myocardial deformation in the canine left ventricle: normal *in vivo* three–dimensional finite strains. *Circ Res* 1985;57:152–163.
3. Waldman LK, Allen JJ, Pavelec RS, McCulloch AD. Distributed mechanics of the canine right ventricle: effects of varying preload. *J Biomech* 1996;29:373–382.
4. Waldman LK, Nossan D, Villarreal F, Covell JW. Relation between transmural deformation and local myofiber direction in canine left ventricle. *Circ Res* 1988;63:550–562.
5. Weintraub WS, Hattori S, Agarwal JB, Bodenheimer MM, Banka VS, Helfant RH. The relationship between myocardial blood flow and contraction by myocardial layer in the canine left ventricle during ischemia. *Circ Res* 1981;48:430–438.
6. LeGrice IJ, Takayama Y, Covell JW. Transverse shear along myocardial cleavage planes privides a mechanism for normal systolic wall thickening. *Circ Res* 1995;77:182–193.
7. Villarreal FJ, Lew WYW, Waldman LK, Covell JW. Transmural myocardial deformation in the ischemic canine left ventricle. *Circ Res* 1991;68:368–381.
8. LeGrice IJ, Smaill BH, Chai LZ, Edgar SG, Gavin JB, Hunter PJ. Laminar structure of the heart: ventricular myocyte arrangement and connective tissue architecture in the dog. *Am J Physiol* 1995;269:H571–82.
9. MacKenna DA, McCulloch AD. Contribution of the collagen extracellular matrix to ventricular mechanics, in Ingels NB, Daughters GT, Baan J, Covell JW, Reneman RS and Yin FC-P (eds): *Systolic and Diastolic Function of the Heart*. Amsterdam, IOS Press, 1996, pp 35–46.
10. Robinson TF, Factor SM, Sonnenblick EH. The heart as a suction pump. *Sci Am* 1988;254:62–69.
11. Guccione JM, McCulloch AD, Waldman LK. Passive material properties of intact ventricular myocardium determined from a cylindrical model. *J Biomech Eng* 1991;113:42–55.
12. Robinson TF, Geraci MA, Sonnenblick EH, Factor SM. Coiled perimysial fibers of papillary muscle in rat heart: morphology, distribution, and changes in configuration. *Circ Res* 1988;63:577–592.
13. Borg TK, Caulfield JB. The collagen matrix of the heart. *Fed Proc* 1981;40:2037–2041.
14. Weber KT, Sun Y, Tyagi SC, Cleutjens JP. Collagen network of the myocardium: function, structural remodeling, and regulatory mechanisms. *J Mol Cell Cardiol* 1994;26:279–292.
15. Borg TK, Rubin K, Carver W, Samarel A, Terracio L. The cell biology of the cardiac interstitium. *Trends Cardiovasc Med* 1996;1996:65–70.
16. Farhadian F, Contard F, Corbier A, Barrieux A, Rappaport L, Samuel JL. Fibronectin expression during physiological and pathological cardiac growth. *J Mol Cell Cardiol* 1995;27:981–990.
17. Yamada KM, Miyamoto S. Integrin transmembrane signaling and cytoskeletal control. *Current Opinion in Cell Biology* 1995;7:681–689.
18. Mamuya WS, Brecher P. Fibronectin expression in the normal and hypertrophic rat heart. *J Clin Invest* 1992;89:392–401.
19. Villarreal FJ, Dillmann WH. Cardiac hypertrophy–induced changes in mRNA levels for TGF–1, fibronectin, and collagen. *Am J Physiol* 1992;262:H1861–H1865.
20. Welch MP, Odland GF, Clark RAF. Temporal relationships of F–actin bundle formation, collagen and fibronectin matrix assembly, and fibronectin receptor expression to wound contraction. *J Cell Biol* 1990;110:133–145.
21. Bashey RI, Donnelly M, Insigna F, Jimenez SA. Growth properties and biochemical characteristics of collagen synthesis by adult rat heart fibroblasts in culture. *J Mol Cell Cardiol* 1992;24:691–700.
22. Eghbali M. Cardiac fibroblasts: function of gene expression, and phenotypic modulation. *Basic Res Cardiol* 1992;87:183–189.
23. Booz GW, Baker KM. Molecular signalling mechanisms controlling growth and function of cardiac fibroblasts. *Cardiovasc Res* 1995;30:537–543.
24. Sadoshima J, Izumo S. Mechanical stretch rapidly activates multiple signal transduction pathways in cardiac myocytes: potential involvement of an autocrine/paracrine mechanism. *EMBO* 1993;12:1681–1692.
25. Eghbali M, Romek R, Sukhatme VP, Woods C, Bhambi B. Differential effects of TGF–1 and phorbol myristate acetate on cardiac fibroblasts. *Circ Res* 1991;69:483–490.
26. Chua CC, Chua BHL, Zhao ZY, Krebs C, Diglio C, Perrin E. Effect of growth factors on collagen metabolism in cultured human heart fibroblasts. *Connective Tissue Res* 1991;26:271–281.
27. Stouffer GA, Owens GK. Angiotensin II–induced mitogenesis of spontaneously hypertensive rat–

derived cultured smooth muscle cells is dependent on autocrine production of transforming growth factor-β. *Circ Res* 1992;70:820–828.

28. Wolf G, Mueller E, Stahl RA, Ziyadeh FN. AII–induced hypertrophy of cultured murine proximal tubular cells is mediated by endogenous TGF–β. *J Clin Invest* 1993;92:1366–1372.

29. Eghbali M. Cellular origin and distribution of transforming growth factor–β1 in the normal rat myocardium. *Cell Tissue Res* 1989;256:553–558.

30. Sadoshima J, Jahn L, Takahashi T, Kulik TJ, Izumo S. Molecular characterization of the stretch–induced adaptation of cultured cardiac cells: an *in vitro* model of load–induced cardiac hypertrophy. *J Biol Chem* 1992;267:10551–10560.

31. Carver W, Nagpal ML, Nachtigal M, Borg TK, Terracio L. Collagen expression in mechanically stimulated cardiac fibroblasts. *Circ Res* 1991;69:116–122.

32. Kim NN, Villarreal FJ, Printz MP, Lee AA, Dillmann WH. Trophic effects of angiotensin II on neonatal rat cardiac myocytes are mediated by cardiac fibroblasts. *Am J Physiol* 1995;269:E426–E437.

33. Burgess ML, Carver WE, Terracio L, Wilson SP. Wilson MA, Borg TK. Integrin–mediated collagen gel contraction by cardiac fibroblasts. *Circ Res* 1994;74:291–298.

34. Ingber DE, Dike L, Hansen L, Karp S, Liley H, Maniotis A, McNamee H, Mooney D, Plopper G, Sims J, Wang N. Cellular tensegrity: exploring how mechanical changes in the cytoskeleton regulate cell growth, migration, and tissue pattern during morphogenesis. *Int Rev Cytol* 1994;150:173–224.

35. Lenoir T. The strategy of life: teleology and mechanics in nineteenth century German biology. Chicago, University of Chicago Press, 1982.

36. Thompson DW. On Growth and Form. New York, Cambridge University Press, 1969.

37. Vandenburgh HH. Mechanical forces and their second messengers in stimulating cell growth *in vitro*. *Am J Physiol* 1992;262 (*Regulatory Integrative Comp Physiol* 31):R350–R355.

38. Mitchison T. Compare and contrast actin filaments and microtubules. *Mol Biol Cell* 1992;3:1309–1315.

39. Beloussov LV, Saveliev SV, Naumidi II, Novoselov VV. Mechanical stresses in embryonic tissues: patterns, morphogenetic role, and involvement in regulatory feedback. *Int Rev Cytology* 1994;150:1–34.

40. Ingber DE, Prusty D, Sun Z, Betensky H, Wang N. Cell shape, cytoskeletal mechanics, and cell cycle control in angiogenesis. *J Biomech* 1995;28:1471–1484.

41. Komuro I, Yazaki Y. Intracelluar signaling pathways in cardiac myocytes induced by mechanical stress. *Trends Cardiovasc Med* 1994;4:117–121.

42. Davies PF. Flow–mediated endothelial mechanotransduction. *Physiol Rev* 1995;75:519–560.

43. Simpson DG, Sharp WW, Borg TK, Price RL, Samarel AM, Terracio L. Mechanical regulation of cardiac myofibrillar structure. *Ann New York Acad Sci* 1995;752:131–140.

44. Davies PF, Tripathi SC. Mechanical stress mechanisms and the cell: an endothelial paradigm. *Circ Res* 1993;72:239–245.

45. Fung YC. Biomechanics: motion, flow, stress, and growth. New York, Springer–Verlag, 1990.

46. Davies PF, Barbee KA, Lal R, Robotewskyj A, Griem ML. Hemodynamics and atherogenesis. Endothelial surface dynamics in flow signal transduction. *Annals NY Acad Sci* 1995;748:86–102.

47. Ingber D. Integrins as mechanochemical transducers. *Current Opinion in Cell Biology* 1991;3:841–848.

48. Kollros PR, Bates SR, Mathews MB, Horwitz AL, Glagov S. Cyclic AMP inhibits increased collagen production by cyclically stretched smooth muscle cells. *Lab Invest* 1987;56:410–417.

49. Lyall F, Deehan MR, Greer IA, Boswell F, Brown WC, McInnes GT. Mechanical stretch increases proto–oncogene expression and phosphoinositide turnover in vascular smooth muscle cells. *J Hypertension* 1994;12:1139–1145.

50. Ando J, Komatsuda T, Kamiya A. Cytoplasmic calcium responses to fluid shear stress in cultured vascular endothelial cells. *in vitro* Cell Dev Biol 1988;24:871–877.

51. Sigurdson W, Rukudin A, Sachs F. Calcium imaging of mechanically induced fluxes in tissue–cultured chick heart: role of stretch–activated ion channels. *Am J Physiol* 1992;262:H1110–H1115.

52. Komuro I, Yamazaki T, Katoh Y, Tobe K, Kadowaki T, Nagai R, Yazaki Y. Protein kinase cascade activated by mechanical stress in cardiocytes: possible involvement of angiotensin II. *Eur Heart J* 1995;16(Suppl. C):8–11.

53. Resnick N, Gimbrone MA. Hemodynamic forces are complex regulators of endothelial gene expression. *FASEB* 1995;9:874–882.

54. Resnick N, Collins T, Atkinson W, Bonthron DT, Dewey CF Jr, Gimbrone MA Jr. Platelet–derived

growth factor B chain promoter contains a cis–acting fluid shear–stress–responsive element. *Proc Natl Acad Sci USA* 1993;4591–4595.

55.   Barbee KA, Macarak EJ, Thibault LE. Strain measurements in cultured vascular smooth muscle cells subjected to mechanical deformation. *Ann Biomed Eng* 1994;22:14–22.

56.   Schaffer JL, Rizen M, L'Italien GJ, Benbrahim A, Megerman J, Gerstenfeld LC, Gray ML. Device for the application of a dynamic biaxially uniform and isotropic strain to a flexible cell culture membrane. *J Orth Res* 1994;12:709–719.

57.   Williams JL, Chen JH, Belloli DM. Strain fields on cell stressing devices employing clamped circular elastic diaphragms as substrates. *J Biomech Eng* 1992;114:377–384.

58.   Wang H, Ip W, Boissy R, Grood ES. Cell orientation response to cyclically deformed substrates: experimental validation of a cell model. *J Biomechan* 1995;28:1542–1552.

59.   Lee AA, Dillmann WH, McCulloch AD, Villarreal FJ. Angiotensin II stimulates the autocrine production of transforming growth factor–β_1 in adult rat cardiac fibroblasts. *J Mol Cell Cardiol* 1995;27:2347–2357.

60.   Lee AA, Delhaas T, Waldman LK, MacKenna DA, Villarreal FJ, McCulloch AD. An equibiaxial strain system for cultured cells. *Am J Physiol* 1996;271:C1400–C1408.

61.   Lee AA, Delhaas T, Villarreal FJ, Leong J, Clemmens J, McCulloch AD. Biaxial mechanical strains in adult cardiac fibroblast cultures. *Mol Biol Cell* 1995;6:278a.

62.   Lee AA, Delhaas T, McCulloch AD, Dillmann WH, Covell JW, Villarreal FJ. Effects of mechanical stretch on extracellular matrix mRNAs and transforming growth factor–β_1 activity in adult cardiac fibroblasts. *Circ* 1995;92:I-526.

63.   Roberts AB, Roche NS, Winokur TS, Burmester JK, Sporn MB. Role of transforming growth factor–β in maintenance of function of cultured neonatal cardiac myocytes. *J Clin Invest* 1992;90:2056–2062.

64.   Carter KC, Bowman D. A three–dimensional view of precursor messenger RNA metabolism within the mammalian nucleus. *Science* 1993;259:1330–1335.

65.   Nicolini C, Belmont AS, Martelli A. Critical nuclear DNA size and distribution associated with S phase initiation. *Cell Biophys* 1986;8:103–117.

66.   Butt RP, Laurent GJ, Bishop JE. Mechanical load and polypeptide growth factors stimulate cardiac fibroblast activity. *Ann New York Acad Sci* 1995;752:387–393.

67.   Bell E. Deterministic models for tissue engineering. *J Cell Eng* 1995;1:28–34.

CHAPTER 20

In Vivo Assessment of Regional Myocardial Work in Normal Canine Hearts Using 3D Tagged MRI

Haim Azhari,[1] James L. Weiss,[2] and Edward P. Shapiro[2]

ABSTRACT

A non–invasive method for assessing regional myocardial work is presented. The method utilizes tagged magnetic resonance images (MRI) obtained from two sets of ortho-gonal planes to mark and reconstruct 24 small myocardial cuboids at end–diastole (ED) and end–systole (ES) in the *in vivo* left ventricle (LV). Regional myocardial work is assessed by calculating the area enclosed by the endocardial wall tension–area (T–A) loop of each studied cuboid. The method was applied to six normal canine hearts. In addition, a global myocardial work index was obtained from the corresponding estimated pressure–volume (P–V) loops. The average work index calculated using the T–A loop was 0.242±0.088 J/100gr/beat, in agreement with the average index obtained from the P–V loop: 0.296± 0.089 J/100gr/beat. The two indices correlate linearly with a correlation coefficient of 0.82.

INTRODUCTION

The heart transforms chemical energy into mechanical work. This work which is manifested in the form of stresses and strains within the myocardium is responsible for the geometrical changes of the heart's chambers which pump the blood. Accurate assessment of regional myocardial work may contribute to better understanding of cardiac mechanics, can lead to the development of improved physiological models of the heart and may potentially serve as a clinical index.

[1]Department of Biomedical Engineering, Technion–IIT Haifa 32000 Israel and [2]Division of Cardiology, School of Medicine, Johns Hopkins University, Baltimore MD, USA

Several methods for assessing global and regional myocardial work have been suggested. The first method utilizes the conductance catheter developed by Baan *et al.* [1], to simultaneously measure the LV pressure (P) and volume (V). Global mechanical work of the LV is then assessed by calculating the area enclosed within the measured P–V loop [2]. Furthermore, the ES elastance line allows to assess mechanical efficiency of the myocardium (e.g. [3]). Others [4] approximate the LV by a thick shell spheroid. The LV pressure is then used to estimate the stresses developed within the myocardium and the change in LV volume is expressed in terms of length changes. Consequently, the external LV work is calculated from the LV force and shortening loop [4].

Another approach used a pair of implanted miniature ultrasonic transducers (sonomicrometers) to measure a segment length within the myocardium. The force developed within the myocardium is simultaneously measured with another implanted miniature transducer. Plotting the force vs. segment length throughout the cardiac cycle yields a characteristic loop. Regional myocardial work is assessed by calculating the area enclosed within this force–length loop (e.g. [5]).

Changes in regional myocardial work of the LV wall have been studied [6] in conscious dogs instrumented with a micromanometer for LV pressure measurement and sonomicrometers for wall thickness and the LV external short and long axes. LV pressure–wall thickness (P–WT) loop area of each region of the LV wall is calculated as an index of regional myocardial external work. These changes of the P–WT loop have been confirmed by calculating stress–strain loop areas as an additional index of regional myocardial external work [6].

In another method [7], regional external work, has been measured by the integral of LV pressure–segment length loop. Although this index does not have true dimensions of work, it can be assumed that the force generated within the myocardium is proportional to the ventricular pressure. Hence, this index can be related to the regional work done by the segment. As shown by McFalls *et al.* [7], this index changes significantly (relative to normalcy) in stunned myocardial regions.

Sugawara *et al.* [8] have implanted two pairs of sonomicrometers within the studied region of the myocardium. The two pairs are roughly perpendicular to each other. The area (A) enclosed within these four transducers was continuously monitored. In addition, other implanted ultrasonic transducers were used to determine the diameter of the ventricle. Using a thick wall spheroid model, the instantaneous wall tension (T) was also calculated. As shown by Sugawara *et al.* [8], the area surrounded by the locus of the tension–area (T–A) loop is approximately equal to the work done by that region.

All the above mentioned methods relate either to the whole heart or require surgical procedures. In this study we have used the conceptual method suggested by Sugawara *et al.* [8], utilizing 3D tagged MRI to define the area enclosed by the T–A loop. This non–surgical procedure is used for estimating the regional mechanical work of the myocardium.

METHODS

Animal Preparation

Six healthy anesthetized dogs (18–22 kg) with re–closed chests were studied. The dogs were anesthetized by intravenous injection of 25–35 mg/Kg of Pentobarbital and 0.05 mg/Kg of Fentanyl. Additional doses were administered when needed. The dogs were artificially ventilated using a Harvard respirator (model 710A). The carotid artery and the jugular vein were cannulated and a pacemaker wire was inserted through the jugular vein to the right atrium. Pacing was applied in order to eliminate beat to beat variability of the heart rate. The aortic pressure was monitored using a catheter with a pressure transducer which was inserted through the carotid artery.

Image Acquisition

Each dog was placed in the MRI scanner (Resonex RX4000, 0.38 Tesla). Following several scout images, the location of the LV and the spatial orientation of its long axis was determined. Two sets of planes were then selected. The first set comprised of four parallel short axis planes (i.e., perpendicular to the LV long axis), about 1 cm apart. These planes were selected to cover the LV from its basal to apical regions. Then, using the LV long axis as a pivot, four equiangular longitudinal planes (45° apart) were selected. The spatial coordinates of each selected plane were registered.

The spin–echo technique was applied with a time to echo (TE) of 30 msec and a repetition time (TR) which equalled twice the cardiac cycle. The electrocardiographic (ECG) signal was transmitted by telemetry to the MRI system using a Hewlett–Packard transmitter (model 78100A). The MRI system was synchronized to the received ECG R–wave for ED gating. Using the tagging technique suggested by Zerhouni et al. [9], an inversion pulse was applied to the set of long axis planes prior to image acquisition along the short axis planes. Consequently, a set of radially tagged short axis images were acquired. Images were acquired at ED and ES.

An inversion tagging pulse was then applied to the short axis planes and images were acquired along the long axis planes. Consequently, a set of longitudinal cross sections of the heart with four parallel tag lines corresponding to the previously imaged short axis planes were obtained. Images were again acquired at ED and ES (for more details see [10]).

Data Processing

The MR images were transferred to an IBM compatible PC. The endocardial and epicardial contours of each slice were manually traced. Papillary muscles and trabeculae were smoothed out during the tracing procedure. The intersection points of each tag line with the endocardial and epicardial contours were digitized, yielding eight endocardial and eight epicardial points per slice.

Fusing the information from the long and short–axis images corresponding to the same cardiac phase, the spatial coordinates (i.e., XYZ) of a set of 64 nodal points (eight tag points at the epicardial and endocardial walls x4 slices) were defined for each temporal point [10]. Combining each set of four endocardial points with its corresponding four epicardial points to define a myocardial cuboid, 24 myocardial cuboids were obtained from each LV at ED and ES. A typical 3D reconstruction of a set of cuboids is depicted in Fig. 1.

Applying the interpolation algorithm suggested by Akima [11], a more accurate geometrical description was obtained by describing the endocardial and epicardial walls as curved surfaces. Using 14 triangular tiles, the endocardial area (A) of each curved cuboid was calculated. In addition, using 42 miniature pyramids, the volume enclosed by each cuboid (V) was calculated. Furthermore, the endocardial radius of curvature (R) was also calculated for each cuboid.

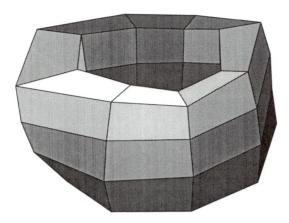

Figure 1. A typical 3D reconstruction of a set of 24 myocardial cuboids obtained from a canine LV.

Assessment of Regional Myocardial Work

Sugawara *et al.*[8] have shown that the area enclosed by the T–A loop is approximately equal to the actual work done by that region, i.e.,

$$\text{Work} = \oint_{\text{cycle}} TdA \tag{1}$$

However, studying their experimental data [8] suggests that the wall tension T ($=PR/2$) is almost constant throughout the cardiac cycle. Hence, the following approximation can be applied:

$$\text{Work} = \frac{P_{es}R_{es}}{2} (A_{ed} - A_{es}) \tag{2}$$

where, P_{es} and R_{es} are the ES pressure and endocardial radius of curvature respectively, and A_{ed} and A_{es} are the ED and ES endocardial area of the studied cuboid, respectively.

Finally, in order to obtain a comparable index, the work done by each myocardial cuboid was normalized to its mass and multiplied by 100 to provide a work index per 100gr tissue:

$$W = \frac{\text{Work}}{V \cdot \rho} \cdot 100 \tag{3}$$

where, W is a normalized work index [J/100gr/beat], V is the volume enclosed by the myocardial cuboid and ρ is the myocardial density.

Assessment of Global Work

In order to obtain some validation for the method, the global hydraulic work (Work$_H$), i.e., the P–V loop area, was calculated using the following approximation:

$$\text{Work}_H = \frac{(P_{es} + P_{ed})}{2} \cdot (V_{ed} - V_{es}) \tag{4}$$

where the average diastolic (P_{ed}) and systolic (P_{es}) pressure at the aorta is multiplied by the LV stroke volume, ($V_{ed}-V_{es}$).

While the calculated regional work relates to a small myocardial cuboid, Work_H represents the global work done by the LV. Thus, in order to enable an adequate comparison between the two, Work_H was normalized to the LV myocardial mass. Global LV mass was calculated by subtracting the volume enclosed by the endocardium from the volume enclosed by the epicardium. Volumes were computed using the set of short axis images, and were calculated by:

$$V = \Delta Z \left(\sum_{i=1}^{NS} A_i + \frac{A_1}{2} + \frac{A_{NS}}{3} \right) \tag{5}$$

where A_i is the cross section area of the ith slice, subscript NS denotes the number of short axis slices and ΔZ is the distance between two consecutive slice centers (about 1 cm). Thus, the work index W obtained from the estimated P–V loop area was:

$$W_H = \frac{\text{Work}_H}{(V_{epi} - V_{endo}) \cdot \rho} \cdot 100 \tag{6}$$

RESULTS

The average regional work index (W) calculated using the T–A loop (Eq. (3)) from 138 myocardial cuboids (six excluded) in the six dogs was 0.242±0.088 (SD) [Joules/ 100 gr/beat] which is comparable with the reported results [8] (after units modification). The average work index derived from the global hydraulic work, i.e., work calculated using the P–V loop via Eq.6, was 0.296±0.089 Joules/100gr/beat for the six dogs studied. The two estimates of myocardial work were correlated by linear regression (Fig. 2), yielding the following line equation:

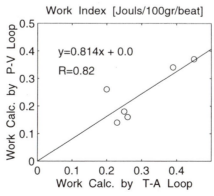

Figure 2. Correlation between the work index obtained for the six dogs using the P–V loop vs. the values obtained using the T–A loop.

$$W = W_H \cdot 0.814 \qquad (7)$$

with a correlation coefficient of R=0.82 (RMS=0.06).

The finding that the work index estimated by the T–A loop is of lower magnitude as compared to the one calculated from the P–V loop (slope=0.84) may be attributed to the fact that this technique is based on measurements which are made only at the endocardium. The inclusion of epicardial area deformations and transmural thickening (both can be obtained from the 3D data) may improve the assessments of the regional myocardial work. However, a reliable mechanical model of the LV wall is required.

CONCLUSIONS

The regional myocardial work index estimated from the T–A loop using tagged MRI 3D data is in fair agreement with that estimated using the P–V loop. This agreement implies that MRI tagging in 3D may be used to assess regional myocardial work *in vivo*. The major advantages of this method are that it is hazardless and non–invasive. Further-more, while myocardial work estimated from the P–V loop corresponds to the entire LV, the work index calculated from the T–A loop corresponds to a defined small myocardial region. Thus, it could be used to study the *in vivo* consumption of energy by various myocardial regions under different physiological conditions. This can be beneficial in basic studies of cardiac mechanics, and can, perhaps, serve as an index of clinical merit.

Comparison to oxygen consumption is still required to validate the method and evaluate its accuracy.

DISCUSSION

Dr. N. Westerhof: Did you find any variability in the work values which you have calculated from the small cuboids?

Dr. H. Azhari: Yes, the standard deviation was 0.088, quite large in fact.

Dr. N. Westerhof: Is this a measurement error or do you think these are real differences?

Dr. H. Azhari: The accuracy of locating a tag point was within 1 mm and the number of cuboids studied was quite large. Therefore, I presume a major portion of the scatter may be attributed to inherent physiological variability.

Dr. N. Westerhof: When you repeat the measurements for several beats, do you find them to be the same?

Dr. H. Azhari: The imaging protocol used here was a "spin–ECHO multi–slice multi–phase" protocol using an old MRI scanner. Therefore, it took us almost an hour to acquire the images required for reconstructing a single heart beat. With more modern scanners, imaging time is much shorter, and one could probably study the variability in several heart beats.

Dr. J.B. Bassingthwaighte: The standard deviation that you are observing fits the kind of standard deviation that we see in flows. Is that a true variation? Let us assume for the sake of argument that it is a true variation and not a methodologic variation. Then the degree of variation also fits what

Dr. McCulloch described (Chapter 19). It may be that what Dr. McCulloch sees as areas of high work are also the areas of high flow, high substrate uptake, and so on.

Dr. H. Azhari: I agree, there is no reason why all myocardial regions should work exactly the same.

Dr. P. Hunter: How do you interpret your tension, T. What does it mean? Have you compared it with the published work on stresses in the heart as a principal stress or fiber stress?

Dr. H. Azhari: This definition of T was applied by Sugawara et al. [8]. We have used it because we wanted to be consistent with their method. I agree that this is probably not the best index in the world. They [8] also refer to it as such, and they use a thick walled spherical model to evaluate their error. However, I would like to emphasize the fact that the real measurements here are geometrical. The other parameters are derived from the assumed model. If a more sophisticated model or a better constitutive law for the myocardium is used, then a more reliable estimate would be obtained. This study was merely a feasibility test.

Dr. N. Westerhof: This T index is of course derived from the simplest form of the Laplace equation, so it is not Sugawara who found it.

Dr. H. Azhari: Correct. Sugawara et al. [8] only used this index in their study. The point is, however, that they used an invasive procedure of implanting ultrasonic transducers. On the other hand, we tried to reproduce the T–A loop with the noninvasive MRI. As we wanted to stay as close as possible to their model, we used the same T index.

Dr. R. Beyar: I do not know how much of the variability is due to the noise of measurement or how much of it is real data. But with this type of imaging, the most problematic measurement is the curvature which comes into this T measurement. The curvature is a very sensitive index. If you miss by one pixel you may get a huge change, like 100%, in the T value. I am sure there is a large variability in the measurement of this curvature which then translates to tension. I would consider the issue of variability in the results here as a point which needs to be better investigated.

Dr. H. Azhari: I agree. Curvature analysis is a pitfall. The approach offered by Miyozaki et al. [6], using the pressure–thickness loop may be less sensitive to tracing error if the volume element method is applied [Beyar et al. Circulation 1990;81:297]. The question is how reliable is it as an index of regional work? That I do not know.

Dr. A. McColloch: There are essentially two types of simplifications that have been made in the estimation of stress in the past. One is to assume that the stress can be computed just by considering the equilibrium of the heart as though it were a membrane, like Laplace did. In that case, the stress becomes only a function of the pressure, which you have to measure. The other simplification is to assume that the stress only depends on the strain and that there is a one–to–one relationship between the fiber stress and fiber strain, which is also a simplification. This is the approach that has been used by Prinzen and Arts [Prinzen et al. J Biomechanics 1984;17:801] and others. Instead of using the pressure directly, they essentially use the strain to estimate the stress and hence get the work. How does your approach compare with that of Prinzen and Arts?

Dr. H. Azhari: It is possible to apply the Prinzen and Arts approach to our MRI measurements [e.g. McGowan et al., Circulation, 1997]. However, we did not compare the two approaches. Again, I would like to emphasize the fact that the only thing one can measure (regionally) here is geometry. There is no gold standard (and we have been chasing it!) for measuring stress within the myocardium. Therefore, it does not matter how sophisticated the model is, as long as there is no gold standard to verify your calculations you will be relying on assumptions. I believe the right way would be to integrate the force–time loop and the force–velocity loop, and see how close one can get to the oxygen consumption, if you can measure it. That might provide a verification to our method in an uncorrelated manner.

REFERENCES

1.   Baan J, Jong TTA, Kerkhof P, Moene R, Van Dijk AD, Van Der Velde E, Koops J. Continuou troke volume and cardiac output from intraventricular dimensions obtained with impedance catheter. *Cardiovasc Res* 1981;15:356.

2.   Takaoka H, Takeuchi M, Odake M, Hata K, Hayashi Y, Mori M, Yokoyama M. Depressed contractile state and increased myocardial consumption for non–mechanical work in patients with heart failure due to old myocardial infarction. *Cardiovasc Res* 1994;28(8):1251–1257

3.   Krams R, Duncker DJ, McFalls EO, Hogendoorn A, Verdouw PD. Dobutamine restores the reduced efficiency of energy transfer from total mechanical work to external mechanical work in stunned porcine myocardium. *Cardiovasc Res* 1993;27(5):740–747.

4.   Kissling G. Mechanical determinants of myocardial oxygen consumption with special reference to external work and efficiency. *Cardiovasc Res* 1992;26(9):886–892.

5.   Kedem J, Lee WW, Weiss HR. An experimental technique for estimating regional myocardial segment work *in vivo*. *Ann Biomed Eng* 1994;22(1):58–65.

6.   Miyazaki S, Goto Y, Guth BD, Miura T, Indolfi C, Ross J Jr. Changes in regional myocardial function and external work in exercising dogs with ischemia. *Am J Physiol* 1993;264(1 Pt 2): H110–H116.

7.   McFalls EO, Duncker DJ, Krams R, Sassen LM, Hoogendoorn A, Verdouw PD. Recruitment of myocardial work and metabolism in regionally stunned porcine myocardium. *Am J Physiol* 1992;263 (6 Pt 2):H1724–H1731.

8.   Sugawara M, Tamiya K, Nakado K. Regional work of the ventricle: Wall tension–area relation. *Heart and Vessels* 1985;1:133–144.

9.   Zerhouni, EA, Parish DM, Rogers WJ, Yang A, Shapiro EP. Human heart: Tagging with MR imaging– A method for noninvasive assessment of myocardial motion. *Radiology* 1988;169:59–63.

10.   Azhari H, Weiss JL, Rogers WJ, Siu C, Zerhouni EA, Shapiro EP. Non–invasive quantification of principal strains in normal canine hearts using tagged MRI images in 3D. *Am J Physiol* 1993;264 (*Heart Circ Physiol* 33):H205–H216.

11.   Akima H. A new method of interpolation and smooth curve fitting based on local procedures. *J Assoc Comp Machinery* 1970;17(4):589–602.

CHAPTER 21

Noninvasive Measurement of Cardiac Strain with MRI

Leon Axel[1]

ABSTRACT

The motion sensitivity of cardiac magnetic resonance imaging (MRI) can be exploited to measure the motion patterns within the heart wall and thus to noninvasively calculate the intramyocardial strain. The resulting large data sets pose a challenge for visualization, but offer the potential of a greatly improved picture of cardiac dynamics. This may have both basic research and clinical applications.

INTRODUCTION

Conventional imaging methods to study heart wall motion have many limitations. Projection methods like contrast ventriculography and radionuclide blood pool imaging show only the motion of the projected endocardial surface. Tomographic imaging, e.g. ultrasound, MRI or fast CT, shows both the endocardial and epicardial surfaces, permitting measurement of wall thickening. However, the lack of identifiable landmarks within the wall prevents any study of nonradial components of motion or of intramural variations of motion. Furthermore, the motion of the curved heart wall through the fixed imaging plane can cause artifactual changes in the apparent motion and thickening of the imaged section. The roughness of the endocardial surface also decreases the reliability of wall thickening as a measure of regional function.

Invasive methods, such as biplane X–ray imaging of embedded metal markers within the heart wall, make it possible to study the motion of specific material points in

[1]Department of Radiology, Hospital of the University of Pennsylvania, 308 Stemmler, 36th & Hamilton Walk, Philadelphia, PA 19104–6086, USA

Analytical and Quantitative Cardiology
Edited by Sideman and Beyar, Plenum Press, New York, 1997

the heart wall. However, the process of implantation and the mechanical effects of the markers themselves may significantly alter the motion of the region to be studied. Furthermore, the technical difficulties of tracking a large number, or density, of such markers have limited the number of such material points that can be tracked in any given subject.

MAGNETIC RESONANCE IMAGING (MRI)

MRI is a useful new method for the evaluation of cardiac function. Conventional MRI can provide high quality tomographic images of the heart, with clear delineation of the myocardium from both blood in the chambers and epicardial fat, without the need for exogenous contrast agents. While image formation typically requires data acquisition over multiple heart beats, the synchronization of data acquisition with the cardiac cycle permits imaging of specific phases of the cycle, provided the heart beat is reasonably reproducible. Imaging in times short enough to suspend respiration, or with further synchronization to the respiratory cycle, permits compensation for respiratory motion.

In addition to its conventional tomographic imaging capability, MRI has intrinsic motion sensitivities that can be exploited to permit the study of intramural heart wall motion. These include magnetization tagging and motion–induced shifts.

Magnetization Tagging

Magnetization tagging to study motion relies on the persistence of any local perturbation of the magnetization for times on the order of the relaxation times; this is a large fraction of a second for myocardium. As the magnetization of the tissue is used to produce the signal displayed in MRI, a local perturbation of the magnetization will be seen as a corresponding visible mark in the resulting MR image. Since the magnetization moves with the underlying tissue, any motion between the time of magnetization tagging and subsequent imaging will be seen as a corresponding displacement of the image of the tag. If the tag is initially created as a plane of altered magnetization perpendicular to the imaging plane, the intersection of the tagged plane with the imaging plane will be seen as a dark stripe in the image. While selective excitation can be used to create small numbers of tags at desired positions, nonselective excitation with spatial modulation of magnetization (SPAMM) can be used to create a whole family of parallel tags simultaneously [1]. Creating a second family of tagging planes orthogonal to the first will result in a tagging grid (Fig. 1). Even with through–plane motion, the starting position of each point on a tagged line is known, at least relative to the normal to the initial position of the tagging plane. When using tagging grids, the initial position of a grid intersection is known in two dimensions. The positions of the centers of the tags or their intersections can be estimated to subpixel accuracy. However, the minimum spacing between tags that will allow them to be independently tracked depends on the resolution of the images. Tracking the positions of the tags thus provides a sampling of the material point displacement field within the heart wall, as a "Lagrangian" picture of the motion.

Motion Induced Phase Shifts

Motion–induced phase shifts provide an alternative way to study myocardial motion. The imaging can be controlled so as to introduce a phase shift in the signal proportional to the velocity along a selected direction. A phase reference image must also be obtained without velocity sensitization, in order to correct for other baseline phase offsets. The phase

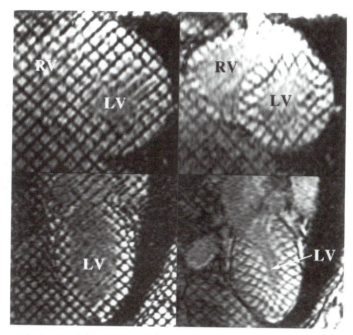

Figure 1. Mid–ventricular short axis **(top)** and long axis **(bottom)** tagged images of the left ventricle (LV) at end–diastole **(left)** and end–systole **(right)**. SPAMM strip deformation can clearly be seen between end–diastole and end–systole.

velocity measurement can potentially be made with greater precision than the tag displace–ment measurement, and with greater sampling density, although noise in the phase mea–surements will produce practical limits to these potential advantages. Additional images can be obtained with velocity sensitization in two other orthogonal directions, in order to find the 3D velocity distribution within the image plane, as an "Eulerian" picture of the motion.

STRAIN ANALYSIS

Strain refers to the differential motion between neighboring material points, normalized for their initial separation. Strain is a tensor property of the motion in a neighborhood. That is, it depends on the orientation of the points being considered. For example, at a given location in the heart wall, the wall may be extending or stretching in one direction, e.g. radially, at the same time as it is contracting or shrinking in another direction, e.g. circumferentially or longitudinally. The values of the strain components are thus generally different in different directions at a given location in the heart wall. The strain at a location can, however, be conveniently described by the principal strains, the direction and magnitude of the greatest stretching and shrinking at that location. The greatest and least principal strains are orthogonal to each other; the third principal strain is orthogonal to both. In general, there will also be shearing except along the directions of the principal strains. Given the principal strains, we can also find the corresponding components of the strains (and shears) in any desired local coordinate system. The strain rate refers to the differential velocity between neighboring points. It is the rate of accumulation of strain and is the tensor corresponding to the time derivative of the strain.

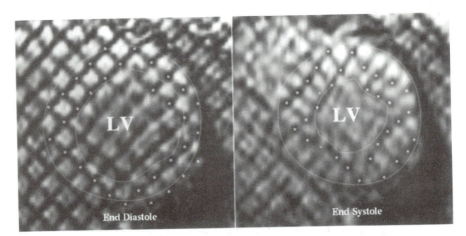

Figure 2. Mid–ventricular tagged images of the left ventricle (LV) at end–diastole (**left**) and end–systole (**right**). Both endocardial and epicardial contours as well as SPAMM stripe intersection points can be seen.

2D Strain

The 2D strain in a given imaged location is analyzed by tracking the positions of the tag grid intersections within the heart wall in successive images over the cardiac cycle (Fig. 2). We can group the grid points as triplets. If we treat the motion in the triangles between these triplets of grid intersections as homogeneous, the motion of the vertices of the triangle will uniquely determine both the homogeneous strain within the triangle and the rigid body components of the motion (displacement and rigid body rotation) [2]. We can integrate the myocardial velocity over the cardiac cycle to find the net displacements and then calculate the corresponding strains. However, integration error will tend to accumulate in the computed displacement due to noise in the phase measurement, decreasing the reliability of the result. Alternatively, we can directly calculate strain rate from the myocardial velocity, although this may be less directly related to the state of the myocardium than the strain itself.

3D Strain

The 3D strain in the heart wall is calculated by combining the wall motion data from multiple image locations. As each 2D tagged image of the heart only provides a 2D sampling of the displacement field within the heart wall, we need to combine data from tagged images acquired in different orientations (e.g. short– and long–axis images) to reconstruct the full 3D displacement field. One approach to such a 3D reconstruction is to use a finite element model to fit the tag motion data to a smoothly varying function of position within each element in the model [3, 4]. The corresponding strain field can then be directly calculated, without the need for assumptions of locally homogeneous strain (Fig. 3). Alternatively, the displacement field can be fit using a parameter function model of the heart wall motion, e.g. with functions such as torsion about the ventricular axis and radial and longitudinal scaling [5]. However, the calculation of the corresponding strains may be less straightforward with this approach.

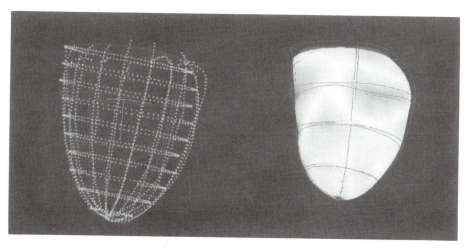

Figure 3. Three dimensional wire model of the left ventricle (FEM). The crosses represent contour data points; the lines represent the element borders (**left**). Three dimensional strain map of the same model (**right**). The variations in shading (when in color) represent different amounts of strain across the heart.

Tracking Structures

Tracking structures in MR images involves manual or more automated methods. The contours of the heart wall itself can be tracked. This will provide conventional global measures of cardiac function such as ejection fraction, as well as local wall thickening measures, and determine the region to be fit for 3D modeling of the wall motion. Unfortunately, the myocardial wall/cavity interface is not always well defined, due to effects such as noise, flow–dependent image contrast and the cardiac cycle–dependent appearance of the trabeculae. The locations of the intersections of tagging grids can be matched up between images to provide a set of material point displacement data. Manually tracing contours or tracking grid intersection points is straightforward but tedious, and is subject to some inter–observer variation. Fully automated approaches to extract position data are subject to error due to the image imperfections mentioned above. However, semiautomated approaches, using human guidance, can considerably speed up the process of extracting position data from the images. A useful semiautomated approach is the use of the active contour model, or "snakes" [6]. In this method, we use splines to track contours or tag lines. Associated with each such spline curve is an energy, determined by a combination of image "forces", spline "stiffness" and user–supplied "forces" (useful for pushing the line away from undesired features and onto the desired ones).

Data Visualization

Data visualization of the results of strain analysis can be difficult, as the data produced has a high dimensionality. Even for 2D strain analysis we have multiple variables of motion to consider, such as rotation and displacement, some of the motion variables are not even vectors (such as displacement) but tensors (strain), and the whole system evolves in time. In 3D strain analysis, we not only add to the dimensions of the motion variables to be considered, we must display them within the thick shell of the heart wall. The task is eased somewhat if we use the capabilities of an interactive workstation for the display, e.g. for dynamic "movie" loops and interactive rotation of the heart. However, hard copy is still restricted to sets of still 2D image displays.

DISCUSSION

Data on normal left ventricular (LV) function provided noninvasively by tagged MRI is now available. Normal LV regional motion data can be used to better understand the mechanisms of cardiac contraction. In particular, the relation between regional strain, provided by MRI, and the local fiber structure of the heart wall can be used to examine phenomena such as the subendocardial cross–fiber shortening.

Potential clinical applications of MRI for regional strain measures may arise from the alterations of regional wall motion seen in a range of diseases of the heart. Global alterations in cardiac function, such as those due to valvular disease, can be reflected in the values of regional measures such as circumferential shortening, even in the presence of normal values of traditional indices such as the ejection fraction. Regional alterations in cardiac function, such as those due to ischemia and infarction or to hypertrophic cardiomyopathy, are also accompanied by corresponding changes in the MRI–derived measures of regional function. The methods described above for the analysis of LV function can also be applied to the study of the right ventricle (RV) [7]. The hypertrophied RV can be treated similarly to the LV. However, even the motion of the relatively thin walled normal RV can be analyzed, e.g. using 3D analysis of the tag motion to reconstruct the contraction patterns in the plane of the RV free wall.

There are several limitations in the current methods used for MRI strain measurements. MR imaging methods, while continuing to improve steadily, still have limitations due to their limited spatial resolution (e.g. limiting the ability to assess the transmural distribution of function) and temporal evolution (e.g. limiting the ability to study more rapid motion such as in early diastole). The current analysis methods also still have some limitations. The speed of the image and strain analysis must be improved in order to make this a practical clinical tool. Ways of registering the motion data between examinations need to be improved, particularly when there may be significant changes in the cardiac morphology between the examinations, as with stress, in serial studies with longer time bases and between different subjects. As mentioned above, the display of the dense data sets produced with these methods is intrinsically difficult. However, progress is being made in all these areas, and it is reasonable to expect there to be significant improvements in MRI strain measurements in the near future.

There are several directions that this work can be extended to. An integrated model of the motion of the LV and the RV will permit analysis of their interaction in health and disease. Combining strain analysis with MRI studies of perfusion will permit study of conditions where there can be mismatches of function and perfusion such as in stunning and hibernation. Performing strain measurements in conjunction with myocardial stress, e.g. with dobutamine loading, can provide a measure of functional reserve, e.g. in ischemic heart disease. Integrating a database of normal strain values into the display program will permit highlighting those regions with abnormal motion. The improved strain measurement provided by MRI methods should lead to improvements in stress–strain modeling of the heart wall. Finally, the strain evolution in the presence of abnormal electrical activation, such as due to aberrant pathways or pacemakers, should provide improved understanding of the electrical/mechanical coupling in such settings.

CONCLUSIONS

The noninvasive measurement of strain with MRI has effectively opened up a new window into the analysis of cardiac function. While limitations still remain, these methods have already provided an unprecedented level of information on regional cardiac function in intact subjects. It is likely that noninvasive strain measurement will become at least an important research tool and, potentially, a useful clinical tool as well.

Acknowledgement

This work was funded by NIH grant R01–HL43014.

DISCUSSION

Dr. D. Noble: What are the criteria for the tissue to be successfully tagged?

Dr. L. Axel: First, you can not have such a short relaxation time that the tag would essentially evaporate before making the image. For example, in fat which has a shorter relaxation time than muscle, the tags fade more rapidly, some 100 ms as opposed to several 100 ms which we find for the muscle. In scarring, where you have replacement by collagen, we have lengthening of the realization time, so that would not be expected to be a problem. In edema, you have lengthened relaxation time so that is not a problem. If you are combining this with a contrast study of perfusion, you would want to do a tagging study first, and then do the perfusion study because the contrast agent will shorten your relaxation time, so you will have less tag persistence. The other criterion is that there have to be enough signals to look at. If you have myocardial scars, they are stiff but they tend to have lower signals because of the longer T1 relaxation time and shorter T2, so a scar may be less suitable for tagging studies.

Dr. D. Noble: Do you have to keep retagging if you are going to pursue something over a period of time?

Dr. L. Axel: Typically, only one portion of the data necessary to reconstruct the image is acquired per heart cycle. In most of the images discussed here, only 1/128 of the image data were acquired per heart beat, so it takes 128 heart beats to acquire an image. If you want to sacrifice a little bit of temporal resolution within a cardiac cycle, you can acquire data in a breath hold. That is the way we do most of our studies; we acquire about 16 heart beats worth of data to reconstruct the full cardiac cycle. You get multiple images corresponding to multiple cycle phases at one location in one breath hold. You can go faster and even do a single heart beat image but you sacrifice having enough resolution to get good tag sampling, so we have not pursued single heart beat imaging.

Dr. H. Strauss: Could you determine the possible effects resulting from a change in activation sequence of the heart on the stress–strain relationships in the ventricle? It has been long appreciated that you see electrical remodeling of the heart (T wave memory) associated with change in pacemaker site from the sinus node to a ventricular site when you pace the ventricle. One of the questions is what has been the transducing mechanisms. Do stress–strain relationships in the ventricle change appreciably with ventricular pacing as opposed to normal sinus activation of the heart?

Dr. L. Axel: We are just getting into the pacing business ourselves. We do not have the experience that the Hopkins group has. What they have found is that, basically, if you have a ventricular pacing site, you get early activation at that region. It starts to move, but then it stiffens up and you do not have the same amount of contraction at the pacing site that you do at the rest of the ventricle. The wave propagates relatively slowly around the ventricle. You would expect that when you hit conduction pathways the wave would spread rapidly, but in fact it does not. It just goes around the muscle. The early activation site does not contract fully; it acts as a stiffened brace that the rest of the heart contracts relative to. This may be part of the reason why when you activate the site of hypertrophic cardiomyopathy with septal predominance early, it keeps it from contracting fully and you do not get the usual kind of collapse of the outflow tract. But in terms of what the underlying stresses are, it just has to be an inference. You know what the boundary conditions are, the blood is pressurized to the same level all around the heart so the heart is being tensed up against the same blood pressure in the chamber, but you do not really know what is in the wall, so it has to be inference.

Dr. D. Adam: Can you elaborate about the way you calculate the exact location of each intersection. The tags are quite wide. How do you chose the location? What kind of techniques do you implement?

Dr. L. Axel: The tags themselves are of the order of one or two pixels wide. We fit the tags with a spline, a smooth curve which has constraints on it so that the curve will settle to the middle, to the bottom of the trough of the intensity, that is, it wants to go to the minimum energy at the darkest part of the stripe and so will tend to settle there, even if the tag is an extended region. There is also a smoothness constraint, in effect a certain amount of stiffness and rigidity that can be controlled interactively. So the curve will tend to move smoothly through the image, even though you have a discrete pixel structure of the image; again you tend to fit it with a smooth line. There is an additional term that you can use to nudge it away from points that you do not want, or towards desired points. For example, at the base of the heart, at the valve plane, there may not be a convenient line to track, so you can pin it down to where your eye guesses is the best estimate of the location of the base of the heart.

REFERENCES

1. Axel, L., Dougherty, L. Heart wall motion: improved method of spatial modulation of magnetization for MR imaging. *Radiology* 1989;172:349–350
2. Axel L, Gonçalves R, Bloomgarden D. Two–dimensional analysis and functional imaging of regional heart wall motion with MR imaging. *Radiology* 1992;183(3):745–750.
3. Young AA, Axel L. Three–dimensional motion and deformation of the heart wall: estimation with spatial modulation of magnetization – a model based approach. *Radiology* 1992;185:241–247.
4. Young AA, Kraitchman DL, Dougherty L, Axel L. Tracking and finite element modeling of stripe deformation in magnetic resonance tagging. *IEEE–TMI* 1995; 14(3): 413–421.
5. Park J, Metaxas D, Axel L. Analysis of left ventricular wall motion based on volumetric deformable models and MRI–SPAMM. *Medical Image Analysis* 1996;1:53–71.
6. Kass M., Witkin A., Tezopoulos D. Snakes: active contour models. *Int J Comput Vis* 1988;1(4): 321–333.
7. Fayad, Z. Magnetic resonance imaging studies of right ventricular regional mechanical function. *Ph.D. Dissertation* 1996, University of Pennsylvania, Philadelphia.

CHAPTER 22

VENTRICULAR REMODELING: FROM BEDSIDE TO MOLECULE

Ronen Jaffe, Moshe Y. Flugelman, David A. Halon, and Basil S. Lewis[1]

ABSTRACT

The multiple mechanisms that bring about the decompensation of the hypertrophic remodeled myocardium are synergistic and not fully understood. Our current hypothesis is that the increased stress on the ventricle is initially offset by compensatory myocardial hypertrophy. In many instances, however, progressive ventricular dilatation and heart failure occur as a result of maladaptive hypertrophy (abnormal myosin–actin production), programmed cell death (apoptosis) and/or changes in the interstitial vasculature and collagen composition. The molecular and genetic background to these processes includes changes in myocardial gene expression, activation of the local tissue renin–angiotensin and other neurohormonal systems, increased matrix metalloproteinase activity (including collagenase), and expression of certain components of the immune system, such as TNF–α. Future research will hopefully provide better methods for limiting the remodeling–ventricular dilatation process by novel pharmacotherapies, gene therapy and, possibly, surgical therapy, and determine the impact of such interventions on survival.

INTRODUCTION

Although congestive heart failure has diverse etiologies with multiple pathophysiologic mechanisms, the common end point is a dilated heart which contracts poorly. The pathogenetic process involved in the development of this state has been termed ventricular remodeling, a concept relating to a complex of anatomic, physiologic, histologic

---

[1]The Department of Cardiology, Lady Davis Carmel Medical Center and the Bruce Rappaport School of Medicine, Technion–IIT, Haifa, Israel

and molecular changes that the myocardium undergoes in response to injury and increased wall stress. Pressure overload, volume overload and cell death increase wall stress and activate compensatory myocardial hypertrophy, an initially adaptive process, but one ultimately resulting in further deterioration of myocardial function.

Our understanding of ventricular remodeling has progressed rapidly from initial bedside observation of large hearts in patients with heart disease to studies of the mechanical consequences of increased volumes, hemodynamic changes and wall stress in the failing left ventricle (LV). Following a description of the neurohormonal mechanisms in heart failure, we have more recently directed our attention to investigating the molecular and genetic alterations that promote further deterioration in the function of the heart and determine the inexorable course to end–stage heart failure. A number of important questions in the remodeling process need to be addressed: 1) The relative interplay between systemic mechanical loading conditions and local myocardial tissue responses to stress, 2) the reason why compensatory adaptive hypertrophy is often inadequate to prevent further deterioration ("maladaptive hypertrophy"), 3) the relative importance of changes in myocardium, interstitium and vasculature, and 4) the molecular and genetic processes underlying and integrating these changes.

Anatomic and Hemodynamic Observations

LV dilatation is a common result of *transmural myocardial infarction*, occurring most frequently after occlusion of the left anterior descending artery [1]. LV volume enlarges initially as a result of infarct expansion [2] but subsequent enlargement occurs in the non–infarcted segments as the result of increased stress on the residual myocardium, with consequent development of eccentric hypertrophy [3, 4]. Hypertrophy is commonly insufficient to normalize the mass:volume ratio; wall stress increases, further dilatation occurs and, according to Laplace's law, stress is again increased, thus establishing a vicious cycle [5]. LV geometry changes from elliptic to spherical [6, 7] and functional mitral regurgitation may appear [8].

Ventricular remodeling also occurs in response to *non–ischemic myocardial injury*, where, at a mechanical level, normalization of wall stress appears to be an important transducer in the biologic processes promoting ventricular hypertrophy (Fig. 1) [9, 10]. Hypertensive cardiomyopathy and aortic stenosis are associated with pressure overload, increased wall stress and concentric hypertrophy [11]. Mitral and aortic regurgitation cause volume overload and eccentric hypertrophy as a mechanism to maintain normal mid–wall stress. In acute myocarditis and idiopathic dilated cardiomyopathy, cell death triggers similar responses [12], but the inability of the diseased myocardium to adapt in this situation results in a higher stress and end–diastolic pressure in many of these patients and an adverse prognosis.

Remodeling after myocardial infarction is associated with increased mortality [13]. For the same degree of ventricular dysfunction, as measured by ejection fraction, a larger end–systolic volume is associated with a poorer prognosis [14]. Prevention or reversal of remodeling is therefore the goal of many therapeutic strategies designed to arrest or reverse progression to heart failure. In the elderly, decreased remodeling has been correlated with a worse prognosis [15], suggesting that in some instances the process may primarily be a compensatory mechanism. Some aspects of the remodeling process may be beneficial and attempts to prevent remodeling may theoretically act as a double–edged sword in some instances.

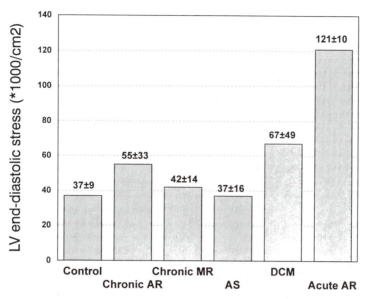

Figure 1. Left ventricular (LV) circumferential end–diastolic stress in control subjects and in patients with different cardiac diseases. End–diastolic stress was relatively normal in all patient groups with chronic mitral (MR) and aortic regurgitation (AR) and aortic stenosis (AS). Stress was increased in dilated cardiomyopathy (DCM), who had a worse prognosis and greater cardiac dilatation and very high in patients with acute AR due to valve rupture, where there was insufficient time for adaptive mechanisms to come into play.

MECHANISMS OF PROGRESSION OF HEART FAILURE

The exact sequence of events by which an injured but functioning heart decompensates remain to be defined. Several aspects should be considered: cellular myocardial changes, interstitial and vascular changes, the renin–angiotensin system and the changes in gene expression underlying these processes (Fig. 2).

Myocyte Structure, Metabolism, Energetics and Gene Expression

Early after transmural myocardial infarction, the infarcted segment expands through thinning and slippage of the necrotic myofibrils, with an acute increase in the surface area [16, 17, 21]. The resulting increase in wall stress activates neurohormonal pathways that induce compensatory myocardial hypertrophy in the non–infarcted segments [1, 4, 18]. This hypertrophy involves a disproportionate increase in the length/width ratio of the sarcomeres [19]. Although myocytes are terminally differentiated cells and theoretically unable to multiply, myocyte hyperplasia has recently been observed in failing hearts [20].

Changes in myocardial metabolism and energetics have been described in the hypertrophic and failing heart. Glucose utilization is enhanced while fatty acid oxidation is decreased [21]. High energy phosphate reserves are compromised [22, 23], adenosine–tri–phosphate (ATP) resynthesis via the creatine kinase (CK) reaction is decreased and CK activity is reduced [24]. Mitochondrial damage has been reported in ischemic [25] and dilated cardiomyopathy [12]. A mismatch between the relative volume of the energy consuming myofibrillar component of the myocytes compared with the number of mitochondria has been described [26]. As a result, the failing heart may be chronically "energy starved" [27].

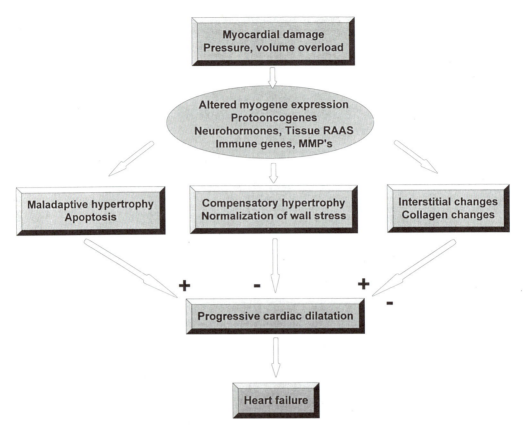

Figure 2. Pathogenetic mechanisms operating in a patient undergoing ventricular damage, pressure and/or volume overload. Changes in gene expression involving the myocardium, interstitium, tissue renin–angiotensin–aldosterone, immune and other system(s) promote myocardial hypertrophy, both compensatory and maladaptive, and changes in collagen and interstitial tissues. The end–result in many patients is progressive ventricular dilatation and advancing heart failure.

Myofibrillar atrophy occurs secondary to interstitial fibrosis [28] and myocyte synthetic activity is depressed under chronic adrenergic stimulation [29]. Changes in gene expression for beta–myosin heavy chain (β–MHC) and cardiac and skeletal actin are observed [30]. Myofilament composition undergoes changes with a decrease in myosin content and myofibrillar Mg–ATPase [22]. Altered sarcoplasmic reticulum Ca^{2+} ATPase gene expression may underlie the prominent diastolic dysfunction that characterizes the hypertrophied failing myocardium [31].

Myocyte loss occurs in chronic heart failure. An important mechanism for cell loss may be through programmed cell death, or apoptosis. In the normal differentiating myocyte, gene expression shifts from production of fetal muscle–specific proteins to the production of adult gene products. Overloading of the adult heart initiates an immediate–early gene response [26] which is characterized by active protein synthesis. However, because the cell cycle remains blocked, the heart undergoes an unnatural growth response. The compensa–tory hypertrophic myocardium may thus be maladaptive (the "cardiomyopathy of overload" described by Katz) [26], with abnormal structure and metabolism and a propensity to programmed cell death (apoptosis) (Fig. 2). The underlying "fetal" genetic program reactivated in patients with heart failure [26, 32] includes protooncogenes such as c–*fos*, c–*myc* and c–*jun* [15], which are known activators of apoptosis. Stretch induced apoptosis, which may be induced by increased wall stress, has been described in animal models [33]. Apoptosis was observed in all of four explanted human hearts with dilated cardiomyopathy [34] but was less widespread in three patients explanted for ischemic heart disease.

Neurohormonal Activation

Activation of both the adrenergic and renin–angiotensin–aldosterone (RAAS) systems plays an important role in the adaptation of the myocardium to increased wall stress. These systems, however, are also involved in the pathophysiology of heart failure and elevated plasma norepinephrine levels predict increased mortality in survivors of myocardial infarction [35].

Adrenergic stimulation has a positive inotropic and chronotropic effect, maintaining adequate stroke volume in the face of an acute decrease in the number of contractile elements [36]. The effects increase myocardial oxygen consumption and may exacerbate ischemia. An increase in preload, which increases cardiac output via the Frank–Starling mechanism, occurs by activation of both the RAAS and adrenergic systems. Aldosterone stimulates salt and water absorption in the kidney, while both RAAS and adrenergic systems induce arginine vasopressin release from the neurohypophysis [37]. Angiotensin II and norepinephrine are powerful vasoconstrictors which maintain tissue perfusion despite reduced cardiac output, but in doing so increase impedance to LV outflow and further increase wall stress.

In the SAVE, ISIS 4, AIRE and SMILE studies [38–41], administration of an ACE inhibitor improved survival in patients recovering from acute myocardial infarction. In the SAVE study, however, where a substudy of echocardiographically determined ventricular geometry was performed, the difference in LV areas between patients treated with the ACE inhibitor captopril and placebo was quantitatively unimpressive [42], amounting to no more than 3 cm^2, or the volume contained in a tea–spoon. This finding suggests that ACE inhibitors improve prognosis by mechanisms other than load and volume reduction, probably by a local tissue paracrine–autocrine mechanism involving changes in cardiac growth. Angiotensin II and norepinephrine are both potent growth factors which promote myocyte hypertrophy [26, 37]. RAAS activates fibroblasts to deposit collagen in the interstitium and causes fibrosis [28], leading to diastolic and systolic dysfunction and progression of heart failure. In transgenic rats, local cardiac renin–angiotensin system activation has been shown to induce ventricular hypertrophy [32]. ACE has been detected in LV myocytes adjacent to the myocardial infarct zone [43] and myocardial angiotensin I synthesis and conversion to angiotensin II have been demonstrated in humans in response to a low salt diet [44]. The role of ACE in maintaining tissue angiotensin II levels has been questioned since the documentation of continued activity of the hormone despite ACE inhibitor therapy [45]. Local angiotensin conversion has been attributed to a chymase–angiotensin system [46] which may upregulate tissue angiotensin II levels despite ACE inhibitor therapy. Angiotensin receptor antagonists such as losartan may therefore act in synergy with ACE inhibitors in prevention of RAAS mediated ventricular remodeling.

Other mechanisms whereby activation of noradrenaline and the renin–angiotensin system play a role in progression of ventricular remodeling and heart failure include the induction by both systems of the "fetal" gene programs implicated in myocyte loss through programmed cell death [47, 48]. Increased levels of catecholamines are associated with β–receptor downregulation, reduced levels of cAMP and depressed myocyte contraction [49, 50]. Catecholamines cause direct myocyte toxicity and can aggravate cell loss [29].

Interstitial Changes

The normal supporting collagen matrix is disrupted early during myocardial infarction [16, 17]. Rupture of intermyocyte collagen struts and myocyte slippage bring about early dilatation of the infarct zone. These changes may be mediated by activation of matrix metalloproteinases of which collagenase is one [51] (Fig. 2). Decreased collagen deposition correlates with increased ventricular remodeling after myocardial infarction in animal models [52].

Type I collagen, which has the tensile strength of steel, is the predominant collagen in the adult heart. During the early healing phase, mature type I collagen is replaced in the infarct zone by type III collagen which is more distensible [28]. The functioning myocardium surrounding the infarct zone subsequently undergoes fibrosis as activated fibroblasts deposit collagen, especially type I [53]. The pattern of types I and III procollagen expression thus differs between the infarct zone and the surrounding myocardium, suggesting that collagen synthesis may be regulated differently between the two zones.

The renin–angiotensin–aldosterone system plays a major role in fibroblast activation. Angiotensin II has been shown to induce collagen formation and to inhibit matrix metalloproteinase activation [54] in cultured rat cardiac fibroblasts. Angiotensin converting enzyme (ACE) inhibitors may exert part of their cardioprotective effect through a reduction in non–infarct zone fibrosis.

Vascular Changes

The myocardial vasculature is an obligatory determinant in the pathophysiology of ventricular remodeling, and angiographic studies show an increase in epicardial coronary arterial diameter which parallels the increase in ventricular muscle mass [55]. The changes in gene expression inherent in the development of ventricular hypertrophy are also relevant regarding vascular growth. Intramyocardial coronary arteries undergo medial thickening [56], which may eventually cause ischemia and further cell death. Coronary perfusion is decreased in the hypertrophied myocardium as a result of fibrosis and structural changes in the capillary network [57], and coronary flow reserve decreased, resulting in tissue hypoxia. Additionally, endothelial function may be impaired in heart failure [58]. These changes may underlie the findings of focal sub–endocardial necrosis secondary to stress induced ischemia [59].

POTENTIAL THERAPEUTIC APPROACHES: FROM MOLECULE TO BEDSIDE

Apart from the classic approaches to treatment of heart failure aimed at decreasing ventricular load (dietary salt restriction, diuretics, digoxin and vasodilators), it has become clear that drugs inhibiting the systemic and local renin–angiotensin system or interfering with angiotensin receptor activation are essential to limit ventricular remodeling and improve survival. A very promising area of research at a molecular level is the possibility of genetic engineering to alter myocardial and interstitial growth and composition. At the other end of the spectrum, at a macroscopic and mechanical level, the results of newer surgical intervention to repair or remove extensive fibrosis (aneurysmectomy), to resect dilated tissue (ventriculectomy) or to use skeletal muscle wrapped around the ventricle (dynamic cardiomyoplasty) are presently under study. These techniques produce abrupt "reversed remodeling" [60] of the ventricle and the long–term results await elucidation.

CONCLUSIONS

Ventricular remodeling following ventricular damage, pressure and/or volume overload, is the beginning of a process of progressive ventricular dilatation which causes end–stage heart failure in a large number of patients. The precise series of events leading to this inexorable course is complex and relates to an interplay of factors at a hemodynamic, mechanical and molecular level. Mechanisms involved include changes in gene expression relating to the myocardium, interstitium, vasculature and neurohormonal systems. Intervention by novel pharmacotherapeutic, surgical and molecular biological techniques may alter the poor prognosis of patients with severe heart failure.

DISCUSSION

Dr. N. Alpert: Dr. Livzboch, a pathologist from Germany, counted cells in hypertrophied hearts and failing hearts and found there was no real reduction in cells. When the heart was much enlarged, the cells seem to split so they were increased in number. Is apoptosis really significant, or does it just happen to a small extent and not making a big difference in terms of the heart?

Another question regarding remodeling. If the heart is truly in failure, can it be remodeled in a positive way, such as you would expect from surgical treatment, or as you would expect from some of the other treatments that are available, like unloading. Dr. Francis [*Francis GS. Left ventricular remodelling: Cellular and morphometric considerations. J Mol Cell Cardiol 1996;28:A137*] from Minnesota presented a very interesting study where they had a heart on an assist device waiting for it to be transplanted. They took biopsies before and after a prolonged period on the assist device. Those hearts seemed to repair themselves, even though they had caused so much damage with the assist device that they had to replace the heart anyhow. Could that simply be myocarditis that then repaired itself instead of Class IV classical failure?

Dr. B.S. Lewis: We really know very little about apoptosis at this time. It is very difficult to study and the techniques for studying it are difficult to set up. Narula *et al.* [*Narula J, et al. Apoptosis in myocytes in end–stage heart failure. N Engl J Med 1996;335:1182–1189*] reported seven patients, a small experience; the findings could well be due to chance. Three had ischemic heart disease and four had end–stage cardiomyopathy. The question is: when duplicating sarcomeres and possibly myocytes, are we getting the maximum benefit, or producing abnormal myocardial proteins due to changes in gene expression in the failing heart? The terminally differentiated myocyte which does not enter the cell cycle may then become apoptopic. I look forward to more data in this regard and to more quantitative data regarding the extent and importance of the phenomenon.

Concerning end–stage heart failure, I agree with you that the end–stage heart is extremely interesting and we know little about the possibilities of "reversed remodeling" by surgery, assist devices or drugs. We recently had the unfortunate opportunity to look at an autopsy specimen of a young patient who died while awaiting transplantation. When you see the size of this gigantic LV, then you appreciate what is involved and wonder whether the recently suggested operation of ventricular resection (ventriculectomy) would make the situation any better. I am very skeptical. It is also surprising that in this situation any of the newer drugs actually improves the prognosis. It is possible that some cases of heart failure are self limiting, such as myocarditis. It is very hard to understand how, for example, a beta–blocker can reduce mortality by more than half in patients who have hearts that are thin–walled and overdilated like an overinflated balloon and do not look as if they are capable of contracting at all. What you have said is very relevant and highlights what we really do not know.

Dr. H. ter Keurs: One of the normal buttresses of the whole heart is the pericardium. What happens to the pericardium in your experience when dilatation takes place? I use the word dilatation because remodeling is many things and thereby lacking definition.

Dr. B.S. Lewis: We learn this from valve disease, where one sometimes gets the most dramatic changes. If one ruptures a valve, the volume of the ventricle, and hence that of the pericardial sac overloads. Dr. Ralph Shabetai of San Diego had very good data on the pericardium, including peri–cardial and transmural pressure, and the type and spatial and directional alignment of the collagen fibers in the pericardium. The pericardium is indeed an important player here. The pericardium has to adapt in some way and if it cannot adapt, then the intrapericardial and end–diastolic pressures go very high and the patient gets into trouble. One of the mechanisms of acute heart failure in acute aortic valve rupture is the inability of the pericardium to adapt quickly enough to the acute volume load, as it does with gradual onset volume overload. I should also mention that the buttressing effect of right heart structures should be taken into account in similar fashion to the pericardium.

Dr. D. Noble: Which T–channel calcium blocker have you used?

Dr. B.S. Lewis: Mibefradil, made by Roche. It is the only one that I know of. It is very interesting that it appears to prevent cell proliferation and hypertrophy in response to various stimuli and growth factors, such as angiotensin II and it seems that the T–channel may be an important transducer in the response of the heart to these stimuli. One of the changes in gene expression in the failing myocardium seems to be the appearance of T–channels (as in the fetus); in the adult heart they are only present in the conducting system and the vasculature. We are involved in a number of clinical trials using mibefradil and look forward to learning more about this very interesting new approach to calcium blockade and in particular to its possible effects in modifying ventricular hypertrophy.

REFERENCES

1.   Warren SE, Royal HD, Markis JE, Grossman W, McKay RG. Time course of left ventricular dilation after myocardial infarction: influence of infarct–related artery and success of coronary thrombolysis. *J Am Coll Cardiol* 1988;11:12–19.

2.   Erlebacher JA, Weiss JL, Weisfeldt ML, Bulkley BH. Early dilation of the infarcted segment in acute transmural myocardial infarction: role of infarct expansion in acute left ventricular enlargement. *J Am Coll Cardiol* 1984;4:201–208.

3.   Mitchell GF, Lamas GA, Vaughan DE, Pfeffer MA. Left ventricular remodeling in the year after first anterior myocardial infarction: a quantitative analysis of contractile segment lengths and ventricular shape. *J Am Coll Cardiol*, 1992;19:1136–1144.

4.   Rumberger JA, Behrenbeck T, Breen JR, Reed JE, Gersh BJ. Nonparallel changes in global left ventricular chamber volume and muscle mass during the first year after transmural myocardial infarction in humans. *J Am Coll Cardiol* 1993;2:673–682.

5.   Pfeffer JM, Pfeffer MA, Fletcher PJ, Braunwald E. Progressive ventricular remodeling in rat with myocardial infarction. *Am J Physiol* 1991;260:H1406–H1414.

6.   Greenberg B, Quinones MA, Koilpillai C, Limacher M, Shindler D, Benedict C, Shelton B. Effects of long–term enalapril therapy on cardiac structure and function in patients with left ventricular dysfunction. Results of the SOLVD echocardiography substudy. *Circulation* 1995;91:2573–2781.

7.   Douglas PS, Morrow R, Ioli A, Reichek N. Left ventricular shape, afterload and survival in idiopathic dilated cardiomyopathy. *J Am Coll Cardiol* 1989;13:311–315.

8.   Kono T, Sabbah HN, Rosman H, Alam M, Jafri S, Goldstein S. Left ventricular shape is the primary determinant of functional mitral regurgitation in heart failure. *J Am Coll Cardiol* 1992;20:1594–1598.

9.   Lewis BS, Gotsman MS. Cardiac hypertrophy and left ventricular end–diastolic stress. *Isr J Med Sci* 1975;11:299–303.

10.   Grossman W, Jones D, McLaurin LP. Wall stress and patterns of hypertrophy in the human left ventricle. *J Clin Invest* 1975;56:56–64.

11.   Anversa P, Ricci R, Olivetti G. Quantitative structural analysis of the myocardium during physiologic growth and induced cardiac hypertrophy: a review. *J Am Coll Cardiol* 1986;7:1140–1149.

12.   Schaper J, Froede R, Hein S, Buck A, Hashizume H, Speiser B, Friedl A, Bleese N. Impairment of the myocardial ultrastructure and changes of the cytoskeleton in dilated cardiomyopathy. *Circulation* 1991;83:504–514.

13.   Cohn JN, Archibald DG, Ziesche S, Franciosa JA, Harston WE, Tristani FE, Dunkman WB, Jacobs W, Francis GS, Flohr KH. Effect of vasodilator therapy on mortality in chronic congestive heart

failure. Results of a Veterans Administration Cooperative Study. *N Engl J Med* 1986;314:1547–1552.

14.   White HD, Norris RM, Brown MA, Brandt PW, Whitlock RM, Wild CJ. Left ventricular end–systolic volume as the major determinant of survival after recovery from myocardial infarction. *Circulation* 1987;76:44–51.

15.   Takahashi T, Schunkert H, Isoyama S, Wei JY, Nadal–Ginard B, Grossman W, Izumo S. Age–related differences in the expression of proto–oncogene and contractile protein genes in response to pressure overload in the rat myocardium. *J Clin Invest* 1992; 89:939–946.

16.   Olivetti G, Capasso JM, Sonnenblick EH, Anversa P. Side–to–side slippage of myocytes participates in ventricular wall remodeling acutely after myocardial infarction in rats. *Circ Res* 1990;67:23–34.

17.   Weisman HF, Bush DE, Mannisi JA, Weisfeldt ML, Healy B. Cellular mechanisms of myocardial infarct expansion. *Circulation* 1988;78:186–201.

18.   Beltrami CA, Finato N, Rocco M, Maurizio GA, Puricelli FC, Gigola E, Quai F, Sonnenblick EH, Olivetti G, Anversa P. Structural basis of end–stage failure in ischemic cardiomyopathy in humans. *Circulation* 1994;89:151–163.

19.   Gerdes AM, Kellerman SE, Moore JA, Muffly KE, Clark LC, Reaves PY, Malec KB, McKeown PP, Schocken DD. Structural remodeling of cardiac myocytes in patients with ischemic cardiomyopathy. *Circulation* 1992;86:426–430.

20.   Olivetti G, Melissari M, Balbi T, Quaini F, Sonnenblick EH, Anversa P. Myocyte nuclear and possible cellular hyperplasia contribute to ventricular remodeling in the hypertrophic senescent heart in humans. *J Am Coll Cardiol* 1994;24:140–149.

21.   Christe ME, Rodgers RL: Altered glucose and fatty acid oxidation in hearts of the spontaneously hypertensive rat. *J Mol Cell Cardiol* 1994;26:1371–1375.

22.   Bashore TM, Magorien DJ, Letterio J, Shaffer P, Unverferth DV. Histologic and biochemical correlates of keft ventricular chamber dynamics in man. *J Am Coll Cardiol* 1987;9:734–742.

23.   Zhang Y, Wang C, Eigelshoven MHJ, Yong, KC, Murakami Y, Ugurbil K, Bache RJ, Arthur HL. Functional and bio–energetic consequences of postinfarction left ventricular remodeling in a new porcine model. *Circulation* 1996;94:1089–1100.

24.   Nascimben L, Ingwall JS, Pauletto P, Friedrich J, Gwathmey JK, Saks V, Pessina AC, Allen PD. Creatine kinase system in failing and nonfailing human myocardium. *Circulation* 1996;94:1894–1901.

25.   Corral–Debrinski M, Stepien G, Shoffner JM, Lott MT, Kanter K, Wallace DC. Hypoxemia is associated with mitochondrial DNA damage and gene induction. *JAMA* 1991;266:1812–1816.

26.   Katz AM. The cardiomyopathy of overload: An unnatural growth response in the hypertrophied heart. *Ann Intern Med* 1994;121:363–371.

27.   Ingwall JS. Is cardiac failure a consequence of decreased energy reserve? *Circulation* 1993;87[suppl VII]:VII–58–VII–62.

28.   Weber KT, Brilla CG. Pathological hypertrophy and cardiac interstitium. *Circulation* 1991;83:1849–1865.

29.   Mann DL, Kent RL, Parsons B, Cooper G. Adrenergic effects on the biology of adult mammalian cardiocyte. *Circulation* 1992;85:790–804.

30.   Schwartz K, Chassagne C, Boheler KR. The molecular biology of heart failure. *J Am Coll Cardiol.* 1993;22[suppl A]:30A–33A.

31.   Mercadier JJ, Lompre AM, Duc P, Boheler KR, Fraysse JB, Wisnewsky C, Allen PD, Komajda M, Schwartz K. Altered sarcoplasmic reticulum Ca^{2+}–ATPase gene expression in the human ventricle during end–stage heart failure. *J Clin Invest* 1990;85:305–309.

32.   Ohta K, Kim S, Wanibuchi H, Ganten D, Iwao H. Contribution of local renin–angiotensin system to cardiac hypertrophy, phenotypic modulation and remodeling in TGR (mRen2)27 transgenic rats. *Circulation* 1996;94:785–791.

33.   Cheng W, Li B, Kajstura J, Li P, Wolin MS, Sonnenblick EH, Hintze TH, Olivetti G, Anversa P. Stretch–induced programmed myocyte cell death. *J Clin Invest* 1995;96:2247–22459.

34.   Narula J, Haider N, Virmani R, DiSalvo TG, Kolodgie FD, Hajjar RJ, Schmidt U, Semigran MJ, Dec GW, Khaw B–A. Apoptosis in myocytes in end–stage heart failure. *N Engl J Med* 1996;335:1182–9.

35.   Benedict CR, Weiner DH, Johnstone DE, Bourassa MG, Ghali JK, Nicklas J, Kirlin P, Greenberg B, Quinones MA, Yusuf S. Comparative neurohormonal responses in patients with preserved and impaired left ventricular ejection fraction: Results of the Studies of Left Ventricular Dysfunction (SOLVD) registry. *J Am Coll Cardiol* 1993;22[suppl A]:146A–153A.

36.   Hasking GJ, Esler MD, Jennings GL, Burton D, Johns JA, Korner PL. Norepinephrine spillover to plasma in patients with congestive heart failure: Evidence of increased overall and cardiorenal sympathetic nervous activity. *Circulation* 1986;4:615–621.

37.   Eichhorn EJ, Bristow MR. Medical therapy can improve the biological properties of the chronically failing heart. *Circulation* 1996;94:2285–2296.

38.   Pfeffer MA, Braunwald E, Moye LA, Basta L, Brown EJ Jr, Cuddy TE, Davis BR, Geltman EM, Goldman S, Flaker GC. Effect of captopril on mortality and morbidity in patients with left ventricular dysfunction after myocardial infarction. *N Engl J Med* 1992;327:669–677.

39.   ISIS-4 (Fourth International Study of Infarct Survival) Collaborative. A randomized factorial trial assessing early oral captopril, oral mono-nitrate, and intravenous magnesium sulphate in 58050 patients with suspected acute myocardial infarction. *Lancet* 1995;345:669–685.

40.   The Acute Infarction Ramipril Efficacy (AIRE) Study investigators. Effect of ramipril on mortality and morbidity of survivors of acute myocardial infarction with clinical evidence of myocardial infarction. *Lancet* 1993;324:821–828.

41.   Ambrosini E, Borghi C, Magnani B, for the Survival of Myocardial Infarction Long-term Evaluation (SMILE) Study investigators. The effect of the angiotensin-converting enzyme inhibitor zofenopril on mortality and morbidity after anterior myocardial infarction. *N Engl J Med* 1995;332:80–85.

42.   St. John Sutton M, Pfeffer MA, Plappert T, Rouleau JL, Moye LA, Dagenais GR, Lamas GA, Klein M, Sussex B, Goldman S. Quantitative two-dimensional echocardiographic measurements are major predictors of adverse cardiovascular events after acute myocardial infarction. *Circulation* 1994;89:68–75.

43.   Hokimoto S, Yasue H, Fujimoto K, Yamamoto H, Nakao K, Kaikita K, Sakata R, Miyamoto E. Expression of angiotensin-converting enzyme in remaining viable myocytes of human ventricles after myocardial infarction. *Circulation* 1996;94:1513–1518.

44.   Serneri GGN, Boddi M, Coppo M, Chechi T, Zarone N, Moira M, Poggesi L, Margheri M, Simonetti I. Evidence for the existence of a functional cardiac renin-angiotensin system in humans. *Circulation* 1996;94 1886–1893.

45.   Mento PF, Wilkes BM. Plasma angiotensins and blood pressure during converting enzyme inhibition. *Hypertension* 1987;9(suppl III):III–42–48.

46.   Urata H, Boehm KD, Philip A, Kinoshita A, Gabrovsek J, Bumpus FM, Husain A. Cellular localization and regional distribution of an angiotensin II–forming chymase in the heart. *J Clin Invest* 1993;91:1296–1281.

47.   Weber KT, Anversa P, Armstrong PW, Brilla CG, Burnett JC Jr, Cruickshank JM, Devereux RB, Giles TD, Korsgaard N, Leier CV. Remodeling and reparation of the cardiovascular system. *J Am Coll Cardiol* 1992;20:3–16.

48.   Simpson P. Norepinephrine–stimulated hypertrophy of cultured rat myocardial cells is an alpha1 adrenergic response. *J Clin Invest* 1983;72 732–738.

49.   Bristow MR, Ginsburg R, Minobe W, Cubicciotti RS, Sageman WS, Lurie K, Billingham ME, Harrison DC, Stinson EB. Decreased catecholamine sensitivity and β–adrenergic–receptor density in failing human hearts. *N Engl J Med* 1982;307:205–211.

50.   Bristow MR, Minobe WA, Raynolds MV, Port JD, Rasmussen R, Ray PE, Feldman AM. Reduced β1 receptor messenger RNA abundance in the failing human heart. *J Clin Invest* 1993;92:2737–2745.

51.   Tyagi SC, Reddy HK, Voelker DJ, Tjahja IE, Weber KT: Myocardial collagenase and tissue inhibitor in dilated, failing human myocardium. *Circulation* 1993(Suppl):88:I–407.

52.   Jugdutt BI, Joljart MJ, Khan MI. Rate of collagen deposition during healing and ventricular remodeling after myocardial infarction in rat and dog models. *Circulation* 1996;94:94–101.

53.   Bishop JE, Greenbaum R, Gibson DG, Yacoub M, Laurent GJ: Enhanced deposition of predominantly type I collagen in myocardial disease. *J Mol Cell Cardiol* 1990;22:1157–1165.

54.   Brilla CG, Zhou G, Matsubara L, Weber KT: Collagen metabolism in cultured adult rat cardiac fibroblasts: response to angiotensin II and aldosterone. *J Moll Cell Cardiol* 1994;26:809–820.

55.   Lewis BS, Gotsman MS: Relation between coronary artery size and left ventricular wall mass. *Brit Heart J* 1973;35:1150–1153.

56.   Brilla CG, Janicki JS, Weber KT. Impaired diastolic function and coronary erserve in genetic hypertension: Role of interstitial fibrosis and medial thickening of intramyocardial coronary arteries. *Circ Res* 1991;69:107–115.

57.   Parodi O, De Maria R, Oltrona L, Testa R, Sambuceti G, Roghi A, Merli M, Belingheri L, Accinni R, Spinelli F. Myocardial blood flow distribution in patients with ischemic heart disease or dilated cardiomyopathy undergoing heart transplant. *Circulation* 1993;88:509–522.

58.   Treasure CB, Alexander RW. The dysfunctional endothelium in heart failure. *J Am Coll Cardiol* 1993;22[suppl A]:129A–134A.

59.   McDonald KM, Yoshiyama M, Francis GS, Ugurbil K, Cohn JN, Zhang J. Myocardial bioenergetic abnormalities in a canine model of left ventricular dysfunction. *J Am Coll Cardiol* 1994;23:786–793.

60.   Kass DA, Baughman KL, Pak PH, Cho PW, Levin HR, Gardner TJ, Halperin HR, Tsitlik JE, Acker MA. Reverse remodeling from cardiomyoplasty in human heart failure. *Circulation* 1995;91:2314–2318.

VI. ELECTRICAL ACTIVATION AND PROPAGATION

CHAPTER 23

CARDIAC EXCITATION: AN INTERACTIVE PROCESS OF ION CHANNELS AND GAP JUNCTIONS

Yoram Rudy and Robin M. Shaw[1]

ABSTRACT

Theoretical simulations were performed to study the interplay between membrane ionic currents and gap–junction coupling in determining cardiac conduction. Results demonstrate that a much slower conduction velocity can be achieved with reduced gap–junction coupling than with reduced membrane excitability. Also, uniform reduction in intercellular coupling increases spatial asymmetries of excitability and, consequently, the vulnerability to unidirectional block.

INTRODUCTION

Success or failure of action potential propagation in cardiac tissue is determined by local source–sink relations. For propagation to succeed, the charge supplied by the source must equal or exceed the charge required to excite the membrane at the sink location. At the cellular level, this condition is determined by the interplay between the state of membrane excitability and the degree and pattern of intercellular coupling at gap junctions. The state of membrane excitability is determined by the kinetics of membrane ionic currents and has been studied extensively (see [1] for a detailed review of experimental work and [2, 3] for theoretical simulations of ionic currents during a ventricular action potential). More recently, increasing efforts have been directed to study the role of the microscopic myocardial architecture in propagation of the action potential [4]. In particular, the role of cell–to–cell coupling at gap junctions has been investigated [5–6].

[1]Cardiac Bioelectricity Research and Training Center (CBRTC), Dept. of Biomedical Engineering, Case Western Reserve University, Cleveland, OH 44106–7207, USA

In this chapter, we use mathematical models to examine the effects of membrane and gap junction factors on propagation of the action potential in the heart. The focus is on changes in membrane excitability and in the degree of cell–to–cell coupling at gap junctions. Altered membrane excitability and reduced cellular coupling are known consequences of various pathologies and can occur together or separately. An example of pathology that influences primarily membrane factors is the early stage of acute ischemia [7, 8]. On the other hand, intercellular decoupling at gap junctions has been demonstrated during the later phases of ischemia [8–10] and in association with various types of injury. This chapter summarizes results from several earlier studies. Details can be found in [11–17].

METHODS

Simulations were conducted in a multicellular one dimensional model that incorporates membrane ionic processes and intercellular gap junctions [11]. The electrical activity of the membrane is represented, in certain simulations, by the Beeler–Ruter (BR) model [18]. In other simulations, the more recent dynamic Luo–Rudy (LRd) model of the ventricular action potential [2, 3] is used. The cells in the fiber are of realistic dimensions (100 μm long) and are connected by gap junctions with 80 Angstroms long resistive channels (connexons) that provide direct cell–to–cell pathways for current flow. The model permits varying the gap junction conductance over a wide range of values, simulating different degrees of intercellular coupling.

RESULTS

Membrane Effects on Propagation

Propagation at various levels of reduced membrane excitability is examined in Fig. 1. Membrane excitability is varied by progressively reducing the maximum sodium conductance, g_{Na}, from 100% (full excitability) to 10%. As excitability is decreased, both $(dv/dt)_{max}$ (the maximum rate of depolarization) and conduction velocity decrease monotonically as a result of decreasing excitatory sodium current, I_{Na}. Over the simulated range of g_{Na}, $(dv/dt)_{max}$ falls from 240 v/s (at 100% g_{Na}) to 19 v/s (at 11% g_{Na}) and the velocity from 54 cm/s to 17 cm/s. Further reduction of g_{Na} results in insufficient I_{Na} to sustain propagation and an abrupt conduction block occurs. Note that by reducing membrane excitability, velocity can only be reduced by a factor of about three before block occurs.

Gap–junction Effects on Propagation

Propagation at various levels of reduced gap junction coupling is examined in Fig. 2. Conduction velocity and $(dv/dt)_{max}$ are shown as a function of the degree of intercellular coupling for a constant myoplasmic resistivity (R_{myo} = 150 Ω cm) and a fully excitable membrane. As cells become progressively less coupled (R_g, the gap–junction resistance, increases and G_j, gap–junction conductance, decreases) velocity decreases monotonically. In contrast, $(dv/dt)_{max}$ displays a biphasic behavior. In the range of R_g from 1.5 Ω cm² to 100 Ω cm² (G_j from 2.5μS to 0.038 μS), $(dv/dt)_{max}$ increases to a maximum value of 360 v/s, reflecting increased confinement of axial current to the activated cell. As the cell becomes less coupled to its downstream neighbors, it is subjected to a reduced electrical load and more current is available for local depolarization. This acts to increase $(dv/dt)_{max}$.

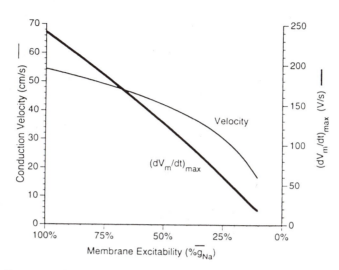

Figure 1. Effects of homogeneous changes in membrane excitability on propagation. Conduction velocity and maximum rate of depolarization, $(dv_m/dt)_{max}$, decrease monotonically with decreasing maximum sodium conductance, g_{Na} (from [17] with permission).

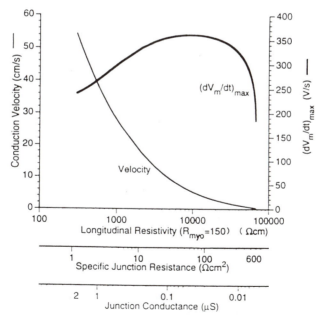

Figure 2. Effects of homogeneous changes in gap–junction coupling on propagation. Velocity decreases monotonically but $(dv_m/dt)_{max}$ displays nonmonotonic behavior as cells become progressively more decoupled. Myoplasmic resistivity, R_{myo}, is held constant at 150 Ω cm. Abscissa shows **Top scale:** effective total intracellular resistivity (contribution from both gap–junction and myoplasm); **Middle scale:** specific gap–junction resistance; **Bottom scale:** gap–junction conductance (from [17] with permission).

At the same time, the reduced coupling creates longer propagation delays in crossing gap junctions and conduction velocity is reduced. The result is "paradoxical" slow conduction that exhibits normal or even high $(dv/dt)_{max}$ (i.e., a highly excitable membrane). Beyond the maximum value, $(dv/dt)_{max}$ decreases with further decrease of intercellular coupling. This is because, for severe uncoupling, the post–junctional charging current becomes very limited and charging time to threshold (i.e the foot of the action potential) is greatly prolonged. The slow charging process allows for greater inactivation of I_{Na} that is reflected in a reduced $(dv/dt)_{max}$. Note (Fig. 2) that very slow conduction (velocity of the order of 1 to 2 cm/s) can be achieved by decoupling of cells at gap junctions. For further gap-junction decoupling, a range of severely reduced coupling is reached for which propagation is decremental, leading to conduction block (Fig. 3).

Unidirectional Block and the Vulnerable Window

The phenomenon of unidirectional block involves successful propagation in one direction and failure of propagation in the other direction. Unidirectional block can occur on the tail of a prior action potential in an otherwise uniform and homogeneous tissue. A directional asymmetry is created by the dispersion of excitability that exists in the wake of the prior action potential. We define the "vulnerable window" (TW) as the time interval in the refractory period (between plateau and diastole) of a propagating action potential during which unidirectional block can be induced (Fig. 4). The vulnerable window can also be represented as a distance in the space domain (SW) or as a range of membrane potentials in the voltage domain (VW). Outside this window, it is impossible to induce unidirectional block; an action potential induced by a premature stimulus either propagates or blocks in both directions. When a premature stimulus is applied inside the window, the membrane generates a critical sodium current, giving rise to an action potential that propagates incrementally in the retrograde direction and decrementally in the antegrade direction. This is because in the retrograde direction the tissue is progressively more recovered as the distance from the window increases in this direction, while in the antegrade direction the membrane is progressively less excitable as the distance from the window increases. Figure 5 provides examples of responses to differently timed stimuli. For stimuli outside the window, bidirectional block (Panel A) or bidirectional conduction (Panel C) occur. When the stimulus falls inside the vulnerable window, unidirectional block develops.

It is clear from the above discussion that the inducibility of unidirectional block and reentry is related to the spatial inhomogeneity (asymmetry) of excitability at the vulnerable window. Figure 6 shows the distribution of excitability properties in the neighborhood of the vulnerable window. Panel A shows the distribution of the maximum fast sodium channel conductance during the action–potential upstroke (g_{Na}) and its spatial gradient dg_{Na}/dx. Panel B and C display the gating parameters m (activation), h (fast inactivation) and j (slow inactivation) of the sodium current and their spatial gradients at the time of peak g_{Na}. The maximum g_{Na} obtained from an isolated cell stimulated at rest with the Luo–Rudy membrane model is 8.36 mS/cm^2 with values of 0.89, 0.55, and 0.94, for the m, h and j gates, respectively. The same parameters computed from a cell in the center of the vulnerable window were 0.844 mS/cm^2, 0.88, 0.30 and 0.18 for g_{Na}, m, h, and j, respec-tively. By separating g_{Na} into its activation (m) and inactivation (h·j) parameters, one observes that the reduction in g_{Na} (89.9%) is determined mostly by unrecovered inactiva-tion (89.6% decrease in h·j). Reduced excitability is therefore not a function of a com-promised m–gate. The dominance of inactivation on the recovery of excitability is further evidenced by a comparison of the spatial gradient of excitability, dg_{Na}/dx in Fig. 6A with the spatial gradient of activation and inactivation of Figs. 6B and 6C. The shape of dg_{Na}/dx

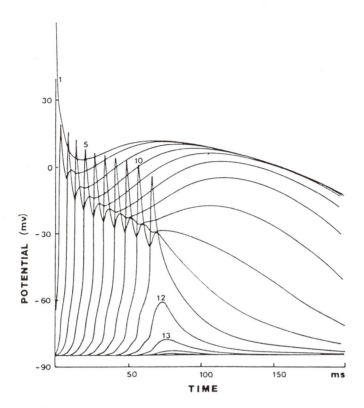

Figure 3. Decremental propagation caused by a very high gap junction resistance (R_g = 380 Ω cm^2). The numbers in the body of the figure indicate the cell number relative to the stimulus site. Beyond cell #13, conduction block occurs (from [11] by permission of the American Heart Association, Inc.).

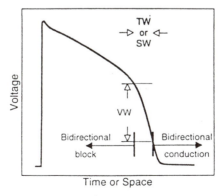

Figure 4. Schematic representation of the vulnerable window during the refractory period of a propagating action potential. TW, SW and VW represent the vulnerable window in the time domain, space domain and voltage domain, respectively (from [16] with permission).

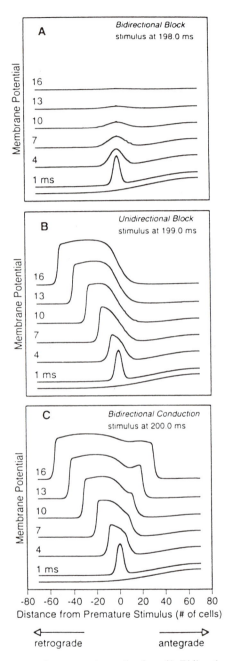

Figure 5. Three types of responses to a premature stimulus. **A)** Bidirectional block occurred when the premature stimulus was applied 198 ms after initiation of the conditioning action potential and resulted from an inability of the premature stimulus to excite the fiber in either direction. **B)** Unidirectional block at 199 ms resulted from successful retrograde, but not antegrade, excitation. **C)** Bidirectional conduction at 200 ms when both retrograde and antegrade fiber were excited. The bottom trace in each panel represents membrane potential immediately prior to stimulus. $R_g = 8 \ \Omega \ cm^2$ (from [14] with permission).

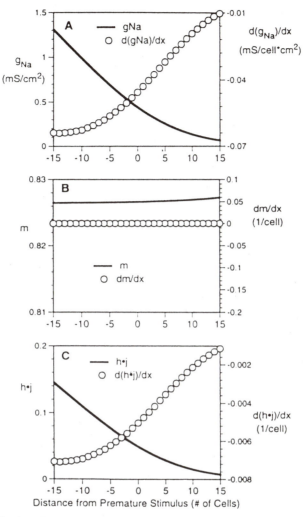

Figure 6. Spatial distribution of excitability, g_{Na}, in vicinity of the vulnerable window. Solid curves represent parameters. Circles represent first spatial derivatives. g_{Na} = peak sodium conductance; m = activation parameter of I_{Na} ; h and j = fast and slow inactivation parameters of I_{Na}, respectively (from [14] with permission).

follows that of d(h·j)/dx. dm/dx is practically zero (and m is constant) throughout the vulnerable window. Therefore, the spatial functional inhomogeneity of excitability is a reflection of the inhomogeneity of h·j and is not influenced by m. An inhomogeneous recovery from inactivation of I_{Na} creates the conditions for unidirectional block by facilitating excitation from a premature stimulus in the retrograde direction while inhibiting excitation in the antegrade direction. As the local spatial gradient of h·j increases, the spatial functional inhomogeneity of excitability increases and unidirectional block is more likely to occur.

Gap Junction and Membrane Factors as Modulators of the Vulnerable Window

The size of the vulnerable window in the time domain (TW) provides a measure of the vulnerability of the tissue to the induction of unidirectional block and reentry. TW is a convenient working definition of the vulnerable window. For a large TW the time interval during which unidirectional block can be induced is long. Therefore, the probability that a premature stimulus (e.g. during clinical electrophysiology study in the catheterization laboratory, or a naturally occurring triggering event in the diseased heart) will fall inside the window and induce reentry is high. In the following simulation we examine the effects of cellular decoupling at gap junctions and of membrane excitability on the tissue vulnerability to unidirectional block. Vulnerability (TW) as a function of gap junction resistance is shown in Fig. 7 (curve 1). As the gap junction resistance increases, vulnerability increases as well, with accompanying decrease in propagation velocity (curve 2). For normal cellular coupling ($Rg=2$ Ω cm^2), the vulnerability is about 0.5 msec. Very precise timing (TW<0.5 msec) of a premature stimulus is required for induction of unidirectional block and reentry. For a high degree of cellular decoupling ($Rg=200$ Ω cm^2), the vulnerability is increased to 30 msec. For such a wide window, unidirectional block can be easily induced. The simulations demonstrate, therefore, that as the degree of cellular decoupling is increased, velocity of propagation decreases (due to long delays at gap junctions) and vulnerability to reentry increases. In the previous section we showed that the vulnerability is determined by the degree of spatial functional inhomogeneity of excitability at the vulnerable window. As regional propagation delay increases, due to long delays at gap junctions, the degree of spatial functional inhomogeneity in the state of the membrane increases we well. As demonstrated in Fig. 6, this increased asymmetry at the vulnerable window reflects an increase in the spatial gradient of the sodium inactivation gates h and j. In contrast to the effect of cellular uncoupling described above, *uniform* reduction throughout the entire fiber in sodium channel conductance (intrinsic membrane excitability) resulted in slow propagation with *decreased* vulnerability to the induction of reentry (not shown). This is because a uniform reduction in membrane excitability produces a shift of the vulnerable window to a more recovered portion of the repolarization phase of the action potential (for a less excitable membrane, similar conditions to those under a non-compromised membrane are produced at a more recovered region). This shift to a less steep

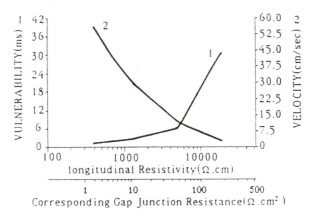

Figure 7. Changes in vulnerability due to changes in gap junction resistance R_g. Curve 1 shows an increase in vulnerability when R_g increases. Curve 2 shows velocity of propagation as a function of R_g. (From Ref. 15 by permission of the American Heart Association, Inc.).

portion of the action potential brings about reduction in spatial gradients and reduces spatial inhomogeneities in the state of the membrane at the vicinity of the window. The result is lower vulnerability to the induction of unidirectional block and reentry. Quantitatively, the effect is small and operatively negligible; 50% reduction of sodium channel conductance brings about a decrease of the vulnerable window from 0.5 msec to 0.1 msec. In comparison, a reduction of cellular coupling that causes similar decrease in conduction velocity is accompanied by a large increase of vulnerability from 0.5 msec to 30 msec (Fig. 7).

DISCUSSION AND CONCLUSIONS

Membrane and Gap–Junction Factors

As stated in the introduction, propagation of excitation in cardiac tissue is determined by the relationship between the availability of depolarizing charge ("source") and the amount of charge required for successful propagation ("sink"). This relationship reflects a complex interaction between the membrane ionic currents which generate the action potential and the microscopic architecture of the tissue which determines the electric load on a depolarizing cell. In particular, the conductance and distribution of gap junctions determines intercellular current flow and conduction. Both membrane factors (e.g. excitability) and gap–junction factors (e.g. conductance and distribution) can be affected by pathologies. In this chapter we have used a theoretical model that contains the elementary building blocks of cardiac tissue (discrete cells connected by gap–junction) to establish certain principles that underlie propagation.

Slow Conduction and Conduction Block

Reduced membrane excitability reduces both conduction velocity and $(dv/dt)_{max}$. By reducing membrane excitability, velocity can only be reduced by a factor of about 3 (from 54 cm/s to 17 cm/s before block occurs. In comparison, reduced intercellular coupling at gap junctions can support very slow conduction velocities (1 to 2 cm/s). This suggests that cellular decoupling plays an important role in very slow conduction that can be observed during reentry [19] while reduced membrane excitability plays a more important role in the development of conduction block. The ability of reduced gap–junction coupling to support very slow conduction is related to the biphasic behavior (increase then decrease) of $(dv/dt)_{max}$ (Fig. 2). This creates conditions for slow conduction with a fully developed rising phase of the action potential.

Unidirectional Block and the Vulnerable Window

Unidirectional block is a necessary condition for the development of reentry. Therefore, the vulnerability to reentry can be expressed in terms of the vulnerability to the induction of unidirectional block. We have quantified the probability of unidirectional block in terms of the vulnerable window. The vulnerable window is characterized by a spatial asymmetry of excitability, brought about by asymmetry of recovery from inactivation of the excitatory sodium current (i.e., d (h·j)/dx, see Fig. 6 and related text). Vulnerability to unidirectional block increases with a uniform increase in the degree of cellular decoupling at gap junctions (Fig. 7). In contrast, uniform decrease of membrane excitability has a small effect on vulnerability (a slight increase or a slight decrease can be observed, depending on the simulation protocol). This last observation seems contradictory to experimental and clinical observations that vulnerability increases when membrane excitability is depressed by sodium channel blocking agents. A likely explanation of this apparent inconsistency is that in the realistic, physiological environment the depression of excitability caused by the drug (or by ischemia, for that matter) can never be uniform and never occurs in a completely uniform substrate since inhomogeneities in action potential duration, refractoriness, and tissue structure are present. These inhomogeneities generate nonuniformities (asymmetries) that enlarge the vulnerable window and facilitate the induction of unidirectional block.

DISCUSSION

Dr. H. Strauss: What happens when you start to change membrane resistance during the plateau and change the relative values of the specific conductances in the membrane. How does that influence the relationship in terms of change in repolarization waveform?

Dr. Y. Rudy: We have modulated the L–type calcium current and the sodium–calcium exchanger. The principles that M–cells are more sensitive (in terms of action potential duration changes) holds true for these interventions.

Dr. H. Strauss: Have you examined the effect of changes in chloride?

Dr. Y. Rudy: No.

Dr. P. Hunter: The cell sodium channel density is greater near the ends of the cells where the gap junctions tend to be. Can you comment on what affect that would have on your safety factor in relation to gap junctions?

Dr. Y. Rudy: The structure–function relationship at the subcellular scale is important and is an area of intense research activity (especially in relation to calcium). We have not considered the effect of sodium channel clustering at gap–junctional regions on propagation. Maddy Spach suggests that this has an "amplification effect" that enhances conduction. This idea sounds attractive but requires careful and quantitative evaluation.

Dr. M.S. Gotsman: If the M cells are different, do we have morphological evidence of this difference? Why should the M cells be different? Why is there not uniform depolarization and repolarization throughout the heart?

Dr. Y. Rudy: There is no morphological evidence that M–cells are different. The difference is in their longer action potential duration, its greater adaptability to rate changes, and higher sensitivity to drugs that prolong the action potential. The etiological question "why should M–cells be different" is difficult to answer. From the electrophysiologic perspective, it is hard to think of a good reason since actin potential differences (dispersion) are associated with arrhythmogenesis. Maybe there is a mechanical reason for these differences.

Dr. P. Hunter: The Auckland work has shown that the cleavage planes and the organization of the sheets across the wall tend to give very large gaps in the middle of the myocardium, which may well have an important mechanical role. The fact that the M cells have a much faster sodium upstroke, you could argue, is that the Purkinje fiber network is rapidly activating the subendo–cardium, and you want the action potential to rapidly propagate transmurally through the wall.

Dr. Y. Rudy: I understand your idea, but why should M–cells have a much longer action potential?

Dr. P. Hunter: Yes. Presumably the gradient of I_{TO} across the wall will be stabilizing the heart in ways which we do not understand yet.

Dr. Y. Rudy: However, guinea pig ventricular myocytes do not have I_{TO}, yet the myocardium contains M–cells and has a similar design to other species that have I_{TO}. It seems that we have another puzzle to solve.

REFERENCES

1.   Spooner PM, Brown AM, eds. *Ion Channels in the Cardiovascular System: Function and Dysfunction.* Armonk, New York: Futura Publishing Company, Inc.; 1994.

2.   Luo C, Rudy Y. A dynamic model of the cardiac ventricular action potential: I. Simulations of ionic currents and concentration changes. *Circ Res* 1994;74:1071–1096.

3.   Zeng J, Laurita KR, Rosenbaum DS, Rudy Y. Two components of the delayed rectifier K⁺ current in ventricular myocytes of the guinea pig type: Theoretical formulation and their role in repolarization. *Circ Res* 1995;77:1–13.

4.   Spach MS, Miller WT, Geselowitz DB, Barr RC, Kootsey JM, Johnson EA. The discontinuous nature of propagation in normal canine cardiac muscle. Evidence for recurrent discontinuities of intracellular resistance that affect the membrane currents. *Circ Res* 1981;48:39–54.

5.   Weingart R, Maurer P. Action potential transfer in cell pairs isolated from adult rat and guinea pig ventricles. *Circ Res* 1988;63:72–80.

6.   Fast VG, Darrow BJ, Saffitz JE, Kléber AG. Anisotropic activation spread in heart cell monolayers assessed by high–resolution optical mapping: Role of tissue discontinuities. *Circ Res* 1996;79:115–127.

7.   Cascio WE, Johnson TA, Gettes LS. Electrophysiologic changes in ischemic ventricular myocardium: I. Influence of ionic, metabolic, and energetic changes. *J Cardiovasc Electrophysiol* 1995;6:1039–1062.

8.   Wit AL, Janse MJ. *The ventricular arrhythmias of ischemia and infarction. Electrophysiological mechanisms.* Armonk, New York: Futura Publishing Company, Inc.; 1993.

9.   Kléber AG, Riegger CB, Janse MJ. Electrical uncoupling and increase of extracellular resistance after induction of ischemia in isolated, arterially perfused rabbit papillary muscle. *Circ Res* 1987;51:271–279.

10.   Wu J, McHowat J, Saffitz JE, Yamada KA, Corr PB. Inhibition of gap junctional conductance by long–chain acylcarnitines and their preferential accumulation in junctional sarcolemma during hypoxia. *Circ Res* 1993;72:879–889.

11.   Rudy Y, Quan W. A Model study of the effects of the discrete cellular structure on electrical propagation in cardiac tissue. *Circ Res* 1987;61:815–823.

12.   Rudy Y, Quan W. Propagation delays across cardiac gap junctions and their reflection in extracellular potentials: A simulation study. *J Cardiovasc Electrophysiol* 1991;2:299–315.

13.   Rudy Y. Models of continuous and discontinuous propagation in cardiac tissue. In: Zipes DP and Jalife J (eds). *Cardiac Electrophysiology – From Cell to Bedside* W.B. Saunders Publishers, 1994; 326–334.

14.   Shaw RM, Rudy Y. The vulnerable window for unidirectional block in cardiac tissue: characterization and dependence on membrane excitability and cellular coupling. *J Cardiovasc Electrophysiol* 1995;6:115–131.

15.   Quan W, Rudy Y. Unidirectional block and reentry of cardiac excitation. A model study. *Circ Res* 1990;66:367–382.

16.   Rudy Y. Reentry: Insights from theoretical simulations in a fixed pathway. *J Cardiovasc Electrophysiol* 1995;6:294–312.

17.   Rudy Y, Shaw RM. Membrane factors and gap–junction factors as determinants of ventricular conduction and reentry. In: *Discontinuities in Cardiac Conduction.* Eds: P. Spooner et al, Futura Publishing Co., 1996; (in press).

18.   Beeler GW, Reuter H. Reconstruction of the action potential of ventricular myocardial fibers. *J Physiol (Lond)* 1977;286:177–210.

19.   Dillon SM, Allessie MA, Ursell PC, and Wit AL. Influence of anisotropic tissue structure on reentrant circuits in the epicardial border zone of subacute canine infarcts. *Circ Res* 1988;63:182–206.

CHAPTER 24

Modeling of Internal pH, Ion Concentration, and Bioenergetic Changes during Myocardial Ischemia

Frederick Ch'en,[1] Kieran Clarke,[2] Richard Vaughan–Jones,[3] and Denis Noble[2]

ABSTRACT

Arrhythmias are caused by the interdependent processes of change in energy metabolism and alterations in sarcolemmal ion gradients that occur during ischemia. Depletion of energy metabolites and increased proton concentrations in ischemic heart may underlie the observed phenomena of reduced contractile force and also of malignant ventricular arrhythmias that can lead to tachycardia and ventricular fibrillation. Recent advances in measuring changes in ion concentrations and metabolites during cardiac ischemia have provided a wealth of detail on the processes involved. Some of the experimental data have been used to construct a computer model that integrates cardiac energetics with electrophysiological changes. This is a novel approach to studying myocardial ischemia, and the resulting model would aid in the prediction of the effects of therapeutic interventions.

INTRODUCTION

Models of the electrical activity of cardiac cells are now highly developed. Starting with the DiFrancesco–Noble model of the Purkinje conducting tissue of the ventricles [1], the latest generation of models include ion concentration changes, the activity of ion pumps and exchangers as well as of ion channels, the buffering, sequestration and release of internal calcium, and the activation of contraction. These developments have already greatly

[1]Balliol College, [2]Department of Biochemistry and [3]Department of Physiology, University of Oxford, Oxford, OX1 3PT, UK

extended the range of application of the models, in particular to an understanding of the cellular basis of many forms of arrhythmia [2]. The cell models have also been incorporated into massive network simulations of cardiac tissue [3]. With the rapid increase in computing power, it has become clear that simulations of the whole heart using biophysically detailed models is feasible. An obvious application of such models is to understand pathophysiological states such as ischemia. We are currently extending the cell models to include the energetic and proton changes that occur in myocardial ischemia and that lead to arrhythmias.

This is a large and ambitious undertaking, requiring a particular combination of experimental and computing methods. In addition to the mechanisms already incorporated into the models, changes in the relevant energy metabolites and ion concentrations must be incorporated. In this progress report, we present two major aspects of the work: the modeling of pH changes and the modeling of metabolite changes.

RESULTS

Modeling of pH Changes

Adequate control of intracellular pH in heart is a fundamental requirement, and deviations from resting levels of around 7.2 result in major changes in contraction and excitability. The pH_i in heart is controlled by at least four sarcolemmal ion carriers, two acid extruders (Na^+/H^+ exchange and Na^+–HCO_3^- symport) and two acid loaders (Cl^-/HCO_3^- exchange and the recently proposed Cl^-/OH^- exchange) [4].

Ventricular myocytes were isolated from guinea–pig, rat, or rabbit hearts using a combination of enzymic and mechanical dispersion, and their intracellular ion activities were measured by intracellular ratiometric ion–microfluorimetry of single superfused cells placed on the stage of an epifluorescence microscope. The dual–emission fluorophore carboxy–SNARF–1 was used to measure changes in internal pH, while SBFI was used to measure internal sodium.

Acid equivalent fluxes were estimated from the time course of pH_i recovery in response to experimentally imposed intracellular acid and alkali loads. The product of dpH_i/dt and β_i (the intracellular H^+ buffering power) gives the flux; the ammonium prepulse technique was used to give an acid load, while the acetate or propionate prepulse technique was used for alkali loading. The various acid–equivalent transporters were dissected by the careful use of buffers. The Na^+/H^+ exchange was described by pH_i recovery from an acid load in HEPES buffered superfusion media; Na^+–HCO_3^- symport was described by a pH_i recovery from an acid load in HCO_3^-/CO_2 buffer in the presence of amiloride in order to inhibit parallel acid extrusion through Na^+/H^+ exchange; the effect of Cl^-/HCO_3^- plus Cl^-/OH^- exchangers was described by pH_i recovery from an intracellular alkali–load measured in HCO_3^-/CO_2 buffered media containing no Na^+, (Na^+ replaced by n–methyl–d–glucamine) to inhibit the acid extruders. At pH_i values close to resting values of pH_o (7.4), the acid extruders are usually pitched against loaders, and so the determination of pure extrusion uncontaminated by import is more complex. Thus the method adopted was first to estimate acid import over the relevant range of pH_i, and then to correct for this when calculating efflux over the same pH_i range.

Data obtained in this way were used to obtain activation curves, and were curve-fitted to polynomial equations to give an expression for the pH_i dependence of acid efflux in terms of mequiv/l/min; this alleviated the need to estimate surface:volume ratios. The theory behind the calculation of acid efflux, J^e, has been described by Lagadic–Gossmann *et al.* [5]. In brief, acid efflux is defined as $\beta_{tot} \cdot dpHi/dt$, where β_{tot} is the total buffering power. Rearranging this equation gives an expression for the rate of change in pH_i with respect to time, i.e., $dpHi/dt = J^e/\beta_{tot}$. The total buffering power has components from intrinsic buffering (β_i) and from buffering due to CO_2 (β_{CO2}), and these have been determined empirically assuming an open system for CO_2.

The equations for proton fluxes have been incorporated in conjunction with modeling work on contraction. Here, the force–Ca^{2+} relationship of myofibrils in skinned cardiac muscles was taken as the basis of proton competition with Ca^{2+} for calcium binding sites on troponin. The end result of this modeling is that the effect of acidosis and alkalosis can be effectively represented. For example, we can impose an acid load of increasing magnitude, from 7.1 to 6.9, 6.7, and 6.5 and observe the effects on contraction and sodium. While the modeling of acid fluxes lacks, at this stage, contributions from metabolic processes such as ATP hydrolysis, creatine phosphate degradation, and glycogenolysis, and the coupling of the pH model with the metabolite model is still in its preliminary stage, the changes observed and the effects on contraction are qualitatively correct. Experiments on single cells have shown the negative inotropic effect of acidosis [6], and this is also seen in the model. Figure 1 shows responses to acid loads of increasing magnitude, leading to sodium overload (and thence to calcium overload) once a pH_i challenge of 6.5 is reached. The recovery in pH_i after acid load, the rise in internal sodium, and the effects on contraction are all very encouraging, and reflect experimental findings. Note that the computation shown in Fig. 1A is run with the constant for calcium binding to its release site (Km_{Ca}) set at 1 μM, whereas in Fig. 1B, to highlight the effect of Na^+/H^+ block, it is set to 4 μM. The value of Km_{Ca} is still very uncertain, in part because the model does not take into account non–uniform distribution of calcium within the cytosol.

Results of the modeling presented in Fig. 1 show that intracellular acidity to a degree that occurs during ischemia might be expected to generate sodium–overload arrhythmias. What is interesting is that drugs which block Na^+/H^+ exchange should attenuate these, as can be seen in the pair of simulations in Fig. 1B when the flux contribution from the Na^+/H^+ exchanger is set to zero. It is noteworthy that Hoe 694, a blocker of the Na^+/H^+ exchanger, has been shown to be cardioprotective and anti–arrhythmic [7].

Modeling of Energetics

Isolated hearts were perfused using the Langendorff method, and total ischemia could be simulated by subsequently restricting the buffer flow. To measure tissue phosphorus metabolite concentrations, a fully relaxed spectrum was acquired using ^{31}P NMR spectroscopy. External standards of methylphosphonic acid (MPA), phenylphosphonic acid (PPA), and dimethylmethylphosphonate (DMMP) were added to determine absolute concentrations of high–energy metabolites and phosphate, extracellular water, and total water respectively. The γ–ATP peak was used as a measure of ATP in the heart. Changes in phosphorus metabolites were determined during the experiments by acquiring consecu-tive 4–minute saturated ^{31}P NMR spectra using a 60° pulse with an inter–pulse delay of 2.15 seconds. Transients were summed, line–broadened, and Fourier transformed. Total phosphate was calculated as the sum of the intracellular inorganic phosphate (P_i), phosphocreatine (PCr), and three times the ATP resonance areas. Intracellular pH was estimated from the chemical shift of the P_i peak relative to the PCr using the equation:

$$pH_{intracellular} = 6.72 + \log\{(X-3.17)/(5.72-X)\} \tag{1}$$

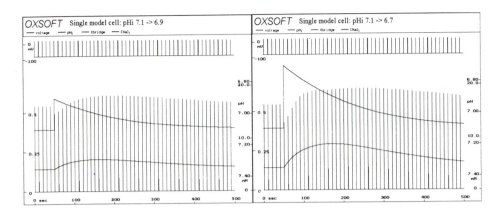

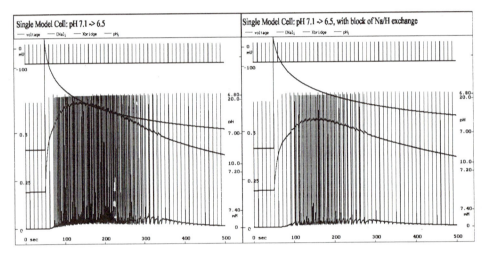

Figure 1. OXSOFT HEART model: computation of the changes in contraction and internal sodium on acid loading in a model cell. Simulations with the constant for Ca binding to its release site set at **(A)** 1 μM and **(B)** 4 μM. Top trace in each panel shows voltage clamping, stimulating at 10 Hz, while the middle trace represents internal pH; the acid load increases successively from the resting pH_i of 7.1 to 6.9, 6.7 (top pair, **A**), and 6.5 **(B)**. The trace that rises suddenly with the acid load is that of internal sodium; the greater the pH_i load, the greater the rise. Finally, the bottom trace represents contraction; note the inotropic effect of acidosis in **A**, and the production of ectopic beats as pH_i is changed to 6.5 in **B**. The lower pair of computations in **B** shows the effect of blocking the Na^+/H^+ exchanger, calculated with a higher value for the constant for calcium binding to its release site (Km_{Ca}). The model predicts an attenuation of the arrhythmic beats when Na^+/H^+ is blocked.

where X = chemical shift of the intracellular P_i peak, and extracellular pH can be similarly calculated using the extracellular P_i peak. Experimental details have been described elsewhere [8]. In this way, changes in the concentration of ATP, PCr, Cr, P_i, and intra– and extracellular pH can be followed in isolated, spontaneously beating hearts under conditions of ischemia. Figure 2 shows typical ^{31}P NMR spectra in conditions of ischemia.

The model of metabolic changes used three basic equations as its basis:

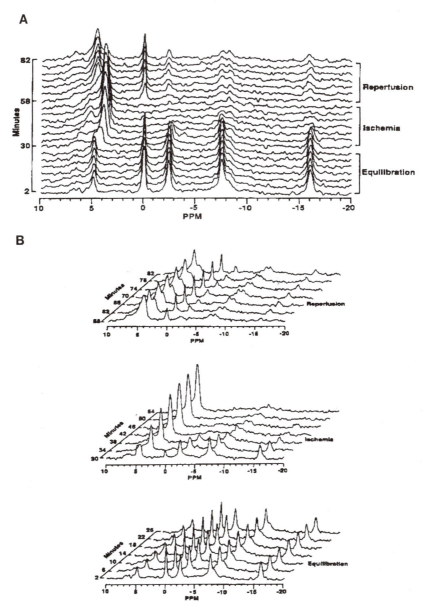

Figure 2. Example of NMR spectra obtained during ischemia. The figure shows ^{31}P NMR spectra from a rat heart subjected to sequential 28–min periods of equilibration, ischemia, and reperfusion. In the top figure (**A**), the peaks correspond, left to right, to P_i, phosphocreatine, γ–ATP, α–ATP, and β–ATP. The upfield movement of inorganic phosphate peak, as pH_i declined, can be clearly seen, whereas the changes in peak areas throughout the experiment are better seen in the bottom set of figures (**B**).

$$\text{ATP} \dashrightarrow \text{ADP} + P_i \qquad (2)$$
$$\text{PCr} + \text{ADP} \longleftrightarrow \text{ATP} + \text{Cr} \qquad (3)$$
$$2\text{ADP} \longleftrightarrow \text{ATP} + \text{AMP} \qquad (4)$$

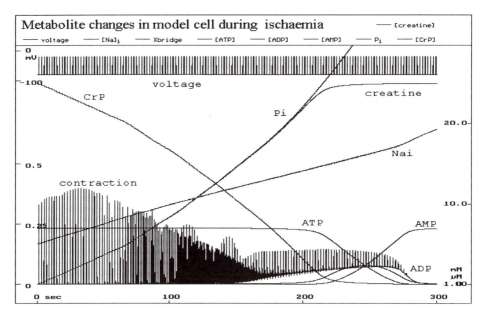

Figure 3. OXSOFT HEART model: computation of the changes in metabolites during five minutes of ischemia. Voltage clamping with stimulation of 10 Hz. See text for details and the equations used for modeling.

If the starting concentrations for all the metabolites are known, then it is possible to create equations for total adenine (5), total creatine (6), total phosphate (7), the creatine kinase reaction (8), and the myokinase reaction (9) as follows (see e.g. [9]):

$$[ATP] + [ADP] + [AMP] = X \text{ mM} \tag{5}$$
$$[PCr] + [Cr] = Y \text{ mM} \tag{6}$$
$$[PCr] + [Pi] + 3[ATP] + 2[ADP] + [AMP] = Z \text{ mM} \tag{7}$$
$$[ATP][Cr] = 200[ADP][PCr] \tag{8}$$
$$[ADP]^2 = [ATP][AMP] \tag{9}$$

These five equations can be rearranged to be solved simultaneously, with the changes in the metabolites a function of the internal phosphate concentration. The modelled changes are plotted in Fig. 3. The model shows the depletion of intracellular phosphocreatine and ATP, while inorganic phosphate, ADP, and Na⁺ concentrations increase. The changes in metabolite levels are qualitatively correct and correlate well with experimental studies [10], though other processes have yet to be incorporated. These include anaerobic glycolysis, changes in contractile function, degradation of AMP, and changes in pH; their effect will be to change both the end point at which the ATP consumption and production are again equal, and also the metabolite concentrations present at this new steady–state.

On reperfusion, the blood flow is restored to a heart. To simulate this, we returned the concentration of metabolites to their original levels, with the model otherwise in the same state as at the end of the period of ischemia, i.e., in a state of sodium and calcium overload. Re–activation of the sarcoplasmic reticulum (SR) Ca²⁺ pump in these conditions leads to increased loading of the SR and thus accentuates the oscillatory release of calcium.

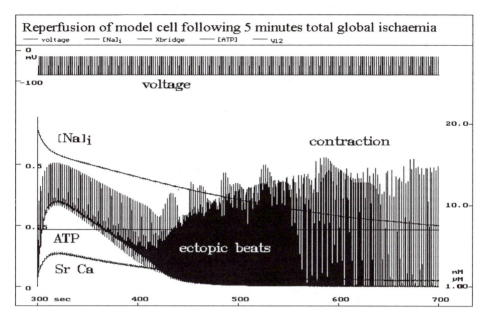

Figure 4. OXSOFT HEART model: computation of the effects of reperfusion following five minutes of ischemia under conditions of voltage clamp.

This effect emerges from the modeling as a possible cause of lethal reperfusion injury, since in Fig. 4 we see that the model shows the arrhythmias to be more severe, in agreement with physiological findings. Other factors which could be involved include the stimulation of adrenergic receptors giving rise to increased cAMP, and disturbances in ionic homeostasis (K^+, as well as Ca^{2+} already mentioned). These additional features have yet to be considered in the modeling.

CONCLUSIONS

The work reported in this paper represents considerable progress towards a comprehensive model of cardiac ischemia. The agreement between experiment and theory on the metabolite changes during total global ischemia and on the proton transporter systems is good. The reconstruction of calcium overload arrhythmias during ischemia and reperfusion and during severe acid load is also very encouraging.

There are, however, several steps in the project still to be undertaken. First, the metabolite and pH modeling have not yet been combined into a single model. This will require adequate representation of the acidity changes consequent upon the metabolite changes during ischemia. Second, there are some major gaps in the metabolite modeling. As indicated above, changes in glycogen have not been simulated, and thus the resultant changes in ATP, lactate, pH, and other metabolites are yet to be incorporated. This is the main reason for which the fall in ATP levels, when they eventually occur in the modeling of ischemia, is too rapid. Third, no account has yet been taken of the variations in external ion concentrations in the restricted extracellular spaces. This is particularly relevant given the importance of extracellular potassium accumulation during ischemia. Finally, the metabolite and pH changes have not yet been connected to the cell electrophysiology. All the simulations shown here employ voltage clamp protocols. We are now working on the incorporation of the effects of the metabolite and pH changes on transporter systems to enable the modeling to be connected to the electrophysiology. When that has been achieved, it will become possible to incorporate models of ischemic regions into the network models of the heart.

Acknowledgements

This work was supported by the British Heart Foundation. The computer modeling used OXSOFT HEART 4.6 and was supported by Physiome Sciences Inc.

DISCUSSION

Dr. L. Cleemann: Relating to the transition into arrhythmia and recovery, what are the exact state parameters that you are considering?

Dr. D. Noble: Perhaps I have given you a false impression in showing these two parts of the attempt to reconstruct ischemia. We have not yet linked together the proton simulations and the metabolite simulations. Before we can do that we need to compute the proton cost of the metabolite changes. That is relatively easy to do and we anticipate that it will produce the known time course of pH change during ischemia when the two parts of the modeling are linked together. We have not yet done that.

Dr. L. Cleemann: What is the rate limiting step in your Na^+/Ca^{2+} exchange mechanism? Do you have empenal equations for the eurik process or do you think that something might be done by considering the one and off–rates of the different partial processes?

Dr. D. Noble: That is a very interesting question because some of the small compounds that are being produced and which are active on the Na^+/Ca^{2+} exchanger act preferentially one mode rather than another, e.g. the compound (No. 7943 or KB–R7943) produced by the Kanebo Company in Japan, act primarily on the outward mode [*Watano et al. A novel antagonist, No. 7943, of the Na^+/Ca^{2+} exchange in guinea–pig cardiac ventricular cells. Br J Pharm 1996;119:555–563*]. Compounds also exist which act primarily on the inward mode [*Watano et al., ibid*]. To answer your specific question, our modeling of the Na^+/Ca^{2+} exchanger is relatively simple and it is based on a reduced form of the equations developed by Mullins [1]. Our justification for doing that, and for continuing to do so, is that it is computationally simple. The exchanger has a single energy barrier to go through, which is voltage sensitive. That generates two exponential components, one each for the inward and outward modes, which when added together give functions similar to the hyperbolic sine function. The second justification is that this turns out to be remarkably close to the experimental current–voltage relations first published by Kimura et al. [*Identification of sodium–calcium exchange current in single ventricular cells of guinea–pig. J Physiol 1987;384:199–222*]. We were very encouraged by that fit. Nevertheless, we now know that the model is too simple because when it comes to asking the question whether we can perturb the system to mimic drugs that act on one mode rather than another, the problem is that we can not do so using the present formulations without breaking fundamental laws relating to thermodynamic equilibrium. If you simply change one mode of the exchanger in the present equations you necessarily change the equilibrium potential, which is thermodynamically impossible. What we are now planning to do therefore is to use one of the complex Hilgemann models [*Hilgemann DW. Numerical approxima–*

tions of sodium–calcium exchange. Prog Biophysics Mol Biol 1988;51:1–45] so that we can plausibly reconstruct drugs that act preferentially on one mode rather than another, perhaps by interfering with sodium inhibition of the exchanger.

Dr. H. ter Keurs: What happens in this very intriguing model if you replace activation of the Na^+/Ca^{2+} exchanger by overexpression of the sarcolemmal calcium pump?

Dr. D. Noble: We have not yet done that. Whether we can up–regulate the sarcolemmal calcium pump and replace the function of the sodium–calcium exchanger is just the kind of question that a model ought to be able to answer. We therefore ought to try it. The usual answer that people give as a *post hoc* justification for what nature has done is that the sodium–calcium exchanger is such a high–capacity transporter that it makes sense for it to be the main mechanism for getting calcium out of the cell rather than the sarcolemmal calcium pump. To get rates that the exchanger is capable of you would have to up–regulate the pump by around two orders of magnitude, since in the present calculations not more than around 2–3% of the total calcium exit from the cell is attributable to the Ca^{2+} pump, which is why we now ignore its contribution in most calculations. The advantage of using the calcium pump of course, were it to work, is that you would avoid the arrhythmogenic current generated by the sodium–calcium exchanger.

Dr. H. ter Keurs: A small technical point. When we look at the recovery from metabolic inhibition by hypoxia via cyanide, we find that during the recovery phase in the period that you see these rather extravagant arrhythmias there is a substantial rise in passive force of the muscles as a result of the spontaneous ongoing calcium release. Did you leave that out intentionally, or is it part of the threshold of the contractile system.

Dr. D. Noble: Are you saying that during this phase you see a considerable degree of contracture?

Dr. H. ter Keurs: Yes.

Dr. D. Noble: That depends on the conditions used in the computations, particularly concerning the level of intracellular free calcium required to induce calcium release. If you repeat the computations with different values for the binding constant for calcium release it is relatively easy to generate arrhythmia and contracture together. Notice, incidentally, that there is some contracture during the acid–induced arrhythmia in the present simulations.

Dr. P. Hunter: Experimentally, what happens during reperfusion arrhythmias when you inhibit the Na^+/Ca^{2+} exchanger? Presumably you can not enhance it.

Dr. D. Noble: There are no experiments on that yet because the only inhibitors of Na^+/Ca^{2+} exchange that we have at the moment are not specific enough. The Kanebo drug, for example, also inhibits calcium current [*Watano et al., ibid*]. IT is only useful for physiological investigations where you have already blocked most other transporters and you want to study the Na^+/Ca^{2+} exchange in those conditions. At present, the only way to do what you are asking would be to use lithium replacement for sodium [*LeGuennec J–Y, Noble D. Effects of rapid changes of external Na^+ concentration at different moments during the action potential in guinea–pig myocytes. J Physiol 1994;478:493–504]*. That would be interesting and I do not know whether anyone has tried lithium replacement for sodium during reperfusion arrhythmias. It would have to be done during that period only, since if you did it during the whole run you would do much damage to the calcium balance before the arrhythmias occur and you would be dealing with a totally different state of affairs. It would still be an interesting question, perhaps using the rapid replacement method that LeGuennec and I used. I do not suggest it as a form of therapy though. You would clearly not want to use 70 mM lithium in a patient!

Dr. H. Kammermeir: There is a sharp pH transition extracellularly, with the transition from ischemia to reperfusion. Does the time course of this transition play a role in your model?

Dr. D. Noble: I do not know what happens if we put on a more gradual transition. It is an interesting question but at the moment I do not know. The effects of extracellular pH have not yet been incorporated, and this is one of the things we will have to do.

REFERENCES

1. DiFrancesco D, Noble D. A model of cardiac electrical activity incorporating ionic pumps and concentration changes. *Phil Trans R Soc Lond* 1985;B307:353–398.
2. Noble D. Ionic mechanisms determining the timing of ventricular repolarisation: significance for cardiac arrhythmias. *Ann NY Acad Sci* 1991;644:1–22.
3. Winslow R, Varghese A, Noble D, Adlakha C, Hoythya A. Generation and propagation of triggered activity induced by spatially localised Na–K pump inhibition in atrial network models. *Proc Roy Soc* 1993;B254:55–61.
4. Allen DG, Ordhard CH. Myocardial contractile function during ischemia and hypoxia. *Circ Res* 1987;60:153–168.
5. Lagadic–Gossmann D, Buckler KJ, Vaughan–Jones RD. Role of bicarbonate in pH recovery from intracellular acidosis in the guinea–pig ventricular myocyte. *J Physiol* 1992;458:361–348
6. Bountra C, Vaughan–Jones RD. Effects of intracellular and extracellular pH on contraction in isolated mammalian cardiac muscle. *J Physiol* 1989;418:163–187.
7. Scholz W, Albus U, Lang HJ, Martorana PA, Englert HC, Scholkenes BA. Hoe 694, a new Na^+/H^+ exchange inhibitor and its effects in cardiac ischemia. *Br J Pharmacol* 1993;109:562–568.
8. Clarke K, Anderson RE, Nedelec JF, Forster DO, Allay A. Intracellular and extracellular spaces and the direct quantification of molar intracellular concentrations of phosphorus metabolites in the isolated rat heart using ^{31}P NMR spectroscopy and phosphonate markers. *Magn Resn Med* 1994;32: 181–188.
9. Sun B, Leem CH, Vaughan–Jones RD. Novel chloride–dependent acid loader in the guinea–pig ventricular myocyte: part of a dual acid–loading mechanism. *J Physiol* 1996;495:65–82.
10. Clarke K, O'Connor AJ, Willis RJ. Temporal relation between energy metabolism and myocardial function during ischemia and reperfusion. *Am J Physiol* 1987;253:H412–421.

CHAPTER 25

GAP JUNCTIONS: FUNCTIONAL EFFECTS OF MOLECULAR STRUCTURE AND TISSUE DISTRIBUTION

Jeffrey E. Saffitz[1]

ABSTRACT

Abnormal conduction is fundamental to the pathogenesis of both atrial fibrillation and ventricular tachycardia/fibrillation. Normal atrial and ventricular myocytes express different combinations of multiple gap junction channel proteins and are interconnected by gap junctions in markedly different spatial distributions. These observations suggest that the disparate anisotropic conduction properties of atrial and ventricular muscle are determined, in part, by both structural and molecular features of gap junctions. Alterations in gap junctional coupling likely contribute to conduction abnormalities underlying reentrant atrial or ventricular arrhythmias.

INTRODUCTION

The heart is not a true electrical syncytium. Rather, electrical activation of the myocardium requires intercellular transfer of current from one discrete cardiac myocyte to another. This process occurs at gap junctions, specialized regions of the surface membranes of adjacent cells containing channels that directly link their cytoplasmic compartments [1]. Individual gap junctions consist of closely packed arrays of tens to thousands of individual channels (Fig. 1) that permit the intercellular passage of ions and small molecules up to approximately 1 kDa in molecular weight [1, 2]. Each individual intercellular channel is created by stable non–covalent interactions of two hemichannels, each located in the plasma membrane of neighboring cells. Each hemichannel is believed to be a multimeric

[1]Department of Pathology, Washington University School of Medicine, 660 South Euclid Avenue, St. Louis, MO 63110, USA

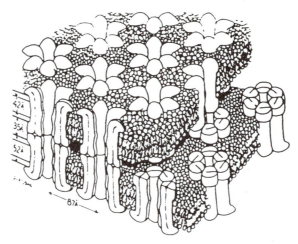

Figure 1. A model of the structure of a gap junction originally proposed by Makowski *et al.* [2] on the basis of X–ray diffraction analysis of isolated junctional membranes. Intercellular channels are created by pairing of hexameric assemblies in the plasma membranes of adjacent cells. Gap junctions may contain tens to thousands of individual channels.

structure composed of six integral membrane protein subunits (connexins) that surround a central aqueous pore and, thereby, create a transmembrane channel [1, 2].

Connexins are members of a multigene family of proteins that form the intercellular channels of gap junctions [3]. Individual connexins contain four hydrophobic domains that span the lipid bilayer, a large but variable hydrophilic carboxy–terminal tail, and three smaller hydrophilic domains separating the hydrophobic domains (Fig. 2). The transmembrane and extracellular domains are among the most highly conserved regions of connexins. In contrast, the cytoplasmic domains differ markedly both in sequence and in length and appear to confer the specific biophysical properties on channels composed of individual connexins [3].

In general, individual parenchymal cells express more than one connexin protein. For example, three individual connexins, connexin43 (Cx43), connexin40 (Cx40) and connexin45 (Cx45), are expressed by cardiac myocytes [4]. However, the pattern of connexin expression and the number, size and distribution of gap junctions vary among functionally distinct excitable tissues [5]. Analysis of single channel events in communication–deficient cells transfected with known connexin sequences has revealed that individual connexins form channels with distinct biophysical properties [6]. Of the cardiac connexins, Cx40 channels have the greatest unitary conductance [7] (mainly 121 or 158 pS) and Cx45 channels have the smallest (29 pS) [8]. Cx43 channels exhibit multiple conductances (50 and 90 pS are most frequently observed) [9]. Cx43 channels are relatively voltage insensitive and highly permeable to anions and cations and fluorescent dyes of different charge densities and molecular weights [6]. In contrast, Cx40 and Cx45 channels are highly cation–selective [6–8]. Cx45 channel gating is highly voltage dependent and the dye Lucifer yellow, used in classical assays of junctional coupling, passes much less freely through Cx40 than Cx43 channels and not detectably throughout Cx45 channels [6–8].

Recognition that individual cardiac myocytes express at least three connexins in different amounts and spatial distributions raises fundamental questions. What are the individual contributions of specific connexin gene products to the conduction properties of

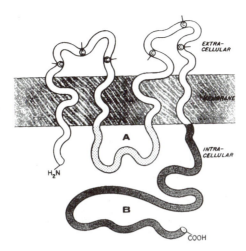

Figure 2. A model of the topology of a connexin molecule in the cell membrane. Six connexin molecules assemble to form individual hemichannels as shown in Figure 1. Each member of the connexin family of proteins has four transmembrane domains and two extracellular loops (each containing three invariant cysteine residues (C)) whose sequences are conserved. However, the intracellular hydrophilic loop (A) and the C-terminal domain (B) have sequences that vary widely among different connexins. These intracellular regions specify some of the biophysical properties unique to channels composed of different connexins.

functionally distinct cardiac tissues in the normal heart? Does expression of specific combinations of connexins confer specific conduction properties on a cardiac tissue? Do hybrid channels (composed of more than one connexin) occur in the heart and contribute to the conduction properties of specific cardiac tissues? Is expression of multiple connexins by individual cells coordinately regulated? Is there a relationship between connexin expression phenotypes and the establishment of tissue-specific patterns of gap junction size, number and spatial distribution? In this report, we review studies designed to characterize the role of molecular and structural features of gap junctions as determinants of the distinct anisotropic conduction properties of atrial and ventricular muscle. The results of these studies suggest the possibility of chamber-specific molecular determinants of conduction that could be targets for new drugs designed to selectively affect atrial or ventricular impulse propagation and, thereby, selectively treat patients with atrial or ventricular arrhythmias dependent upon reentrant mechanisms.

METHODS

Tissue Acquisition and Preparation

Samples of crista terminalis and subepicardium of the anterior left ventricular (LV) free wall were dissected from hearts excised from five mongrel dogs. Some tissue samples were frozen and stored at −70°C for subsequent immunocytochemical analysis and extraction of total RNA for Northern blot analysis. The remaining tissue samples were fixed for high resolution light microscopy and analysis of the spatial distribution of intercellular connections.

Light Microscopic Reconstructions of the Spatial Distribution of Intercellular Connections

Small fragments of myocardium were embedded in epoxy resin and sectioned in a plane longitudinal to the long fiber axis. A series of 40 consecutive sections, each approximately 1 μm in thickness, was prepared from each tissue block and mounted sequentially on slides. The sections were stained with toluidine blue and examined by light microscopy. Under these conditions, the outlines of individual cell profiles could be easily discerned and the locations of intercalated disks connecting adjacent cells were also readily identified. Two individual index cardiac myocyte profiles were randomly selected in the 20th section of each set of 40 serial sections, and these index cells and all neighboring myocytes to which they were connected by intercalated disks were delineated and counted by identifying, in their entirety, profiles of these cells in sections 19 and below and sections 21 and above. A cellular interconnection was tabulated only after an intercalated disk between the adjacent cells was identified unequivocally. It was assumed that the presence of one or more intercalated disks connecting two cells identified at the light microscopic level of resolution indicated electrical interconnection at gap junctions. This assumption is based on observations by us and others that at least one and usually several gap junctions occur at each intercalated disk [1, 10–12].

In addition to measuring the number of cells connected to each index cell in each set of serial sections, we characterized the spatial distribution of each interconnection on the basis of its relative side–to–side or end–to–end orientation according to a system devised in our previous studies [10,11]. Four classes of interconnections were defined as follows:

Type I, >75% of the lateral borders of the two cells overlap.
Type II, 25% – 75% lateral border overlap.
Type III, <25% lateral border overlap and <50% end–to–end overlap.
Type IV, <25% lateral border overlap and >50% end–to–end overlap.

The maximum length and width of each index cell was also measured in selected sections.

Northern Blot Analysis

Total cellular RNA was extracted from samples of crista terminalis and LV epicardium as previously described [4, 13]. RNA was separated by electrophoresis on formaldehyde/agarose gels, transferred to nylon membranes, and cross–linked with ultraviolet light. Specific [^{32}P]–labeled DNA probes, shown in previous [4] studies to hybridize specifically with mRNA for the three mammalian cardiac connexins, were synthesized by the random primer technique. The blots were hybridized for approximately 18 hrs, washed stringently and analyzed by autoradiography as previously described [4, 13].

Immunofluorescence Analysis

Sections (12 μm in thickness) of frozen, unfixed crista terminalis and LV subepicardium were prepared in the cryostat and mounted on gelatin–coated slides. Sections were washed in phosphate buffered saline (PBS) and preincubated for 30 min in a blocking buffer do reduce non–specific binding of primary antibody as described [13,14]. Sections were incubated with monospecific antibodies against Cx43, Cx40 and Cx45. The primary antibodies used in immunocytochemical studies have been extensively characterized in previous work and shown to be monospecific [14]. Sections were incubated overnight with

1:400 dilutions of primary antibodies mixed in blocking buffer. Normal non–immune mouse and rabbit sera were used as negative controls. After being incubated with primary antibodies, sections were rinsed in PBS and incubated with appropriate rabbit or mouse secondary antibodies conjugated to CY3.

RESULTS

Spatial Distribution of Intercellular Connections and Atrial and Ventricular Muscle

    The number and spatial orientation of myocyte interconnections, determined by three–dimensional reconstructions in serial sections of crista terminalis and LV, are shown in Fig. 3. In the LV, randomly selected ventricular myocytes were found to have 11.3 ± 2.2 neighbors to which each was connected at intercalated disks. Approximately 29% of interconnected cells were juxtaposed in a purely side–to–side orientation (Type I connections) and 34% were oriented end–to–end (Type IV junctions). If Type I and Type II junctions are considered to represent interconnections between cells in a pure or predominant side–to–side orientation, and Type III and Type IV junctions occur between neighbors in a pure or predominant end–to–end orientation, then approximately half of the total cellular interconnections in ventricular muscle occurred between cells oriented side–to–side and the remaining half occurred between cells oriented end–to–end.

    In contrast to the architecture of the LV, a markedly different pattern of intercellular connections was observed in the crista terminalis. Randomly selected myocytes of the crista were connected by intercalated disks to 6.4 ± 1.7 individual cells (p<0.05 vs. LV myocytes). The great majority of interconnections occurred between cells oriented in end–to–end apposition. Of the 6.4 neighbors to which the average crista terminalis myocyte was connected, 3.8 (60%) of these neighbors had Type IV connections and an additional 1.1 (19%) had Type III connections. Thus, more than three–fourths of the interconnections in the crista terminalis occur between myocytes juxtaposed in a purely or predominantly end–to–end orientation. Even though ventricular myocytes are connected to twice as many

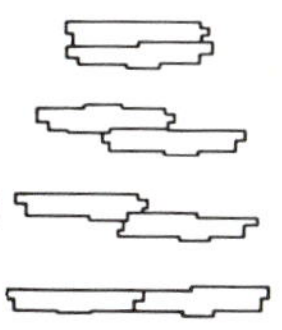

		LEFT VENTRICLE	CRISTA TERMINALIS
I		3.3 ± 1.4 (29)	0.8 ± 0.6 (12)
II		2.0 ± 0.7 (18)	0.7 ± 0.6 (11)
III		2.1 ± 0.9 (19)	1.1 ± 0.7 (17)
IV		3.9 ± 1.1 (34)	3.8 ± 0.7 (60)
		11.3 ± 2.2 CELLS CONNECTED TO EACH MYOCYTE	6.4 ± 1.7 CELLS CONNECTED TO EACH MYOCYTE

Figure 3. Comparison of the total number and spatial orientation of cells interconnected by gap junctions to individual randomly selected myocytes in normal canine left ventricular (LV) epicardium and crista terminalis. The values are the mean (± SD) number of cells connected to each individual cell in each of four different orientations. Type I connections are purely side–to–side. Type IV connections are purely end–to–end, and Types II and III exhibit variable side–to–side and end–to–end orientations. The numbers in parentheses indicate the percentage of each connection type in the two tissues. Ventricular myocytes are extensively interconnected by gap junctions that link cells in both side–to–side and end–to–end orientations. In contrast, myocytes of the crista are connected to fewer neighbors but most connections occur between cells oriented end–to–end (reproduced from [13] with permission of the American Heart Association).

neighbors as crista terminalis myocytes, the number of interconnections between cells in end–to–end orientation (Type IV connections) is equivalent in the two tissues (3.9 ± 1.1 Type IV connections per myocyte in the ventricle and 3.8 ± 1.1 Type IV connections to each myocyte of the crista terminalis, p=NS).

The mean maximum length and width of index ventricular and crista terminalis myocytes were measured. Ventricular myocytes were approximately 27% longer (122 ± 14 vs. 96 ± 18 μm) and 21% wider (23 ± 4 vs. 19 ± 5 μm) than crista terminalis myocytes (p<0.05 for both) but the length–to–width ratios were the same: 5.3 for ventricular myocytes and 5.2 for atrial myocytes.

Connexin Expression Phenotypes in Atrial and Ventricular Muscle

Figure 4 is a representative Northern blot showing the relative abundance of mRNA transcripts for the three mammalian gap junction proteins, Cx43, Cx40 and Cx45. Both crista terminalis and LV myocytes contained abundant Cx43 mRNA transcripts. Under comparable gel loading and film exposure conditions, the Cx45 signal was weak, although it appeared that the crista contained slightly more Cx45 mRNA than in the ventricle. In contrast, abundant Cx40 mRNA was observed in atrial samples whereas Cx40 transcripts were nearly undetectable in the ventricle.

Results of immunohistochemistry on frozen sections of the crista terminalis and LV revealed abundant Cx43 and Cx45 immunoreactivity in both tissues (Fig. 5). In contrast, Cx40 staining was far more intense in the crista terminalis than in the LV muscle. More-over, the pattern in the LV was confined almost exclusively to the endothelial cells of intramural coronary arteries and microvessels, consistent with previous observations [15, 16]. No detectable Cx43 immunoreactive signal was present in ventricular myocytes. As shown in Fig. 5, junctions between atrial myocytes occurred in relatively simple, straight intercalated disks that connected cells in a predominant end–to–end fashion. In contrast, the pattern of immunostaining in the ventricular muscle reflected the far more extensive gap junctions between ventricular cells juxtaposed in side–to–side as well as end–to–end orientation.

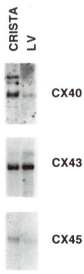

Figure 4. Northern blots of connexin mRNAs in canine LV myocardium and crista terminalis (reproduced from [13] with permission of the American Heart Association).

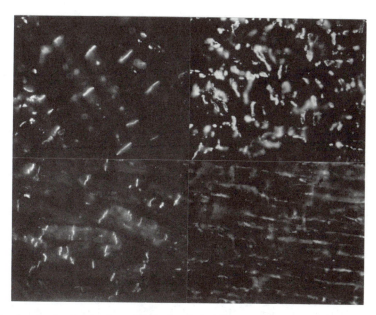

Figure 5. Photomicrographs showing immunohistochemical delineation of Cx43 (**top** half) and Cx40 (**bottom** half) expression in the LV (**right** half) and crista terminalis (**left** half). Cx43 and Cx40 immunoreactivity are readily apparent in the crista terminalis in a pattern consistent with the predominant end–to–end orientation of intercellular connections in this tissue. The staining pattern of ventricular junctions seen in the Cx43 preparation is more complex, consistent with the extensive side–to–side and end–to–end interconnections. However, Cx40 immunoreactivity in the ventricle is considerably less than that in the crista and is associated primarily with microvessels (reproduced from [13] with permission of the American Heart Association).

DISCUSSION

The results of this study indicate that myocytes of the canine crista terminalis and the LV subepicardium differ markedly in the number and spatial distribution of their intercellular junctions and in the molecular composition of their gap junction proteins. These findings are consistent with the disparate anisotropic conduction properties of the crista terminalis and the LV. Longitudinal propagation in defined atrial fiber bundles such as the crista terminalis is not only extremely rapid but also highly anisotropic. Conduction velocity in the crista terminalis is approximately 10 times more rapid in the longitudinal direction (parallel to fiber orientation) than in the transverse direction (perpendicular to the long cell axis) [17]. In contrast, a directional difference of only approximately 3:1 has been observed in ventricular muscle. Although atrial and ventricular muscle differ in their active sarcolemmal membrane ionic currents, these properties cannot account for their disparate tissue anisotropy. The results of the present study suggest that both molecular and structural features of gap junctions are important determinants of the anisotropic properties of atrial and ventricular muscle.

Our observations suggest that 1) the conduction properties of atrial and ventricular muscle are determined, in part, by the specific types of connexins they express and the number, size and spatial distribution of their gap junction connection; and 2) altered intercellular coupling due to changes in connexin expression and/or gap junction distribution contribute to arrhythmogenesis. Although these hypotheses are supported by a large body of indirect evidence, there has been no direct analysis of the functional roles subserved by multiple connexins expressed in individual cardiac myocytes.

To elucidate the functional contributions of individual connexins in myocardial conduction, we have begun studying Cx43 knockout mouse originally produced by Reaume *et al.* [18]. We have discovered that adult mice heterozygotes for the Cx43 null mutation (Cx43 −/+ mice) exhibit a marked slowing of ventricular conduction [19]. We also analyzed three lead electrocardiograms and observed significant prolongation of the QRS interval in heterozygotes compared to wild type animals. Taken together, the results of conduction studies and ECG measurements indicate that neonatal and adult mice hetero−zygotes for a Cx43 null mutation exhibits slow ventricular conduction.

CONCLUSIONS

Because ventricular myocytes express both Cx43 and Cx45, the marked slowing of ventricular conduction in Cx43 −/+ mice suggests that Cx43 is a significant conductor of intercellular charge whereas Cx45 may or may not play a significant role in this function. Because atrial muscle expresses Cx40 in addition to Cx43 and Cx45, and because Cx40 is not expressed in the ventricle, we hypothesize that the presence of Cx40 in atrial muscle may prevent the development of slow conduction in mice with a single null allele for Cx43 even though Cx43 is expressed in the atrium. If this hypothesis can be substantiated, then this will provide the first evidence for chamber−specific molecular determinants of conduction in atrial and ventricular myocardium. These results would also provide a rationale for the development of new drugs designed to target specific gap junction channel to selectively modulate atrial or ventricular conduction and, thereby, selectively treat conduction abnormalities in patients with either atrial or ventricular arrhythmias.

Acknowledgements

Supported by National Institutes of Health Grant HL50598.

DISCUSSION

Dr. H. Strauss: I relate to the ECG in the animals that are heterozygotes for connexin 43. Although the P wave duration is not changed, the P wave amplitude looks like it is significantly greater in those mice than in the wild type. Also, the end−to−end distribution of connexin 43 in the crista terminalis is estimated to be about 60%. In the heterozygote mice you show no change in the distribution of connexins at the gap junction. Therefore, the connexin isoform at that end−to−end site is all connexin 40 in the crista terminalis. Is that correct?

Dr. J. E. Saffitz: No. There are, in fact, three connexins present in the crista terminalis and they co−localize in individual gap junctions, at least as determined with confocal microscopy. Those straight end−to−end junctions in the immunofluorescence preparation contained Cx43, Cx40 and Cx45.

Dr. H. Strauss: Do you think there is a redundancy in terms of the number of proteins needed for intercellular communication? You show no change in conduction velocity in the crista terminalis, and that is the dominant connexin between cells. If that is the case, then how do you explain the increase in P wave amplitude that you see in your records?

Dr. J. E. Saffitz: We have not seen a consistent increase in P wave amplitude. We have only studied three animals of each genotype. At this point, we have not done enough experiments to reach any definitive conclusions. Based on what we have done so far, there is a significant increase in QRS interval and no change in any other parameter. The question of redundancy is a major question. What are the functions of the three connexins present in individual gap junctions that connect myocardial cells? Is this merely redundancy or are these proteins fulfilling different functions? Our results so far suggest that Cx43 plays a major role in the ventricle. If half of the Cx43 is removed, as is the case in the Cx43 −/+ animals, there is a large effect on ventricular conduction. Cx45 may not play a major role in ventricular conduction. In the Cx43 −/+ animals, Cx45 expression is not changed although there is still a marked ventricular conduction phenotype. Atrial muscle expresses not only Cx43 and Cx45, like the ventricles, but also Cx40. We do not know the exact proportions; rigorous quantitative measurements have not been performed. However, there appears to be abundant Cx40 and abundant Cx43 in atrial muscle. Our preliminary results suggest that if approximately half of the atrial Cx43 is removed, there seems to be no effect on atrial conduction. This suggests that Cx40 functions as a principal conductor of intercellular current in atrial muscle. We have not yet characterized the distribution of junctions in atrial and ventricular tissues in these mice. We have also not yet defined the conduction pathways. It is possible that some alterations in the patterns of intercellular connectivity occur in these genetically altered mice that could contribute to the ventricular conduction abnormalities identified in heterozygotes. All of this remains to be done in the future.

Dr. H. ter Keurs: Coming back to the homozygote knockout. You have indicated that you could not measure conduction in the ventricle. That leads to the question, did these ventricles contract at all while you were looking at them? If they did or if they did not, is that a cause of death at birth? Are they living in utero only on atrial contractions, and, in general, why did they die?

Dr. J. E. Saffitz: These are very important questions. I have very little data to answer them with. First, I should point out that Cx43 is widely expressed throughout the animal. Thus, the knockout of Cx43 could affect not only the heart but many other organs as well. The only gross abnormality that can be seen at autopsy in the knockout animals is a malformation of the right ventricular outflow tract. As a pathologist who performs autopsies, I can tell you that human infants who are born with more profound degrees of right ventricular outflow tract obstruction than that seen in these animals do not die immediately after birth. For example, pulmonary atresia is not a fatal malformation. Therefore, I am not convinced that the right ventricular outflow tract obstruction is the sole cause of death in these animals although it could play a significant role. There may be a combination of many effects. For example, Cx43 is abundantly expressed in the adrenal cortex. Perhaps these animals have some defect in cortisol secretion or something of this sort. It appears that the fetus can survive and develop when it is connected to the maternal circulation but as soon as the fetal–maternal circulation is disrupted and the neonate is on its own, it may suffer from multiple organ problems. At this point, however, this is purely speculative. With regard to your question about contractions, the answer is yes. These hearts do contract occasionally but the contractions appear to be very weak. Because of the amount of manipulation involved in removing the hearts, placing them in the tissue bath, and putting the electrode array on to the surface of the heart, we have not been able to reliably measure electrical activity in the homozygous Cx43 null hearts. In fact, when we discovered that the heterozygotes had a ventricular conduction phenotype, we stopped our attempts to analyze conduction in Cx43 −/− neonates and studied heterozygote adults instead. However, we plan to continue studies of the Cx43 knockout neonates in the future.

Dr. H. ter Keurs: Is the contraction that you see occasionally synchronous in the ventricle, and if so, why?

Dr. J. E. Saffitz: Although they are weak and irregular, the contractions do appear to be synchronous. The mice homozygous for the Cx43 null mutation express Cx45 in their ventricles. We speculate that Cx45 may be able to provide sufficient coupling of ventricular myocytes to allow these hearts to beat. Certainly, these hearts beat in utero so the ventricular muscle must be electrically coupled in some way.

Dr. Y. Rudy: I realize that the heart is only 2 mm long and difficult to handle, but have you tried to measure velocity in different directions to evaluate the effect on anisotropy?

Dr. J. E. Saffitz: We have not yet done these studies, but we plan on performing this type of analysis. We anticipate observing directional differences and predict that conduction in the ventricle will be more anisotropic in the heterozygotes than in wild type animals. Our preliminary results would also suggest that there would be no difference in anisotropic conduction properties in the atria of wild type and Cx43 −/+ animals.

Dr. Y. Rudy: The other obvious question is whether the reduced coupling is due to smaller conductance of individual connexons or due to decrease in the number of functional connexons. Also, you mentioned that Kathryn Yamada is conducting whole–cell experiments. Has she tried obtaining cell–pairs to measure the intercellular conductance?

Dr. J. E. Saffitz: I would suggest that the number of channels is reduced because the total amount of Cx43 in cells is reduced. Whether the properties of the channels are also changed is not known. With regards to cell pair studies, we are just beginning to do these. However, your question raises another issue that is worth thinking about. This concerns the question of whether hybrid channels form. One potential outcome in cells that express multiple connexins is formation of individual intercellular channels made of more than one connexin. This could happen in several ways. One possibility is the creation of a heterotypic channel in which each cell's contribution to a complete channel is composed of a different protein. Alternatively, there might be heteromeric channels in which an individual hemichannel is composed of more than one protein. The latter situation could theoretically occur in many different stoichiometries. Results of studies in expression systems suggest that some connexins can form hybrid channels where as others cannot. For example, if you take two Xenopus oocytes, one transfected with Cx43 and the other transfected with Cx45, and physically hold them together, you can detect formation of functional channels that must be created by the heterotypic association of Cx43 hemichannels and Cx45 hemichannels. However, if this experiment is repeated using oocytes transfected with Cx40 and Cx43, no functional channels are detected.

What happens if we diminish the expression of one protein, for example Cx43? How does this affect the assembly of all the remaining connexins into gap junction channels? This is a very complicated question about which we have very little data. However, as you indicate, one way to get at this question is to perform cell pair studies to measure junctional conductances and delineate the spectrum of single channel currents under different conditions in which expression of individual connexins is manipulated. In this way, one can begin to get some insight into the important questions you raised.

Dr. L. Gepstein: Did you try to look at the dispersion of repolarization in this ventricle? People have shown that the electronic interaction can also affect repolarization.

Dr. J. E. Saffitz: This is an obvious thing to do but we have not yet performed these studies.

Dr. G. Kessler–Icekson: I would like to come back to the malformation of the heart in the knockout mice. How would you explain this malformation? What are the roles of connexins and how are they expressed in the embryo or the developing heart? Is there anything known regarding the regulation of expression?

Dr. J. E. Saffitz: It is not understood how this malformation occurs. Cx43 is expressed very early on during embryogenesis. Cx43 mRNA can be detected as early as the four–cell embryo stage and Cx43 in gap junctions can be identified immunohistochemically in eight–cell embryos. It seems likely that these intercellular connections may play an important role in the spread of morphogenetic information. However, knocking out Cx43 has no demonstrable effect on early events in development. Presumably, other connexins that are expressed in early embryos can fulfill required roles in mediating intercellular communication. With respect to how the malformation occurs in the knockout mice, I do not know. Cx43 is expressed throughout the development of the heart. It appears to be expressed uniformly and not regionally. Therefore, it remains a mystery as to why there is a malformation involving one specific region of the heart. It is possible that this malformation could be secondary to some other problems which could lead to the hypertrophy of the right ventricular outflow tract. At this point, one can only speculate.

REFERENCES

1. Page E. Cardiac gap junctions. In: The Heart and Cardiovascular System (Fozzard HA, Haber E, Jennings RB, Katz AM, Morgan HE, eds). New York: Raven Press, 1992;1003–1047.
2. Makowski L, Caspar DL, Phillips WC, Goodenough DA. Gap junction structure: analysis of X–ray diffraction data. *J Cell Biol* 1977;74:629–645.
3. Beyer EC, Goodenough DA, Paul DL. Connexin family of gap junction proteins. *J Membr Biol* 1990;116:187–194.
4. Kanter HL, Saffitz JE, Beyer EC. Cardiac myocytes express multiple gap junction proteins. *Circ Res* 1992;70:438–444.
5. Davis LM, Kanter HL, Beyer EC, Saffitz JE. Distinct gap junction protein phenotypes in cardiac tissues with disparate conduction properties. *J Am Coll Cardiol* 1994;24:1124–1132.
6. Veenstra RD. Size and selectivity of gap junction channels formed from different connexins. *J Bioenergetics Biomembranes* 1996;28:317–337.
7. Dillon SM, Allessie MA, Ursell PC, Wit AL. Influences of anisotropic tissue structure and reentrant circuits in the epicardial border zone of subacute canine infarcts. *Circ Res* 1988;63:182–206.
8. Veenstra RD, Wang H–Z, Beyer EC, Brink PR. Selective dye and ionic permeability of gap junction channels formed by connexin45. *Circ Res* 1994;75:483–490.
9. Moreno AP, Saez JC, Fishman GI, Spray DC. Human connexin43 gap junction channels. Regulation of unitary conductances by phosphorylation. *Circ Res* 1994;74:1050–1057.
10. Hoyt RH, Cohen ML, Saffitz JE. Distribution and three–dimensional structure of intercellular junctions in canine myocardium. *Circ Res* 1989;64:563–574.
11. Luke RA, Saffitz JE. Remodeling of ventricular conduction pathways in healed canine infarct border zones. *J Clin Invest* 1991;87:1594–1602.
12. Severs NJ. The cardiac gap junction and intercalated disk. *Int J Cardiol* 1990;26;137–173.
13. Saffitz JE, Kanter HL, Green KG, Tolley TK, Beyer EC. Tissue–specific determinants of anisotropic conduction velocity in canine atrial and ventricular myocardium. *Circ Res* 1994;74:1065–1070.
14. Kanter HL, Beyer EC, Green KG, Saffitz JE. Multiple connexins colocalize in canine cardiac myocyte gap junctions. *Circ Res* 1993;74:344–350.
15. Bastide B, Neyses L, Ganten D, Paul M, Willecke F, Traub O. Gap junction protein connexin40 is preferentially expressed in vascular endothelium and conductive bundles of rat myocardium and is increased under hypertensive conditions. *Circ Res* 1993;73:1138–1149.
16. Chen S, Davis LM, Westphale EM, Beyer EC, Saffitz JE. Expression of multiple gap junction proteins in human fetal and infant hearts. *Ped Res* 1994;36:561–566.
17. Spach MS, Miller WT III, Geselowitz DB, Barr RRC, Kootsey JM, Johnson EA. The discontinuous nature of propagation in normal canine cardiac muscle: evidence for recurrent discontinuities of intracellular resistance that affect the membrane currents. *Circ Res* 1981;48:39–54.
18. Reaume AG, de Sousa PA, Kulkarni S, Langille BL, Zhu D, Davies TC, Jeneja SC, Kidder GM, Rossant J. Cardiac malformation in neonatal mice lacking connexin43. *Science* 1995;267:1831–1834.
19. Guerrero PA, Schuessler RB, Beyer EC, Saffitz JE. Mice heterozygous for a Cx43 null mutation exhibit a conduction defect. *Circulation* 1996;94:I–8.

CHAPTER 26

3D Cardiac Imaging of Electromechanical Coupling

Lior Gepstein[1] and Shlomo A. Ben–Haim[1,2]

ABSTRACT

A novel method for three dimensional (3D) electromechanical mapping of the heart is presented. The new method is based on utilizing special magnetically locatable catheters connected to a mapping and navigation system. The 3D electromechanical map of the chamber is reconstructed by sampling the location of the catheter tip throughout the cardiac cycle at a plurality of endocardial sites together with their local electrograms. The ability to spatially combine electrical and mechanical information may provide a useful tool for both research and clinical cardiology.

INTRODUCTION

The heart is characterized by two major functional phenomena: electrical excitation and the resulting myocardial contraction. Consequently, numerous methods have been developed to evaluate these functions in health and disease, both for the cardiac scientist investigating the heart as well as for the practicing cardiologist. Nevertheless, a single method which can combine quantitative information regarding both the electrical, mechanical, and hemodynamic properties of the heart is still lacking.

Cardiac electrical mapping was reported as early as 1915 [1] and implies registration of the electrical activation sequence by recording extracellular electrograms. One of the objectives of cardiac electrical mapping is to analyze the activation wave fronts emerging

---

[1]Cardiovascular System Laboratory, The Bruce Rappaport Faculty of Medicine, Technion–Israel Institute of Technology, Haifa, Israel, and [2]Harvard–Thorndike Electrophysiology Institute and Arrhythmia Service, Beth Israel Hospital, Boston, Massachusetts 02215, USA

from those structures that are involved in the genesis of arrhythmias [2]. The exact local–ization of such structures is a prerequisite for understanding the pathophysiological mech–anisms that underlie the arrhythmia, for evaluating the effects of drugs, or for directing surgical or catheter ablation procedures [3–5]. Cardiac mapping is a broad term that covers several modes of mapping, such as body surface, endocardial, and epicardial mapping [6–9]. Electrogram acquisition can be simultaneous from many sites, usually during sur–gery, with the use of fixed–shape electrode arrays such as epicardial socks and endocardial balloons or, more commonly, using catheters that are introduced percutaneously into the heart chambers, and sequentially record the endocardial electrograms [2]. These electro–physiological catheters are navigated and localized with the use of multiplanar fluoroscopy.

A major limitation in the currently used methods is the inability to accurately associate the electrophysiological information with its exact spatial orientation in the heart. Thus, the localization of the recording sites with fluoroscopy is inaccurate, cumbersome, and associated with considerable X–ray exposure for both the patient and the physician.

Similarly, a number of techniques have been developed to evaluate heart mechanical function, including echocardiography, ventriculography, CT, and MRI. One of the limita–tions of these clinical methods is that the assessment of cardiac mechanics is usually extra–polated from two dimensional (2D) images. Furthermore, these methods cannot associate the local electrical and mechanical functions.

We present here a new method for nonfluoroscopic, catheter–based endocardial mapping of the heart that enables 3D mapping of cardiac electromechanics [10, 11]. This method is based on utilizing a new locatable catheter connected to a mapping system. The system uses magnetic technology to accurately determine the location and orientation of the roving mapping catheter and simultaneously records the intracardiac local electrogram from its tip. The chamber 3D geometry is reconstructed in real time as a function of the time during the cardiac cycle, with the electrical information color–coded and superimposed on the geometry.

The mapping technology, the *in vitro* and *in vivo* accuracy, the initial results of evaluating the heart's mechanics, and the possible contribution of this methodology to both basic and clinical cardiology, are discussed.

METHODS

System Components

A real–time, high–resolution, miniature passive magnetic sensor has been developed and incorporated into a standard 7F electrophysiological catheter, just proximal to its tip. Ultralow magnetic fields (5×10^{-6} to 5×10^{-5} T) are radiated from three radiators placed under the operating table. The amplitude, frequency, and phase of the sensed magnetic fields contain the information needed to solve a set of overdetermined algebraic equations yielding the location (x, y, and z) and orientation (roll, yaw, and pitch) of the tip of the catheter. The mapping system reports in six degrees of freedom the location and orientation of the mapping catheter tip. This information enables tracking the tip of the mapping cath–eter while it is deployed within the heart. All the information is displayed on a graphic workstation.

Mapping Procedure

Two locatable catheters are introduced into the heart. The first catheter is placed in the coronary sinus or the right ventricular (RV) apex and serves as a reference catheter.

The second, the mapping catheter, is then placed in the chamber to be mapped. The location of the tip of the mapping catheter while inside the heart is recorded relative to the fixed intracardiac reference catheter. This relative location determination enables correction for subject motion and the movements of the heart within the subject due to breathing. The locations of the mapping and reference catheters are gated to a fiducial point in the cardiac cycle selected by the user. For instance, gating to the ECG R wave results in detection of the catheter tip at end diastole (ED) and reconstruction of an ED map. In this setting the ED location and orientation of the catheter are continuously shown on the mapping computer's screen. By moving the catheter inside the heart, the mapping system continuously analyzes its location and presents it to the user, thus enabling navigation without the use of fluoroscopy.

The mapping procedure is based on dragging the mapping catheter randomly over the endocardium and sequentially acquiring the location of the tip while in contact with the endocardium. The set of points collected comprises an irregularly sampled data set of location points that are members of the endocardial surface. Chamber geometry is then reconstructed, in real time, using the sampled set of location points (Fig. 1). The endocardial surface is presented as a set of polygons (triangles) whose vertices are the sampled points. The local activation time (LAT) at each site is determined from the intracardiac electrogram. The reported results were collected from unipolar recordings filtered at 0.5 to 400 Hz. The LAT at each site was calculated as the interval between a fiducial point on the body surface ECG, or a fixed intracardiac electrogram, and the steepest negative intrinsic deflection from the mapping catheter unipolar recording. The activation map was color-coded and superimposed on the 3D chamber geometry (electroanatomical map).

Electroanatomical Mapping

The location capabilities of the new method were first tested in both *in vitro* and *in vivo* studies and were found to be highly reproducible (standard deviation, 0.16 ± 0.02 mm and 0.74 ± 0.13 mm [mean $\pm$ SEM]) and accurate (mean errors, 0.42 ± 0.05 and 0.73 ± 0.03 mm). We then proceeded to map the different heart chambers in 15 healthy male pigs (30 to 40 kg). A 7F reference catheter was positioned in the coronary sinus or the RV apex. Using fluoroscopic guidance, the mapping catheter was introduced into the left ventricle (LV). From our initial experience we found that after taking the first three points (two at the base and one at the apex) under fluoroscopic guidance, the rest of the mapping procedure could be achieved relatively quickly without the use of fluoroscopy. We also learned that about 30 to 50 evenly spaced points were needed to reconstruct the chamber geometry. The quality of the catheter–wall contact was evaluated at every site by examining the location stability (the difference in ED location between two consecutive beats) and the LAT stability (measured as the difference between the LATs of two consecutive beats). A point was added to the map only if the ED stability was less than 2 mm and LAT stability was less than 2 msec.

Electromechanical Mapping

In this part of the experiments the system was modified to determine the mapping catheter's tip at a frequency of 125 Hz. Hence, the local trajectory of each endocardial site throughout the cardiac cycle could be tagged in space and analyzed by synchronizing the set of locations of each endocardial site with the final fiducial point on the ECG. We were thus able to create a dynamic beating image of the 3D reconstructed map. The center of mass of the reconstructed chamber was automatically calculated from the set of the surface

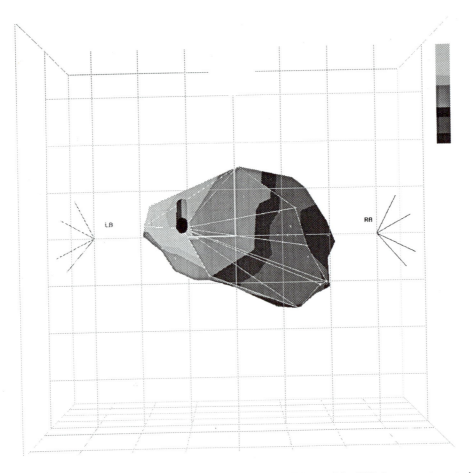

Figure 1. Initial reconstruction (27 sampled points), showing the left ventricle (LV) from a posteroanterior view. Note that the catheter icon is pointing posteriorly.

points at ED and was updated upon acquisition of each new site. The volume of the chamber could be calculated at each time step (8 msec) from the sum of the volumes of all tetrahedrons formed when connecting the center of mass to all triangles forming the reconstructed surface.

RESULTS

Electroanatomical Maps

Figure 2 is a black and white representation of a typical anteroposterior view of an activation map of the LV during sinus rhythm, reconstructed from 50 sampling points. The geometries and activation patterns were similar in all maps. Note that the LV apex in the pig points towards the right and the base is located superiorly, with the mitral valve located posterolaterally. The earliest site of activation (the darkest area) was located on the

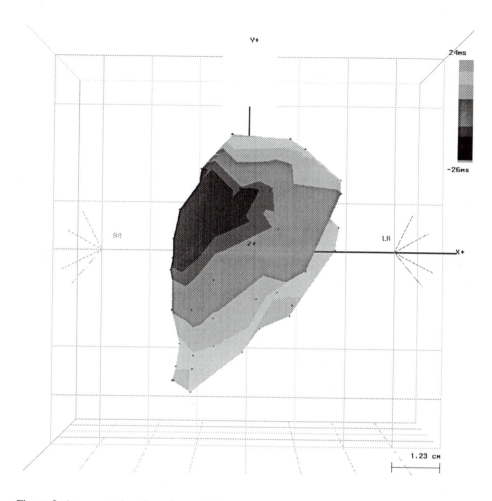

Figure 2. Anteroposterior view of an activation map of the left ventricle (LV) during sinus rhythm.

anterosuperior portion of the septum. In some cases a second endocardial breakthrough was noted more posteriorly. The activation then spread to the rest of the ventricle (activation colors changing from dark to light), with the posterobasal and lateral walls (lighter areas) activated last. Total activation time of this ventricle was 50 msec.

Accuracy of the Electromechanical Maps

Electromechanical maps were obtained in 12 healthy male pigs. In some of the experiments, a 5F solid–state pressure catheter (Millar Instruments, Houston, Texas, USA) was positioned in the LV cavity for simultaneous pressure recording, and in others a 6F Swan–Ganz thermodilution catheter was advanced to the pulmonary artery for simultaneous calculation of cardiac output.

The mapping procedure was similar to that described earlier. The LV was mapped a total of three times by two different users, and the intra– and interobserver variabilities were calculated. The mean ED and end–systolic volumes were 50.6 ± 3.1 and 29.5 ± 1.7 ml, respectively, with the mean stroke volume (SV) and ejection fraction (EF) being 21.1 ± 2.1 ml and 41.3 ± 2.3%, respectively. Intraobserver variability was found to be relatively small (SV, 4.6%; EF, 6.8%). Similarly, interobserver variability was also relatively small (SV, 11.6%; EF, 8.1%). SV measurements highly correlated with those determined by thermodilution (r = 0.94; slope = 0.95; Y intercept = −0.12 ml). The average deviation between the two methods was found to be 8.1 ± 2.2%.

Electromechanical Coupling

Figure 3 is a typical graph displaying all the relevant information regarding the electromechanical function of a specific site in the map. The volumetric changes of the global heart during the cardiac cycle are illustrated by the dashed line. The regional mechanical function (dotted line) is calculated as the change in the areas of all polygons connected with this specific site and normalized by the area at ED. Note that this plot correlates nicely with the global volumetric plot, indicating a normally contracting zone. The solid line shows the unipolar electrogram recorded at that site and represents the local electrical event, which can be characterized by its timing, amplitude, and configuration.

DISCUSSION

Importance of Electroanatomical Mapping

The unique ability of the new mapping method to combine, for the first time, endocardial electrophysiological and spatial geometrical information improves our insight regarding the pathophysiological mechanisms that are involved in the genesis of various arrhythmias. Features like dispersion of repolarization, conduction abnormalities, and

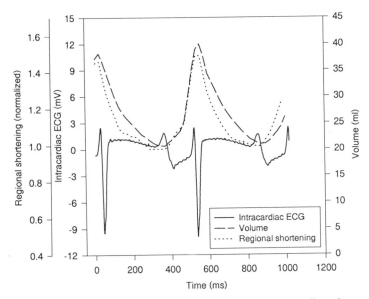

Figure 3. Global volumetric measurements, regional shortening, and intracardiac electrogram changes throughout the cardiac cycle.

conduction anisotropy, which form the pathologic substrate of various arrhythmias, can now be examined in a spatially oriented fashion, and the relationship between the anatomy and the initiation of arrhythmias can be examined.

Moreover, the new mapping method offers several advantages for clinical electrophysiology: (1) high spatial resolution that enables the formation of a very detailed activation map; (2) the ability to navigate the catheter without the use of fluoroscopy, which should reduce X–ray exposure and procedure time; and (3) the ability to relocate accurately in 3D the tip of the mapping catheter superimposed on the electroanatomical map, which may bring a unique value to ablation procedures. Thus, this new mapping method enables to first perform the mapping procedure, then design ablation strategies, and finally return accurately to the desired site for the delivery of radiofrequency energy.

Mechanical Maps

This study presents our initial experience in using a new mapping method for evaluating mechanical heart function. As described here, the initial results show that the volumetric measurements of pig LVs are reproducible and correlate well with thermodilution measurements. The regional mechanical properties calculated by this new procedure still have to be defined and correlated with other methods such as MRI tagging. Nevertheless, the new method may possess some important clinical and research advantages: The ability to calculate accurate volumetric measurements, together with the assessment of the 3D dynamic geometry of the chamber without extrapolation from 2D images, injection of contrast media, or edge–detection algorithms, provide useful information regarding the heart's systolic and diastolic functions. Moreover, the ability to tag the motion of specific endocardial sites throughout the cardiac cycle can provide valuable information regarding regional endocardial mechanics.

Electromechanical Information

The simultaneous evaluation of both the global and regional electrophysiological and mechanical properties may stimulate research in a number of fields. There is growing interest in the role of asynchronous activation, as occurs during ventricular pacing from different sites, in the synchronization of the mechanical activities and global performance. The ability to combine data on ventricular electrical activation together with regional and global mechanical performance can provide valuable knowledge about the interaction between these two processes during ventricular pacing. This may consequently be clinically important; recent work has suggested that the position of the pacing electrode may significantly change cardiac performance in health and disease [12–14]. Improved LV performance during certain pacing regions has been shown to occur in hypertrophic obstructive cardiomyopathy [12, 13] and in patients suffering from dilated cardiomyopathy [14].

Electromechanical coupling may also be important in examining the tissue characteristics during ischemia and infarction. It has long been known that normal mechanics change during ischemia as well as in infarcted areas. Similarly, it is widely accepted that infarcted tissue is characterized by very low amplitude and fractionated electrograms. Thus, the ability to spatially combine information regarding the mechanical and electrical properties of the tissue may improve our knowledge of the tissue characteristics during ischemia, hibernation, and infarction.

CONCLUSIONS

Our experience in mapping the heart's electrical activity and our initial results in evaluating the cardiac mechanical function with a novel method for 3D electroanatomical mapping of the heart has been presented here. The ability to accurately combine detailed information regarding cardiac mechanics and electrophysiology in a spatially oriented fashion may provide a useful tool in both clinical and basic cardiology.

DISCUSSION

Dr. P. Hunter: What is the spatial resolution of the magnetic sensor when you use it on a pig? Also, what is the size of the sensor, and how accurately can you locate where the tip is?

Dr. L. Gepstein: The spatial resolution outside the heart is about 0.2 mm. Inside the heart it is around 1 mm. The size of the sensor is about 1 mm. It can fit into a 7 Fr catheter. For electro–physiological reasons, the tip electrode is 4 mm; it actually averages electrograms from this area. Thus, the location resolution is greater than the electrophysiologic one.

Dr. P. Hunter: Is there enough flexibility in the catheter tip to ensure that when you position it in the wall it stays at its material point, or is it sliding on the wall?

Dr. L. Gepstein: This is a very good question that leads to the issue of tissue contact. We have six ways of defining stable contact of the catheter with the endocardium: 1) Location stability, which is defined as the difference in location of the catheter tip at two consecutive EDs. If the catheter tip is in stable contact, this difference should be less than 1–2 mm. 2) Local activation time (LAT) stability, which is defined as the difference in LATs in two consecutive beats. Again, if the catheter is in stable contact with the endocardium, this difference should be less than 1–2 ms. 3) Morpholo–gies of the local electrogram at two consecutive beats. If the catheter is in stable contact with the same endocardial site it should record the same local electrogram. 4) Differences in impedance measurement when the catheter is in contact with the endocardium as compared to blood. 5) The orientation of the catheter. Initially when navigating the catheter and touching the wall the catheter icon is pointing down. If we apply a little bit more pressure, the tip is stuck but the shaft is free, so it moves to a horizontal position. 6) We can also examine the local trajectories of each endocardial site at two consecutive beats. If these displacement loops are repeatable than the catheter was in stable contact.

Dr. J. Downey: Your criteria require three beats per contact. How long does it take to get a map?

Dr. L. Gepstein: It depends on the map you want. If you want one for electrophysiological reasons and only need to concentrate on a small area, you can get a rough idea of where the arrhythmia is originating from and then try to go there and look at a very small area in detail. If you want to look at the mechanics of the whole heart, it usually takes about 40–50 sample points, requiring about 5–10 minutes.

REFERENCES

1.   Lewis T, Rothschild MA. The excitatory process in the dog's heart. II. The ventricles. *Philos Trans R Soc Lond B Biol Sci* 1915;206:181–226.
2.   Josephson ME, Horowitz LN, Spielman SR, Waxman HL, Greenspan AM. Role of catheter mapping in the preoperative evaluation of ventricular tachycardia. *Am J Cardiol* 1982;49:207–220.

3. Josephson ME. Use of electrophysiological testing to select antiarrhythmic drug therapy for ventricular arrhythmia. In: Rosen MR, Janse MJ, Wit AL, eds. *Cardiac Electrophysiology: A Textbook*. Mount Kisco, NY: Futura; 1990:1137–1158.

4. Gallagher JJ, Kasell JH, Cox JL, Smith WM, Ideker RE, Smith WM. Techniques of intraoperative electrophysiologic mapping. *Am J Cardiol* 1982;49:221–240.

5. Jackman WM, Wang XZ, Friday KJ, Roman CA, Moulton KP, Beckman KJ, McClelland JH, Twidale N, Hazlitt HA, Prior MI, Margolis PD, Calame JD, Overholt ED, Lazzara R. Catheter ablation of accessory atrioventricular pathways (Wolff–Parkinson–White syndrome) by radiofrequency current. *N Engl J Med* 1991;324:1605–1611.

6. Flowers NC, Horan LG. Body surface potential mapping. In: Zipes DP, Jalife J, eds. *Cardiac Electrophysiology: From Cell to Bedside*. 2nd ed. Philadelphia, Pa: WB Saunders; 1995:1049–1067.

7. De Bakker JMT, Janse MJ, Van Cappelle FJL, Durrer D. Endocardial mapping by simultaneous recording of endocardial electrograms during cardiac surgery for ventricular aneurysm. *J Am Coll Cardiol* 1983;2:947–953.

8. Hafala R, Sarvard P, Tremblat G, Page P, Cardinal R, Molin F, Kus T, Nadean R. Three distinct patterns of ventricular activation in infarcted human hearts. An intraoperative cardiac mapping study during sinus rhythm. *Circulation* 1995;91:1480–1494.

9. Eldar M. Percutaneous multielectrode endocardial mapping and ablation of ventricular tachycardia in the swine model. In: Sideman S, Beyar R (editors) *Analytical and Quantitative Cardiology: From Genetics to Function*, Plenum Publ, New York, 1997, Chapter 27.

10. Ben–Haim SA, Osadchy D, Schuster I, Gepstein L, Hayam G, Josephson ME. Nonfluoroscopic, *in vivo* navigation and mapping technology. *Nature Med* 1996;2:1393–1395.

11. Gepstein L, Hayam G, Ben–Haim SA. A novel method for nonfluoroscopic catheter–based electro-anatomical mapping of the heart: *in vitro* and *in vivo* accuracy results. *Circulation* 1997;95:1611–1622.

12. Fananapazir L, Cannon RO 3d, Tripodi D, Panza JA. Impact of dual–chamber permanent pacing in patients with obstructive hypertrophic cardiomyopathy with symptoms refractory to verapamil and beta–adrenergic blocker therapy. *Circulation* 1992;85:2149–61.

13. McAreavey D, Fananapazir L. Altered cardiac hemodynamic and electrical state in normal sinus rhythm after chronic dual–chamber pacing for relief of left ventricular outflow obstruction in hypertrophic cardiomyopathy. *Am J Cardiol* 1992;70:651–656.

14. Hochleitner M, Hortnagl H, Hortnagl H, Fridrich L, Gschnitzer F. Long–term efficacy of physiologic dual–chamber pacing in the treatment of end–stage idiopathic dilated cardiomyopathy. *Am J Cardiol* 1992;70:1320–1325.

CHAPTER 27

Percutaneous Multielectrode Endocardial Mapping and Ablation of Ventricular Tachycardia in the Swine Model

Michael Eldar, Dan G. Ohad, Arnold J. Greenspon, Jeffrey J. Goldberger, and Zeev Rotstein[1]

ABSTRACT

A basket shaped catheter carrying 64 electrodes was deployed in the left ventricle (LV) of 53 pigs which had undergone induction of myocardial infarction. Pacing during sinus rhythm, or echocardiographic and hemodynamic measurements as well as pathological studies revealed no significant damage due to the basket catheter. Eighty one episodes of ventricular tachycardia (VT) were mapped and analyzed, requiring only several beats and less than 10 seconds to complete. We were able to successfully ablate ventricular tachycardias in four pigs.

INTRODUCTION

Nonpharmacological treatment of sustained VT by catheter ablation requires recording of endocardial electrograms from multiple ventricular sites during the arrhythmia (1–7). Percutaneous catheter mapping techniques usually use a conventional catheter carrying a relatively small number of electrodes which is sequentially moved around the endocardium during VT (8–11). This method is time consuming and limited to the mapping of patients with hemodynamically stable sustained monomorphic VT which lasts a relatively long time. Methods that allow simultaneous recording from multiple endocardial sites

---

[1]Neufeld Cardiac Research Institute, Tel Aviv University, Israel

could shorten the mapping procedure. They could also ensure more accurate identification and ablation of VT, theoretically increasing the number of patients eligible for ablation.

We describe here a multielectrode basket shaped catheter which was used for endocardial LV recording and as a guide for VT ablation, in a pig model of post myocardial infarction sustained monomorphic VT.

MATERIAL AND METHODS

Animal preparation

Female domestic pigs (n=53) weighing between 25–35 kg underwent a closed chest induction of myocardial infarction under general anesthesia (12). The animals were returned 2–6 weeks later for induction of VT.

Characteristics of multielectrode basket catheter

The catheter (EP Technologies, Sunnyvale, CA) consists of an 8 Fr flexible, 110 cm long shaft carrying eight 7 cm long nitinol super elastic splines in the shape of a basket (Fig. 1). These splines are collapsible so as to fit inside a specially designed guiding sheath for introduction into the heart. When released from the guiding sheath, the splines expand and conform to the shape of the cardiac chamber. Each spline has eight electrodes (a total of 32 bipolar pairs per basket) which are individually connected to insulated thin electrical wires. Catheter introduction into the LV was done through a long specially designed sheath, and lasted less than 5 min in all animals.

Measurements During basket deployment

Sinus rhythm: Intracardiac electrograms were recorded during sinus rhythm following deployment of the basket catheter. Surface 12 lead electrocardiograms and signals from each of 32 bipolar pairs of electrodes were recorded.

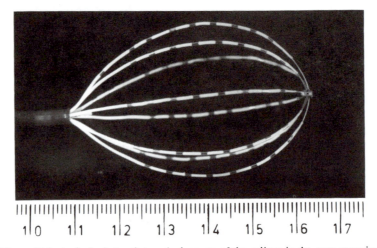

Figure 1. The multielectrode basket catheter. A close–up of the splines in the open mapping position.

Unipolar pacing was performed from each of the 64 electrodes at 3 and 10 mA to evaluate electrode–tissue contact. The hemodynamic effects of the expanded basket were evaluated by measuring LV and aortic pressure (n=9) and right heart pressures (n=5) before and after deployment of the catheter. The catheter was left in the ventricle for 0.5 to 7 hr.

Ten pigs underwent transthoracic Doppler echocardiographic study (Hewlett Packard, Androver, MA). The parasternal long and short axis views were measured during the predeployment study. During catheter deployment, 2D echocardiograms allowed visual evaluation of the basket's conformity to the ventricular shape and its effects on ventricular contraction. Pulsed and color Doppler were used to assess aortic and mitral valve function.

Pacemapping was performed from bipolar basket catheter electrodes, or the ablation catheter tip, recording the earliest presystolic or diastolic potentials at a rate similar to the VT rate. "Good" maps were defined as showing very similar surface electrograms to those during VT in 9–10 leads, "identical" maps as being similar in 11–12 leads and "poor" maps being similar in less than eight leads.

Measurement During Ventricular Tachycardia

VT induction: Induction of VT was attempted 2–6 weeks after the induced myocardial infarction (12). Overdrive pacing and programmed electrical stimulation were performed from the right ventricular apex or from bipolar pairs of electrodes on the basket catheter. Presystolic activity was defined as endocardial electrode activity preceding the beginning of the surface electrocardiogram. Entrainment was performed from the bipolar basket electrodes, or the ablation catheter tip, recording the earliest electrograms by pacing during VT at a cycle length of 20–70 msec shorter than the VT cycle length. VT was defined as either manifest or concealed according to acceptable criteria (13).

The ablation procedure: Ventricular tachycardia was targeted for ablation if it was induced or spontaneously occurred at least twice. Potential ablation sites were identified by demonstrating early, mid or continuous diastolic activation, plus either "identical" pacemaps with long stimulus to QRS interval and/or demonstration of transient concealed entrainment, achieved by pacing from the tip of the ablation catheter.

An 8 Fr, 8 mm thermistor embedded deflectable tip ablation catheter was directed to the desired target using a "homing" device. The homing device presents on its surface 64 miniature light emitting diodes arranged in an array similar to the arrangement of the 64 MMC electrodes. Each spline was given a letter (A to H) and each electrode a number, "1" being the most distal and "8" the most proximal on the spline. When the ablation catheter tip electrode contacts one of the MMC electrodes, the respective light emitting diode lights up, indicating which electrode is contacted. The ablation catheter is thus moved inside the ventricle under fluoroscopic guidance and directed towards the target with the aid of the "homing" device.

The power source used for catheter ablation was a commercially available generator with temperature feedback capabilities (EP Technologies) that delivered continuous unmodulated radiofrequency current at a frequency of 500 kHz. Radiofrequency energy was delivered between the catheter tip and a skin patch for a maximal duration of 120 sec per application, to achieve a tip–tissue interface temperature of 80°C.

Following each radio–frequency energy application, induction of sustained monomorphic VT (SMVT) was attempted again using the induction protocol previously described. In some pigs, when SMVT was non–inducible, isoproterenol was administered intravenously with the end–point being a 20% increase in the basal sinus heart rate, and the induction protocol was repeated. Successful ablation was defined as the inability to reinduce the same SMVT after ablation. If SMVT was still inducible, the above procedure was repeated until non–inducibility was achieved.

At the end of the experiment the pigs were killed under general anesthesia by intravenous injection of 20 ml KCl 15%. The hearts of 12 pigs were subjected to macroscopical examination; four weeks later an additional six pigs were sacrificed and their hearts examined.

Statistical analysis: Values are given as a range and mean ± 1 standard deviation, or as median and interquartile (25%–75%) range. The statistical tests include: 1) the two tailed, (two sample, unequal variance) Student's t–test; 2) Chi–Square test. Significance was prospectively defined as p≤0.05.

RESULTS

The first 43 pigs served to assess electrode tissue contact, the effects of the basket catheter on the ventricular function, and possible endocardial or myocardial damage. Four VT morphologies were considered for ablation (see below) in an additional 10 pigs in which VT was induced.

Sinus Rhythm

Electrode–tissue contact: Unipolar ventricular pacing at 3 mA, from each of the basket catheter electrodes, was performed in 27 animals during sinus rhythm. Ventricular capture, indicating electrode–tissue contact, was achieved in 78±15% (mean ± standard deviation) of the electrodes. Ventricular capture at 10 mA was evident in an additional 13±7% of the electrodes. Failure to capture occurred primarily in electrodes located below the aortic valve.

Hemodynamic, echocardiographic and morphologic evaluation: The systolic LV mean aortic and right heart pressures were not affected significantly during basket deployment (Table 1). Fluoroscopy and echocardiography revealed stable contact of the basket with the ventricular wall, with no apparent impairment of wall motion by visual inspection. This was confirmed by measurements of LV fractional shortening and systolic and diastolic dimensions before and during catheter deployment (Table 1). No significant aortic or mitral valve dysfunction (neither insufficiency nor obstruction) could be detected, although a mild degree of either may have been missed due to difficulties in obtaining optimal echocardiographic views.

Mapping of VT: Complete activation recordings from 32 bipolar sites and during 118 episodes of VT took less than 10 seconds to acquire and generally provided good quality electrograms. Endocardial mapping using the multielectrode basket catheter was

Table 1. Hemodynamic and echocardiographic parameters before (baseline) and during basket catheter deployment

	Hemodynamic (mmHg)				ECHO (cm)			
	LVs	AOm	RVs	PAs	PCWm	SF(%)	LVs	LVd
Baseline	142±31	101±12	32±13	33±12	15±10	28±10	2.8±1.0	3.9±0.4
Basket	120±6	98±14	33±10	33±10	10±7	30±4	2.6±0.8	3.7±0.6

LV = left ventricle; AO = aorta; RV = right ventricle; PA = pulmonary artery; PCW = pulmonary capillary wedge; SF = shortening fraction; d = diastolic; m = mean; s = systolic.

analyzed during 81 induced episodes of sustained or non–sustained monomorphic VT (40 baseline and 41 post antiarrhythmic drug). Pre–systolic electrograms were recorded during 47 episodes (58%). The earliest presystolic activity was recorded 10 to 46 msec (27.6±13.2) prior to the QRS complex.

Ablation of VT: Four pigs out of 10 considered for VT ablation had the same VT morphology induced or occurring at least twice (1 VT in each) (Table 2).

Table 2. Data recorded during ventricular tachycardia (SMVT), pacemaps and concealed entrainment in the four out of 10 pigs which underwent ablation

Pig No.	SMVT			Pacemap		Entrainment
	Location of Earliest ES/MD Activity	V–Q (msec)	S–Q (msec)	Matching Pacemap/SMVT		S–Q (msec)
1	RV/D 5–6	34	37	11/12		–
2	G–1–2	48	48	–		46
3	C–1–2	38	28	11/12		34
4	E–5–6	18	46	11/12		–

ES = end–systolic; MD = mid–diastolic; RV = right ventricle; S–Q (pacemap) = interval between pacing artifact and surface QRS during pacemap; S–Q (entrainment) = interval between pacing artifact of the last paced beat and the first surface QRS of the SMVT. V–Q (SMVT) = interval between earliest endocardial electrogram and surface QRS during SMVT.

Presystolic or mid–diastolic electrograms were recorded in all SMVTs requiring a median mapping time of 8 sec (2.5–25 sec). Pacemaps were identical in three SMVTs with a similar stimulus to QRS interval to the electrogram to QRS interval during SMVT (Fig. 2). Concealed entrainment was achieved in two VTs (Fig. 3).

Guiding the ablation catheter to the target using the homing device required a median time of 120 sec. The target VT morphology in three pigs could not be reinduced at the end of the ablation procedure and the ablation was considered successful. One pig died during the ablation procedure and success could not be assessed.

DISCUSSION

The study demonstrates for the first time the feasibility of percutaneous LV mapping and ablation of VT in the pig model using a basket shaped multielectrode catheter. The catheter could be safely deployed in the LV without hemodynamic compromise, providing stable simultaneous multielectrode endocardial recordings, rapid endocardial mapping and enabled ablation of SMVT.

The Basket Catheter

The multielectrode basket catheter has been developed to solve some of the problems which limit VT mapping by the roving catheter technique. The specially designed introduction system allows retrograde transaortic deployment of the basket within a few minutes of the femoral artery cannulation. Since this is a flexible 8 Fr catheter it could conceivably be introduced by atrial transseptal puncture when necessary, e.g. in patients with tortuous aorta and prosthetic aortic valve.

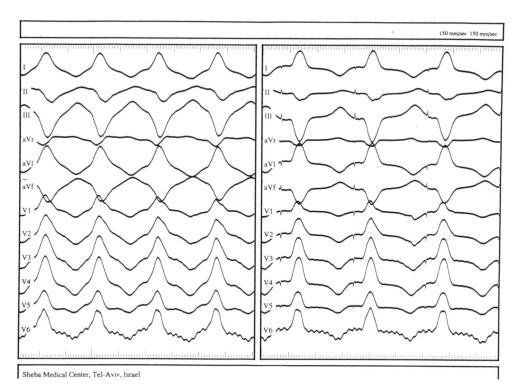

Figure 2. Left: Induced monomorphic VT. **Right:** 12–lead electrogram during pacing from the basket catheter bipole that recorded the earliest systolic electrogram during VT.

The deployed catheter conformed to the LV geometry, and echocardiographic and hemodynamic examinations failed to reveal significant interference with ventricular function. Moreover, there was no evidence of aortic or mitral valve obstruction or regurgitation during the introduction, deployment and following the retraction of the catheter. Although minor valvular and subendocardial hemorrhage were noted acutely following the mapping procedure, none were present 4 weeks later.

Mapping of VT using the basket catheter was rapid and easy. The quality of the endocardial electrograms was similar to that obtained using standard electrode catheters. Early systolic or mid diastolic electrograms can be identified in a majority of VTs. The very short VT mapping time allows mapping of short and hemodynamically unstable VT.

VT Ablation

Choosing the appropriate target site for catheter ablation of VT may be possible using this system. Activation mapping detected presystolic electrograms in the four targeted VTs. Pacemaps from bipolar electrodes recording early electrograms proved to be very similar to the target VT and quite effective for identification of the ablation target. This suggests that ventricular depolarization in the pig may be different than in humans, since pacemapping is usually of only limited use in the post myocardial infarction in man (14–17). The similarity between stimulus to QRS and electrogram to QRS of identical pacemap and SMVT, respectively, suggests that the diastolic potentials are from area of slow conduction which is an integral part of the reentry circuit. Concealed entrainment seems

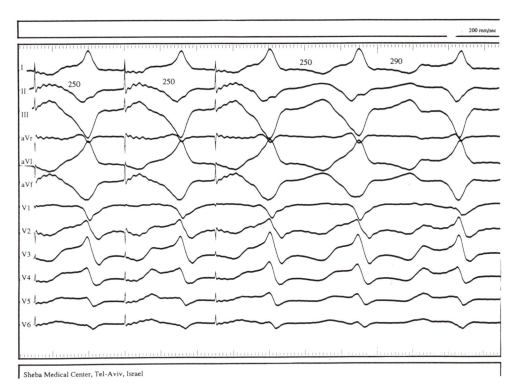

Figure 3. Concealed entrainment. Bipolar pacing at a cycle length of 250 msec from the bipole that recorded the earliest mid–diastolic potential during VT. The 12–lead electrocardiogram during pacing is identical to the VT morphology with the last beat entrained at the pacing rate and a long stimulus to QRS interval.

to identify an area of slow conduction critical to the VT circuit and to guide ablation successfully.

Although the number of attempted ablations is small, it was felt that the combination of early potentials, plus either identical pacemaps and/or concealed entrain–ment, can be obtained rapidly, accurately and guide the ablation procedure. The use of the homing device allowed rapid maneuvering of the ablation catheter to the target ablation sites, without the need for spatially locating the basket bipole inside the ventricle.

CONCLUSIONS

We have developed a new catheter which allows simultaneous multielectrode mapping of the LV in a relatively fast and safe fashion during induced VT. The catheter allows direction of an ablation catheter to the presumed target and seems to facilitate successful ablation of SMVT.

DISCUSSION

Dr. L. Gepstein: It seems that the pig model is an ideal model for the induction of VT because you can have a patchy infarct in which you have areas of dead and living tissue together, which is an ideal substrate for reentry. Also, if it is true, then more than one reentry circuit may occur. Did you look at the density of the infarct? Did you notice more than one morphology of VT in each pig?

Dr. M. Eldar: Pathologically, the infarction area is transmural and patchy. Most of the pigs had more than one morphology induced. However, only a few had the same morphology induced more than once. We induced three to five different morphologies in many pigs, and at some point the pig would just die. Four pigs out of 10 were unique in that we were able to reinduce the same VT at least twice so it served as a baseline. We felt that if we cannot reinduce VT after ablation, it probably, but not definitely, means that we had a successful ablation.

Dr. Y. Rudy: If you wanted to map the details of a reentry pathway with higher spatial resolution, could you collect data from more points by rotating the basket? Of course, this will be possible only in sustained monomorphic VT. Also, what happens in areas of irregularities of the ventricular wall, where contact can not be established? For example, in aneurysms or papillary muscles.

Dr. M. Eldar: We can easily rotate the basket inside the ventricle. We insert it into the ventricle inside a sheath that goes over a pigtail catheter through the aortic valve. Then we pull the sheath back and the basket opens because it is preshaped. If needed, we can push the sheath inside the ventricle so it collapses the basket, rotate the sheath and then reopen the basket. It is easy to get more electrograms using the same basket during sustained monomorphic VT. As to your other question, the pigs have no aneurysms, only areas of akinesis and of hypokinesis. Aneurysms pose a mapping problem.

Dr. R. Beyar: From the shape of the catheter I cannot see how it can access high places like LV outflow tract or even above the papillary muscle. How often in clinical set–up do the arrhythmias come from these places? This would be a practical question: when can you use your basket?

Dr. M. Eldar: I believe that most infarctions involve the apex and maybe the distal two–thirds of the ventricle. Only a few will involve the subaortic area. You are right that the areas where we have the worst contact is really the outflow tract. Fortunately, this is not a big problem in the clinical setting.

Dr. S. Sideman: Have you tested it on human patients?

Dr. M. Eldar: Yes. The results are no different from what we have seen with pigs. We experienced a successful VT ablation. Mapping lasted 3 sec after we placed the catheter, and placing the catheter does not take more than 2 min. This is a straight forward transaortic approach using a pigtail catheter.

Dr. L. Axel: If you are looking for RV arrhythmogenic dysplasia, you are going to have trouble getting to the outflow tract placing through the tricuspid.

Dr. M. Eldar: I agree. There are two things we should do to get to the outflow tract of the RV. First, shape a guiding catheter that will direct it to the RVOT and second, we need a smaller size basket. Theoretically, this is feasible.

REFERENCES

1.   Josephson ME, Harken AH, Horowitz LN. Long–term results of endocardial resection for sustained ventricular tachycardia in coronary artery disease patients. *Am Heart J* 1982;104:51–57.
2.   Josephson ME, Harken AH, Horowitz LN. Endocardial excision: a new surgical technique for the treatment of recurrent ventricular tachycardia. *Circulation* 1979;60:1430–1439.
3.   Horowitz LN, Harken AH, Kastor JA, Josephson MA. Ventricular resection guided by epicardial and endocardial mapping for treatment of recurrent ventricular tachycardia. *N Engl J* Med 1980;302:589–593.

4. Brodman R, Fisher JD, Johnston DR, Kim SG, Matos JA, Waspe LE, Scavin GM, Furman S. Results of electrophysiological guided operations for drug–resistant recurrent ventricular tachycardia and ventricular fibrillation due to coronary artery disease. *J Thorac Cardiovasc Surg* 1984;87:431–438.

5. Platia EV, Griffith LSC, Watkins L Jr, Mower MM, Mirowski M, Reid PR. Treatment of malignant ventricular arrhythmias with endocardial resection and implantation of the automatic cardioverter-defibrillator. *N Engl J Med* 1986;314:213–216.

6. Garan H, Nguyen K, McGovern B, Bukley M, Ruskin JN. Peripoerative and long–term results after electrophysiologically directed ventricular surgery for recurrent ventricular tachycardia. *J Am Coll Cardiol* 1986;8:201–209.

7. Kron IL, Lerman BB, Nolan SP, Flanagan TL, Haines DE, DiMarco JP. Sequential endocardial resection for the surgical treatment of refractory ventricular tachycardia. *J Thorac Cardiovasc Surg* 1987;94:843–847.

8. Josephson ME, Horowitz LN, Farshidi A, Spear JF, Kastor JA, Moore EN. Recurrent sustained ventricular tachycardia. 2. Endocardial mapping. *Circulation* 1978;57:440–447

9. Josephson ME, Horowitz LN, Farshidi A, Spielman SR, Michelson EL, Greenspan AM. Recurrent sustained ventricular tachycardia. 4. Pleomorphism. *Circulation* 1979;59:459–468.

10. Miller JM, Kienzle MG, Harken AH, Josephson ME. Morphologically distinct sustained ventricular tachycardias in coronary artery disease. Significance and surgical results. *J Am Coll Cardiol* 1984;4:1073–1079.

11. Fitzgerald DM, Friday KJ, Yeung Lai Wah JA, Lazzara R, Jackman WM. Electrogram patterns predicting successful catheter ablation of ventricular tachycardia. *Circulation* 1988;77:806–814.

12. Eldar M, Ohad D, Bor A, Varda–Bloom N, Swanson DK, Battler A. A closed chest pig model of sustained ventricular tachycardia. *PACE* 1994;17:1603–1609.

13. Stevenson WG, Khan H, Sager P, Saxon LA, Middlekauff HR, Natterson PD, Wiener I. Identification of reentry circuit sites during catheter mapping and radiofrequency ablation of ventricular tachycardia late after myocardial infarction. *Circulation* 1993;88:1647–1670.

14. Stevenson WG, Sager PT, Natterson PD, Saxon LA, Middlekauff HR, Wiener I. Relation of pace mapping QRS configuration and conduction delay to ventricular tachycardia reentry circuits in human infarct scars. *J Am Coll Cardiol* 1995;26:481–488.

15. Morady F, Kadish A, Rosenheck S, Calkins H, Kou WH, De Buitleir M, Sousa J. Concealed entrainment as a guide for catheter ablation of ventricular tachycardia in patients with prior myocardial infarction. *J Am Coll Cardiol* 1991;17:678–689.

16. Hamlin RL, Smith CR. Categorization of common domestic mammals based upon their ventricular activation process. *Ann NY Acad Sci* 1965;127:195–203.

17. Hamlin RL, Burton RR, Leverett SD, Burns JW. Ventricular activation process in minipigs. *J Electrocardiology* 1975;8:113–116.

VII. THE CARDIONOME: CONCEPTS IN MODELING

CHAPTER 28

Design and Strategy
for the Cardionome Project

James B. Bassingthwaighte[1]

ABSTRACT

The Physiome Project has the goal of providing the quantitative description of the integrated functions of the living organism. This is too large an undertaking to be begun all at once. What needs to be developed first are large comprehensive databases containing genomic, biochemical, anatomical and physiological information that can be searched and retrieved via the Internet. A more modest and achievable goal is the Cardiome Project, whose goal is to describe the functioning heart. Since it is impractical to develop this from the genetic and molecular level, we begin it as a multicenter collaborative effort at the level of the functioning organ. The work of Hunter, Noble, and others provides a central scheme, a description of the spread of excitation and contraction through an anatomically detailed cardiac model with fiber directions. This will be augmented by the additions of regional blood flows, substrate uptake and metabolism, and energy production and utilization in serving contraction and ionic balances. Later stages will involve cellular regulation and responses to interventions. The organization of such projects is by the assembling of components whose linkages one to another are first minimized and then augmented to improve the approximation to reality.

INTRODUCTION

"From Genomics to Physiology and Beyond. How do we get there?" is the title of a workshop held in early 1997 at Coldspring Harbor, New York. The idea is clear. It is now recognized that the genome, while holding the code for the proteins, does not provide

---

[1]Department of Bioengineering, University of Washington, Seattle, WA 98195–7962 USA

a complete instruction set on how to build, operate and maintain the human organism over a period of three score and ten years. It is fair to say that few held to the theme of Gunther Stent's 1969 book [1], "The Coming of the Golden Age", that when the genome was sequenced all scientists could sit in the sun, for all would then be known. But it is, contrarily, also fair to say that too few recognized that molecular biology, its methods and its teachings, was failing to provide investigators with the tools that are needed to unravel the physiological mysteries uncovered by the discovery of new, uncharacterized, proteins whose functions are not identified, whose phenotypic expression is unrecognized, and whose deletion or enhanced expression might not be translated into phenotypic physiolog-ical behavior for decades after the birth of the organism.

What the genome will provide is the sequence of CGAT's, and after some struggle, the localization of the genes, and the sequence of the amino acids in the proteins. How the proteins fold, their physical and chemical characteristics, and their chemical reactions will become the foci of work by biophysicists and biochemists. Figuring out how the proteins serve the organism is to be the task of the integrative physiologists and the biosystems engineers.

Boyd and Noble's 1993 collection of essays [2], "The Logic of Life" is a translation of physiology, physio = life, logy = study or logic. Since the logic is not all in the genome, where is it stored? Can the logic of life be reconciled with the observations that life forms are complex and that living organisms are masterpieces of complexity and unpredictability. Since simple low order systems are not predictable, as Newton observed with respect to the interactions of three planets, what should we expect of large complex homeodynamic systems. I have chosen the word "homeodynamic" to replace the idea of physiological "homeostasis". Stasis is the wrong idea, for nothing remains exactly static. Only with death does the body achieve thermodynamic equilibrium, and, with it, "stasis".

THE PHYSIOME PROJECT

The Physiome Project is perhaps the grandest of the Grand Challenges of modern science. Let's define "physiome" as life as a whole, physio = life, and −ome = the whole, paralleling the definition of "genome" as the whole of the assemblage of the genes in the chromosomes. Then, if the genotype defines the information contained in the genome, phenotype defines the anatomy and the physiology of the intact organism in its functioning state. The physiome is therefore the quantitative description of the integrated functions of the living organism.

The Physiome Project, following the style of the Genome Project, is to develop the databases of physiological data, to archive and document these data, to make the data available for investigators around the world via the Internet, and to build, little by little, ever more comprehensive models describing those data sets of physiological phenomena. By these means, the Project would provide vehicles for defining hypotheses about the systems, foster the design of ever more revealing experiments to test these hypotheses, and to provide ever deeper insight into the behavior of the system so that the effects of physiological stress or therapeutic intervention may be understood or even predicted.

The principle components of the Physiome Project are therefore databasing and modeling. By databasing, we mean the gathering of the physiological information, associating it with genomic information wherever possible, finding the means of preserving this information so that it is searchable from diverse points of view, while preserving measures of the reliability and reproducibility of the data, and preserving the methods by which the data were analyzed and interpreted. Given that the "raw" data are well preserved, one enters the realm of analysis, of logic, of interpretation and of modeling. Mathematical models provide summaries of data, describing the data in a form that is interpretive and self–consistent. The development of the mathematical models may be regarded as the ultimate goal of integrative physiology.

A self consistent model is one that has been freed of internal contradictions. By extrapolating this logic, the larger, more comprehensive models, describing larger sets of physiological observations remain self–consistent only because there has been a selection. It is inevitable that there are conflicting sets of data. Quite often the conflicts are more apparent than real, and are resolved in the larger models by recognizing differences in conditions or variation in parameters. A central goal of the modeling is therefore to seek resolution of conflict, regarding the modeling as a vehicle of arbitration. Likewise it will be a vehicle for the elimination of artifact. But no model is "truth" and can at best be regarded as a description of the "working hypothesis", and a transient descriptor of "under–standing" or at least consensus. The risk to be avoided is that the model should be regarded as a final truth. The physicists of the twentieth century have succeeded in making theoretical physics an honored and respected part of their discipline. A part of their success has been that skepticism about their favorite models has always remained high.

FROM THE GENOME TO THE PHYSIOME

Thomas Henry Huxley's statement, "The tragedy of science is the slaying of a beautiful hypothesis by an ugly fact," [3] sets the stage for quantitative modeling. A mathematical model is a refutable hypothesis, simply because it is quantitative and precise. One gets away with verbal hypotheses only too readily, because they are usually sufficiently vague that refutation is difficult or impossible. Hypotheses are predictors, not mere descriptors, and mathematical models have the advantage over verbal hypotheses that they can be used to predict the results of a proposed experiment, a result which can be tested statistically against the experimental data and evaluated for goodness of fit. Large data sets provide an overabundance of constraints on the ranges of parameters in mathematical models, so one need not be handicapped by underdetermination.

Platt's admonition [4] to us was to develop the alternative hypothesis. Make it as beautiful as the original hypothesis yet let it be a true alternative, not just a straw man to be knocked over all too easily. Then the process of experimental design begins: find, from the models or from logic, the experiment that clearly distinguishes between the two hypotheses. Do the experiment. The result must produce an advancement of the science: one of the hypotheses must be proven wrong. Since disproof of the hypothesis is the only way by which science advances, such an advance will be made with each such carefully designed experiment.

Scientists try not to make foolish hypotheses, but often do so unknowingly. Some try to be vague enough so that they can not be proven wrong. A few of these have led productive and stimulating careers, but most are wanderers in the swamp. The mathematical modeling approach is therefore a vehicle for clarifying the ideas and the goals of experimentation.

Modeling analysis is also a vehicle for description. The parameters of a model that is fitted to sets of observations are a summary of those data. The summaries, the parameter values, can be compared from laboratory to laboratory; there is nothing new in this. Parameter values such as cardiac output, renal creatinine clearance, hepatic clearance of bromsulfalein, visual recognition of letters down to line 4 of the eye chart, and so on, have been a part our language in clinical medicine now for decades. They are summaries of quantitative evaluation; they are parameters of mathematical models. They serve as vehicles for databasing information on populations and for deciding on treatment.

So if we are going to end up having to put together large models with many components, what is the path to doing so without getting lost in the swamp? How does one make the modeling manageable?

MANAGEABLE MODELING: THE CARDIOME PROJECT

The process is already begun. The literature abounds with models of relatively small systems. Noble's [5] and Rudy's [6] models of the action potential of the heart describe a couple of dozen paths for ionic regulation in the myocyte during excitation and recovery from it. The voltage– and time–dependent kinetic models for myocardial ionic exchanges (See Chapters 23 and 24 by Y. Rudy and D. Noble, respectively, in this book) are based on large numbers of experiments, including the measurement of action potentials at varied extracellular and intracellular ionic concentrations, voltage clamp and patch clamp studies under varieties of preconditoning voltage steps, rate changes, etc., so that the models summarize years of experimental work in computationally fast, easy to operate, programs. Upon these models others will design their experiments and add their results. Models for excitation–contraction coupling, for the production of energy from metabolism, for the delivery of substrate by flow and transmembrane transport can all be linked, conceptually, to these currently available models. These classes of models for transport, metabolic reaction, ATP production and utilization, ionic fluxes, myofilament shortening are all at a common level, that of the sarcomere or cell. Each is more or less circumscribed, but has links to the others, so it is fairly obvious how one would put all of these models into one larger model of sarcomere or cellular behavior.

The next stage has also begun, namely that of incorporating such cellular models into tissue and organ models. Winslow and Varghese [7] have incorporated Noble's ionic currents into a tissue model of the myocardium. This integrates the information to the next level, namely the spread of excitation across the myocardium, taking into account the anisotropy of the spread, faster along fiber directions than perpendicular to the cell axes. Linking this effort with that of Peter Hunter and collaborators [8] was the key to develop– ing a model of a functioning contracting heart, which can now be displayed in its three– dimensional glory on the computer screen for a full contraction (Chapter 18). This level of success has required some years of intensive work, but the result now represents the sum– mary of what has been learned in the accumulated output of thousands of published studies; this beginning model incorporates electrophysiology, excitation–contraction coupling, mechanical deformation of tissues, the torsion and contraction of the heart, the pressure development and ejection of the volume of blood contained in the ventricle under normal physiological circumstances. It represents a "Theory of Heart", to take the title of the book edited by Glass and Hunter [9], that is not merely picturesque, but accurately descriptive and insight producing. This accomplishment is represented by the three boxes in Fig. 1 labeled 3D heart, excitation–contraction coupling, and electrophysiology.

The components of this "Cardiome" model so far encompass a minimal number of hierarchical levels, proteins (channels and pumps and motors), sarcomeres or cells (trans– membrane potentials, ionic concentrations, sarcomere shortening), the syncytium of cells forming a tissue (excitatory spread, tissue deformation, tension development, compression), and organ (shape change, pressure generation, valvular action). One might say that there are four hierarchical levels covered here, all relating to the normal physiology of the adult organ. The organ is unconnected to the body, to neural influences or to its history of growth and development.

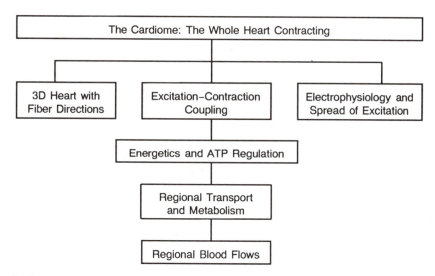

Figure 1. Diagram of the Cardiome Project at its simple beginnings. The modeling of Hunter, McCulloch, Noble, and Winslow is represented by the three boxes on the second row. The next components to be added concern ATP sources and sinks, transport and metabolism, and blood flow.

Further development can occur without spreading the range of hierarchical levels. To the Hunter–McCulloch–Noble–Winslow model one needs now add the elements needed to sustain it: blood flow, the delivery of substrate and oxygen, the machinery for metabolism of fatty acids and glucose for energy production, the removal of metabolites, the formation and utilization of ATP, and purine balance in myocytes. These are represented in the bottom three boxes of Fig. 1.

Necessarily, there will need to be interactions between the various main groups of elements in the model. The utilization of ATP depends on the contraction and on the needs of the pumps, particularly for calcium cycling. The formation of ATP depends on the delivery of substrate and oxygen by blood flow, and this to some extent depends on the degree of compression of the intramural arteries.

THE ROLE OF MODELING

The modeling developed so far has been tightly coupled to reality. Models that are not so coupled, not tested and evaluated against data, can be the entry into a world of science fiction. To prevent this it seems best to do the experimentation and modeling together, for it is the experimentalist who has the deepest understanding of the sources of error in the experimental measurements and the reliability and reproducibility of the particular studies being used to evaluate the models, and it is the modeler who has the best understanding of the sensitivity of the model functions to error in the parameter estimates.

It is accepted that simple models can be adequate to explain or describe simple biological systems, but does this work when systems are much more complex? The acceptance of the Hodgkin–Huxley expressions for the action potential of neurons was due in part to the close similarity between model behavior and experimentally observed action potentials and ionic currents. Hodgkin and Huxley [3] did not actually fit the model solutions to the data, but did show the behavioral similarity. By more precise experimenta–

tion in a variety of tissues, the number of ionic channels now recognized is much greater than they had found, but their descriptions of the sodium and potassium currents have pretty well stood the test of time. In this case the biophysical behavior of single ion channels and of assemblages of ion channels were described by the model. The model was simple, and understandable in both kinetics and physical terms.

More complex models are less readily understood and more easily rejected by scientists. The first problem is that they are commonly found to be incorrect, and even if not proven incorrect, they are seen to be incomplete, in the sense that there other attributes of the system that are not included in the model. The larger they are the easier it is to find the faults. So if a fault is found, one tends to reject the model, even if its overall behavior is apparently acceptable. The other side of the coin is that biological systems are remark-ably redundant, and therefore tend to preserve their proper behavior even when a component is not operating. The same will apply to the more complex models. This means that it will be difficult to find definitive tests of all of the components from an *in vivo* study, and that there will continue to be dependence upon information gained from incomplete systems or *in vitro* studies.

Biological control systems are sloppy. There are no set points, there are no proportional controllers in the traditional engineering sense. The systems are in continu-ously fluctuating balance, influenced by controllers that are combinations of derivative, integral and proportional control. Stability is homeodynamic, not homeostatic: this means that the system is not obviously chaotic and that fluctuations are generally moderate. The reason is that the controllers are highly redundant and the connections are several rather than few. Ari Goldberger [10] has a good idea, namely the hypothesis that when the number of controllers is reduced from many to a few or to one, then the system becomes stable, rather than fluctuating. The failure of the various controllers or linkages allows the dominance of a single controller, leading to regularity. He proposed further, that when this occurs the stability may be regarded as a portent of doom, or high risk; the example is that when heart rate variability is reduced to nothing, a purely periodic rhythm, than not only are the controllers gone, but there may be reason to predict a higher likelihood of sudden death due to arrhythmia. This may not be proven, but the principle makes sense.

DISCUSSION

The Tools for the Physiome Project

Focusing on the modeling as the endpoint of the Physiome Project is asking for trouble. Such a goal is too distant and too esoteric to be appealing to the average bench scientist. What is more important and more immediately useful is the development of databases of genomic, biophysical, biochemical, structural, physiological, pharmacological, and pathophysiological information. The toolkit therefore includes: 1) Databases, structured for free access, and relatively free entry. 2) Modeling toolkits and interfaces for investi-gators to run models. 3) Computer models and parameter sets for various cells, tissues, organs, species. 4) Resource facilities specializing in particular topics. 5) Tutorial systems for self learning and for classroom demonstration. 6) Mechanisms for the distribution of models over Internet.

Physiome Resource Centers

No Center, not even the National Library of Medicine, can be a resource for all of the databases on different topics, different species, and different models. Consequently it makes sense to consider establishing a large set of resource facilities each of which has a particular span of expertise and interest. Their responsibilities might be summarized: 1) Establish the databases of information on a focal topic, in the style of EcoCyc, the database for *E. Coli*, or for the tricarboxylic acid cycle, or for the arachidonate cascade, or for coronary vascular regulation. 2) Develop and maintain sets mathematical models related to the topic. 3) Develop model tutorials, provide parameter sets for particular situations, maintain exemplary data sets of physiological information, and make all of these available over the Internet. 4) Maintain multimedia connections for bringing together groups of investigators for Internet conferences, database structuring, committee meetings, discussions of models and tutorials. 5) Develop training programs in integrative physiology, experimental and analytical studies, especially in areas related to phenotyping abnormalities of the genome. 6) Organize a "patchwork" structure amongst resource facilities, so that each resource has established connections and responsibilities with respect to the foci of the related resources. By this means, each resource will develop their databases and models in a fashion suited to those most closely connected.

Why Should We Undertake the Physiome Project Now?

As the Genome project winds down in the next 5 years or so, the main emphasis will be on finding out what each gene is intended to do. Some knockouts are lethal while others have no apparent phenotype, but many important ones lie in between these extremes. Many autosomal dominant diseases of man are not clinically evident until mid–life. Further, their phenotypic expression is not necessarily clearly related to the genetic disorder. What this means is that phenotyping will be difficult.

To design therapy, phenotyping will be critical. Gene replacement is a long way off. Thus developing strategies for relatively rapid phenotyping and for sorting out the complex behavior of the organism is important for the pharmaceutical industry and for the physician.

The complexity of biology frustrates understanding. Relatively simple systems with only a few non–linear components cannot be understood a priori; even the direction of a response to an intervention is often predicted incorrectly, yet predicting quantitatively is what is needed for patient therapy. While it will take highly sophisticated models to predict reasonably accurately, the possibility of doing so is now real. What could not be done a decade ago is now in the realm of the possible.

Effective research is getting more difficult because the information swamp is so large. The literature is difficult to search; the manuscripts are not on line, not retrievable over the Internet, and the information deep within the articles is not often indexed by the key words. Try to find out the value for the diffusion coefficient of your favorite solute in plasma or inside cells! Or the V_{max} of your favorite enzyme in cardiac versus mesenteric capillary endothelial cells!

Even when one has the specific information, one does not usually have a solid context for it. This is where the modeling will be of benefit, even in incomplete models. The user can explore the model to determine the effects of parameter changes; since very often a user will have data relating to the topic, he will be able to ascertain when the incompleteness of the model renders its solutions incompatible with reality. In the absence of conflicts with data, one will tend to be more accepting of a model. Even knowing that they are always wrong, either incomplete or inexact, there is still the risk that one will be too accepting of what the model predicts. Beware!

What the modeling does offer then is a basis for sorting out behavior in a complex system with many interacting components. This can only be done if the database is complete enough to provide self–consistent sets of parameter values, so the databasing is the highest priority component of the Physiome Project. Databases established at resource facilities distributed around the globe will therefore be invaluable long before detailed, large models are available.

CONCLUSION

Because biological systems are complex, having aids to experimental design and analysis is obviously beneficial to advancing the field. Today the realization that most of the proteins coded in the genome are not yet identified with respect to their function has led to renewed interest in integrative physiology. The molecular biologists who make up most of the faculties of academic departments of physiology, pharmacology, bacteriology, immunology, pathology, and genetics have not been trained in integrative biology. They lack training in physical chemistry, physics, instrumentation for physiological measurement, mathematics, statistics, systems analysis, signal analysis, and modeling. The leaders of the pharmaceutical corporations are concerned that there is no pool from which they can hire employees with the skills to unravel the consequences of the genome. Some good reasons for starting the Physiome Project now are:

- To initiate training programs in integrative biology.
- To enhance investigator productivity.
- To provide vehicles for quantitative analysis.
- To gain understanding of complex systems.
- To help determine causation of disorder in human disease.
- To predict the effects of intervening in the functioning of a biological system.
- To aid in designing effective therapy.

Acknowledgment

Research has supported by NIH grant RR 1243 from the National Center for Research Resources, and from experimental programs supported by the National Heart Lung and Blood Institute, HL19139, and HL50238.

DISCUSSION

Dr. S. Sideman: Let me start by asking if the physiome, or the cardionome which is a relatively small part of it, is a feasible dream. Do we need it and can we ever reach it? These are difficult questions. The physiome is conceptually an intelligent and effective construction of interrelated models, allowing an integrated approach to particular problems concerning human physiology in health and disease. Models, any model, should give us both insight into the present and foresight into the future: In other words, better understanding of the system as well as predictions about unknown and untested regions of potential interest.

Let me relate here only to the cardionome. The Heart System Research Center began naively some 15 years ago, thinking that we can develop an integrated single quantitative engineering model of the cardiac system. Today, I do not see a reasonable model that will include all the parameters making up the cardionome. However, the important result of our efforts, if we may take some credit, is that modeling is now a legitimate tool in studying cardiac phenomena. When we started we heard arguments on the need for models in cardiology, kind of like "I can see the heart is sick, so why do I need models?" It was almost impossible to publish modeling efforts some 10 years ago. This has changed since then and models are now accepted as building blocks in the development of tools to understand the cardiac physiology and/or design new experiments. This is one answer as to why we need models.

I do not think that we will have a single all inclusive cardiac model in the foreseeable future. But we can develop building blocks for it. For example, the model that Dr. Rudy presented here (Chapter 23). I believe that he is surprised at what he has achieved in 10 years. The picture is clearer and broader now. More elements went in and more understanding came out. The same applies to our own modeling efforts, briefly discussed in Chapter 30. If we use imagination and are bold enough to introduce new ideas, we may eventually realize the cardionome, or at least part of it, made up of many elements that should be there.

Dr. E. Ritman: When you talk about models and you review the huge list of parameters involved in the cardionome (Chapter 29) that strikes fear in our hearts, it reminds me of an Arthur Guyton production. He worked on a model that filled a whole wall with interconnecting boxes. Each little box captured something of our knowledge, but I am not sure how their interconnections really helped us go beyond the knowledge already available. An element that we do not seem to be talking about much is: are there any general rules that we should be paying attention to? You get nothing for nothing: if an organism evolves to generate a new function or new capability it usually gives up something. Is that the sort of general rule which should be used to formulate a much more fundamental model? In other words, what sort of model are we looking for? just an archive of everything we know, or do we want the model to point out areas of missing information, somewhat like the "gaps" in the elemental periodic table.

Dr. D. Noble: I would like the opportunity to react to what I regard as a kind of *cri de coeur*. This is the first of these workshops I have attended and I am extremely excited by what I see coming together. Let me react to some of the things that have been said. I would like to echo them, but in slightly different words.

First, the physiome is surely much bigger than the genome. So, we should not be surprised by the audacity in even the presumption that one can even remotely successfully tackle it. After all, the genome project, when it was first proposed, was regarded as a totally audacious proposal. The physiome is a multi–layered problem. It needs not only to satisfy its own goals, but also to inform and interpret the genome project itself. That is an aspect we should not forget. The genome project is a useless one if it is not interpreted. I like to use the analogy that if the genome is the machine code for setting the system up, then the physiome is the understanding of its interactions, both with its environment and within the phenotype itself. All of that is both complex and, most importantly, constraining. If I may correct one of the modern biological philosophers from my own country for a moment, I would like to say that genes are far from "selfish". They are rather "captives" within the successful physiological systems that contain them [*Noble D, Boyd CAR. The challenge of integrative physiology. In: The Logic of Life (Boyd CAR, Noble D, editors). Oxford Univ. Press, Oxford; 1993: pp 1—13*]. I am not implying anything here that would necessarily differ from what Richard Dawkins is saying with regard to the facts of evolution and the way in which the biological mechanisms work. I am just using a different way of coloring the picture. I am putting the point in a different way, using purple prose, like him, to emphasize a point. But I also think that the way I have just put it captures more of the truth from the point of view of how difficult it is going to be to understand the overall situation than is his particular way of putting it.

I want to react to the question: why so many models? It seems to me that this is not surprising and that we need them. It is not surprising because they capture different subsets of reality. We need that for validation because we need to be sure that what any particular model shows is not itself so model–dependent that it is not reliable, or applicable. To have different subsets of reality extracted from the totality is in fact a great virtue. We should not be worrying too much about the fact that there are so many models coming up, even if they are aiming at the same goals. We should regard that as a strength.

I like to use the analogy of the radio producers who in days gone by set themselves up by first designing a perfect radio, which they built at great cost. They then pulled out one component after another until it failed to work. The last component to be removed was then put back in and the radio was produced at a much lower cost. The point I am making, and this is the relevance to using many different models representing different subsets of reality, is that if one used a different route in pulling the components out, one would end up with a different conception of what is the crucial component. That is one use of having many different models.

Dr. H. Strauss: Although the genome project and the physiome project overlap conceptually, their perceived goals are really quite different at this point. The genome project was introduced because of the absence of knowledge about much of the human DNA sequence in the body. The idea was to provide scientists with information about the DNA sequence as it came on line. It has been extremely useful because it has been kept up to date. As the journals have required publication of structure coincident with publication of articles, people can routinely and easily access that information in data banks and utilize it for examining similarities in DNA or RNA sequence, analyzing potential protein–protein interaction and predicting tertiary structures that have been helpful and instrumental in designing experiments. The data banks in which all these sequences have been entered are of great and continual use to scientists.

The question is, what are you going to be able to do with the physiome project that is going to be of comparable interest and use to the scientific community? I would agree with Dr. Noble that you can not incorporate everything. Obviously, in attempting to model a particular set of experiments, you are going to have to start selecting components of models that you think are of interest to try and explain your data. The other issue is how to move from the cell to the whole organism? For example, there is great interest in events occurring at the cell level to reconstruct, as Dr. Rudy is doing, the cellular action potential. However, there will also be great interest in going from such a cellular system to determine how the whole heart performs in a variety of perturbed states such as heart failure, conditions wherein one sees upregulation, downregulation, or changes in protein expression that effect cardiac performance. The question is: can you go from the molecule to the integrated system in a meaningful and realistic manner using sophisticated computer models?

Another issue pertains to access to databases that can be accessed to enable scientists who want to download components that they want to incorporate into a small model in which they have interest. This would minimize the time needed to set up a model. Although the emphasis will be different, the needs are clearly there to those of us who worry about both questions from both sides of the street; questions that pertain to the structure of the gene, function of the gene product, changes in its expression and what is its contribution to integrated system function, whether it be at the cell level or *in vivo*. Whatever you set up should be given some careful thought because if it is set up right, it can be of great use to the scientific community. In addition, you are going to need to try to convince authors to archive the codes for their models in data banks so that people can access that information in a way that is reasonable and timely.

Dr. J.B. Bassingthwaighte: The evolution of this discussion is following along the lines that I had hoped for. We need to raise these questions. We cannot answer them all, but the goal of this discussion is to get the questions on the table. Returning to Dr. Ritman's comment on Arthur Guyton's model of hypertension, which was a short–term and a long–term model [*Guyton AC, Coleman TG, Granger HJ. Circulation: overall regulation. Annu Rev Physiol 1972;34:13–46*]. It was generally unacceptable to physiologists because every element of that model was considered by some expert in the area of that element to be incorrect. In fact, as people looked at that model they pulled it apart piece by piece and said, if this little piece is incorrect, the whole must be incorrect. Yet the remarkable thing about that model (and this is a comment on Dr. Sideman's comment on how several different models can fit the same data rather well), surprisingly, is that the overall behavior of the Guyton model was really rather good, despite the seeming inadequacy of its components. So there was something in the integrative behavior that was captured by the simplicity of the elements.

Guytonian modeling never caught on, partly because others could not use the model as well as he and Tom Coleman. It was distributed as the model, Human, but it never really caught on; it was too complicated to use, it was not intuitive, and the computation was too slow. However, we are now in a different era where a model of that level of complexity is actually probably not as complex as Dr. Rudy's or Dr. Noble's models, and certainly not nearly as complex as Dr. Hunter's models. So obviously, times have changed. One can manipulate and explore and gain an understanding of such models [*Montani JP et al. A simulation support system for solving large physiological models on microcomputers. Int J Biomed Comput 1989;24:41–54 and Knopp TJ, Anderson DU, Bassingthwaighte JB. SIMCON–Simulation control to optimize man–machine interaction. Simulation 1970;14:81–86*]. Complex integrated models do what you really want models to do: they arm your intuition so you can think about the system. So with the new computational power and the larger scale models that pull things together, we are entering a new era and can think of modeling quite differently from 20 years ago.

Dr. R. Beyar: A comment on the genome and the physiome: The genome is made of factual data which contain a lot of information. The physiome is an interpretation of facts. Models are a way of interpreting reality, and for any interpretation there will be another interpretation. This is something which has to be considered in the physiome project. How would you select one model over another in describing a phenomenon? Is this based on consensus, or should you use different types of models so that you can replace one with another and see how the overall system behaves?

Another thing which bothers me: We have heard a great deal about molecular biology, for example on techniques like knockout genes and overexpressed genes. How do you create models that can actually take you from the genetic level to the cellular level, and then to the development level of organ function. There are many things missing in the transition between the genome and the physiome. In fact, the genome must have all the information of the physiome, in spite of its much lower complexity level compared to the physiome.

Dr. D. Noble: Dr. Beyar has said that the genome has all the information for the physiome. I would like to rephrase it and say that, with equal truth, the physiome has all the interpretation of the genome. What is the difference between these statements? I suggest nothing from the point of view what we all have in mind about the relationship between the system that sets it all up and the interpretative system (the physiome) required to understand it. The trouble, though, is that it actually matters how you describe the relationship. This is where language can get in the way. Starting from the same basic assumptions, you get a totally different picture depending on how you choose to express it. We are in trouble if that is the case. We need to be aware that our language is often not as neutral as scientists would like it to be.

Dr. J.B. Bassingthwaighte: One of the issues that I would enjoy coming back to is how we can develop even broader levels of collaboration amongst the members of this society of cardiac scientists of all kinds, in order to achieve the ends that we all dream of. Dr. Strauss brought up that if we are going to archive by publication and dispersal on the Web the information that we gather, how should we collaborate on this? I wonder what mechanisms are available in various agencies and research agencies in different countries that might allow us to set up data bases so that they can be used as vehicles for communication and keeping the knowledge that has been presented to us closer to our finger tips. We would love to have all this information available on a more nearly daily basis. Dr. Strauss has been making extensive use of the genome data base on a more or less daily basis. The convenience with which one can access the genome data base is a lesson to us. We can not do that in normal physiological or bioengineering cardiology. We need to see some ways toward doing that. We need to address that issue, either at the national funding level, or at the mechanistic level on how to put it together.

Dr. H. Strauss: The issues are the accessibility, the timeliness of information and yet the right to protect the interests of the person providing the information, who want to maintain their own research interests in that area. There are going to be some areas that will not be covered. The responsibility of the individual towards making sure that the information that is provided is usable vs the responsibility of the individual who wants to use it to be familiar enough with programming and not be dependent on the source. My entry into the molecular biology field, in which I am not an expert, was by a variety of people in the laboratory. It was very clear to me that many of the programs that were used repeatedly were very user friendly, and it did not take very long to determine how to access data bases and get the information needed, such as homology or similarity in nucleotide sequence. This required minimal instruction. As I look around my institution, I see that there are very few of the molecular biologists who have an interest in physiology, who are also very familiar with the physical sciences and the quantitative approaches. I am worried that the information that will be dispersed will not be as user friendly to them as the molecular biology information is to us.

This is an opportunity for us to introduce more measurements on the molecular level to the integrated system function, whether it be the ECG or contractile function *in vivo*. It is now within our grasp to start to figure out how to put the system together in a way that we can really address, at each step, the questions and incorporate the answers that are derived from these questions in a meaningful way and their solutions into integrated function at the cell level or at the whole organ level.

Dr. E. Ritman: The National Library of Medicine has this visible human project that is readily accessible, though you will sit there all day collecting the data. Maybe that is a good model to start out with, and maybe that is even a financial mechanism for getting help with this sort of project.

Dr. J.B. Bassingthwaighte: That is right on target. There will be a meeting in Cold Spring Harbor called "From Genomics to Physiology." One of the speakers at that meeting will be Francis Collins of the U.S. National Library of Medicine, who has put together the genome data base, and his associate Bob Lindbergh, who is running a whole variety of related programs that are available at the National Library of Medicine, which are directed more closely to medical school teaching rather than to research. Maybe there is another class of program which could be more research oriented than those, but those provide a very good starting base. They have a wealth of experience. In that instructional media center they have some 40 professional programmers and guardian angels of the code presented to them working there.

Dr. D. Noble: I agree that the demand for software will grow as projects like the physiome take off, that the software should be accessible, user friendly and so on. But those of us who do a lot of programming know that is asking a lot. The occasional individual scientist is capable of doing it, but by and large the scientists who create the programs are not very good at doing the kind of job we are talking about. It think this is going to require that one brings in professional programmers. That is certainly what we have to do now because the programs, and the projects on which they are being used, have developed way beyond what we can cope with ourselves. This is also going to be very expensive, and this is a comment on the cost of the physiome project as a whole. I doubt very much if the funding agencies of national governments are going to be able to fund what is required, not just because there are fashions in science (and the present fashion is very much a reductive one), but also because even if the physiome does become very fashionable and such priorities change, this is a time of extreme difficulty in interesting governments in funding research. I do not know who will do it unless we also tap commercial resources. I do not think we should be afraid of that. Exploitation of the physiome could be one of its sources of funding. Handled properly, it is also a source of protection. There are a lot of issues here, and I am only just pushing them up above the surface, but this funding issue will be a very big one.

Dr. L. Axel: Part of the problem with the National Library of Medicine's Visual Human Program is not just the simple size of the database which has to be sorted through and then downloaded, but that there are no convenient programs to deal with it. There are some commercial companies that have produced little subsets that have precanned renderings of those datasets that you can look at; it is a minor industry in universities and now in meetings on visualization there is always a separate section on dealing with that dataset. But there are no convenient and visually powerful and mobile programs to deal with it. We are talking about images which are 10^9 voxels. That is a large dataset to deal with and that is just one specimen. If you are going to make that kind of data available, say on a national repository, it is going to be difficult to move over the information on the not–so–super highway and then deal with it on your own computer once you have got it.

With the advance of processors, all this will become easier in the future but somebody will have to do the actual work of writing the programs to make this run, even if they are written as something portable like JAVA. For example, with some of the software that we developed for dealing with our datasets, which are fairly large, we spent more time doing the user interface than we did doing the internal algorithms.

Dr. S. Sideman: There is no question in my mind that data is crucial to whatever we are going to do. Yet, one wonders, have we exhausted the questions? Do we know all we want to know and now we want the data to prove it? I would like to interject a question on the future of our work. Assuming that we have the data, what are we looking for in the real world?

Dr. J.B. Bassingthwaighte: I was thinking about Dr. Noble's (Chapter 24) and Dr. Rudy's (Chapter 23) models and of the way they have presented their models. Dr. Rudy's model showed channels and pumps. I have my own tentative example. I can do the same kind of thing with an interface for models of blood–tissue exchange processes. One can go from one model to the next. For example, one may have the capillary blood–tissue exchange unit and the transporter model. To use the interface as a vehicle for carrying the information, one might like to click the button for the transporter and display the database underlying it. The database would provide information on the affinities, the values of the K_m for different species, and the enzyme abundances in different cell types and species. This would be a magnificent expansion of the Enzyme Handbook for each particular purpose. One could do the same thing for intracellular enzymes in the metabolic chains and so on. One could devise the models so that they are approached visually. One could explore them at the surface or more deeply. There may be a lot of submodels or little models we can develop in this kind of fashion. We will not develop the all encompassing model for maybe hundreds of years, but we can do little models and make them visually useful. This, however, is but one approach to the complex problem of how to make an enormous body of information available to biological researchers.

Dr. N. Westerhof: When needed, it is better to go to where the desired model works, do the experiments and collaborate with the people in that particular place. In general, computer models are written in such a manner that others cannot use them. A completely other approach suggested a number of years ago, is to adapt biomedical research, the approach used by physicists. They work altogether in one location and write publications with contributions of many authors. This approach does not work in our field. We are either too individualistic or our experiments are too far away from each other. It is good that we know each other from meetings like this, know the reasonably updated literature, and if somebody does an experiment or he has an interesting model, it is best just to call him and say, "can we spend a couple of weeks or months together."

Dr. D. Noble: The problem with that is that, in the present generation of cardiac models of the kind we are using, and which started with the paper with DiFrancesco [*DiFrancesco D and Noble D. A model of cardiac electrical activity incorporating ionic pumps and concentration changes. Philosophical Trans of the Royal Soc 1985;B307:353—398*], we were swamped with precisely that kind of request. We simply could not cope. What do you do when you have 100 other people in the world writing to get access to a model and who suddenly want to collaborate with you? That is the main reason why we commercialized that particular program. There is a dilemma here, which is going to come up more and more frequently because the models are becoming vastly more useful than they were 10 years ago. Five years down the line at a meeting like this, in order to have the relevant people, you may have to be 10 times bigger. This is going to grow explosively. If that happens, then the problems are even bigger.

Dr. N. Westerhof: To write your model for others who want to use it requires an enormous amount of work. So it is a trade–off between the number of people you want to collaborate with and the number of hours, or years, you spend to program it in a way that others can use it.

Dr. D. Noble: Its a mixture of the two. One has to be the response of the other.

Dr. H. Strauss: Would the NIH through NCRR pick out a few areas that it may want to develop, as a pilot project, to see whether or not it would be possible to do what Dr. Noble did with the pacemaker model that he developed with Dr. DiFrancesco, and make a user–friendly model accessible to all people. Such models would enable people to incorporate the appropriate variables thereby permitting them to use it in a variety of different physiological circumstances. It should focus on two or three models that people thought would be important in their particular areas thereby making it accessible throughout the community. Would that be something of interest to the scientific community at large? It would not impose the burden on the individual who initially described the model. It would not require the investigator to provide source code. The NCRR would obviously have to undertake the responsibility of funding somebody to put this model in a user–friendly format that would enable its wider use. Obviously, the investigator would be contacted to be sure that what was being done was appropriate and correct.

Dr. U. Dinnar: Is it a repeat of the Guyton model? How can you prevent another Guyton model?

Dr. J.B. Bassingthwaighte: Do we want to? I think there are some intermediate stages where Guytonian models are truly valuable. I am very alert to the point that Dr. Strauss has made, that you would like to have models in a targeted area. Well, we work in a targeted area. So this is a good discussion for us to have. If we load everything we have discussed over the last three days into the model that Drs. Hunter, Noble, McCulloch and Rudy are putting together, that is a model that we will find difficult to use. The reason I am worried about it even at the smaller level model is that in our group where we are supported by the National Center for Research Resources of NIH for coding models and delivering them to other users, we find that about 90–95% of our coding effort is done after the model has been developed, proven to be useful, used to fit data, analyzed and maybe even published. To make useful this 90% of the heavy duty labor to other people includes the development of manual pages, tests, datasets, experimental observations that can be used to run against the model, and descriptions of the experiments. It is tedious and is very heavy investment to take it from that initial phase of modeling to a phase of modeling that can be archived and utilized by other people. Thus, I am not too worried about being overwhelmed by having the big model, for I do not think that it will come for a while. I am more worried about getting a battery of relatively local smaller models together so they can be, in the long range, put together in super computers for a specific task. But they are not going to be in daily use.

Dr. A. McColloch: The National Center for Research Resources is interested in funding this kind of venture because of the benefits that can clearly accrue. In the case of our center in San Diego, the NIH has funded the resource and one of the major objectives of that resource was to take a large molecular dynamics code that was already commercialized and fairly widely used, and make it even more accessible to bench biologists, structural biologists, and others by making an equally usable form available on parallel super computers because one of the problems with those particular models is that you need to have a massive infrastructure in order to run them in a reasonable amount of time. The comment about the funding agencies and Dr. Noble's comment about commercializing some of the software that arises from these efforts reflect the underlying fact that it does take a lot of time and effort and money that takes away from the time and effort and money. If we do not want to diminish the science and the experimental work for the egalitarian purpose of making our codes more widely available, there needs to be a way of recovering the cost.

REFERENCES

1. Stent GS. The Coming of the Golden Age; A View of the End of Progress. Garden City, NY: Natural History Press, 1969, 146 pp.
2. Boyd CAR, Noble D. The Logic of Life: The Challenge of Integrative Physiology. New York: Oxford University Press, 1993, 226 pp.
3. Hodgkin AL, Huxley AF. A quantitative description of membrane current and its application to conduction and excitation in nerve. *J Physiol* 1952;117:500–544.
4. Platt JR. Strong inference. *Science* 1964;146:347–353.
5. DiFrancesco D, Noble S. A model of cardiac electrical activity incorporating ionic pumps and concentration changes. *Philos Trans R Soc Lond B Biol Sci* 1985;307:353–398.
6. Luo CH, Rudy Y. A dynamic model of the cardiac ventricular action potential: II: Afterdepolarizations, triggered activity, and potentiation. *Circ Res* 1994;74:1097–1113.
7. Winslow RL, Varghese A. Generation and propagation of ectopic beats induced by spatially localized Na–K pump inhibition in atrial network models. *Proc R Soc Lond B Biol Sci* 1993;254:55–61.
8. LeGrice IJ, Smaill BH, Chai LZ, Edgar SG, Gavin JB, Hunter PJ. Laminar structure of the heart: Ventricular myocyte arrangement and connective tissue architecture in the dog. *Am J Physiol* 269 (*Heart Circ Physiol* 38):H571–H582, 1995.
9. Glass L, Hunter P, McCulloch A. Theory of Heart: Biomechanics, Biophysics, and Nonlinear Dynamics of Cardiac Function. New York: Springer–Verlag, 1991, 611 pp.
10. Goldberger AL, Rigney DR, Mietus J, Antman EM, Greenwald S. Nonlinear dynamics in sudden death syndrome: Heartrate oscillations and bifurcations. *Experientia* 1988;44:983–987.

CHAPTER 29

Integrative and Interactive Studies of the Cardiac System: Deciphering the Cardionome

Samuel Sideman and Rafael Beyar[1]

ABSTRACT

The cardiac system, denoted as the Cardionome, represents one of the most exciting challenges to human ingenuity. Critical to our survival, it consists of a tantalizing array of interacting phenomena, from ionic transport, membrane channels and receptors through cellular metabolism, energy production, fiber mechanics, microcirculation, and electrical activation to the clinically observed global functions. These are measured by pressure, volume, shape, coronary flow, heart rate, and other changes. It is a complex interactive system requiring the intense efforts of capable scientists in the life sciences, including medicine, exact sciences, engineering and biomedical technology devoted to address these multivariable, multidisciplinary challenges, so as understand and control the pathologies involved. Here we present some of our past interactive studies and highlight two new models, one demonstrating micro to macro integration, and one involving tissue–organ interaction of various parameters. These models yield new insights into cardiac performance.

BACKGROUND

Necessity, imagination, ingenuity and persistence sustain our attempts to understand and overcome heart disease, which accounts for over 50% of human mortality. The enormity of the task of deciphering the cardiac "codes" is evident in Table 1 [1], which lists the major elements in the various physiological elements, arranged in hierarchies, or levels, of the cardionome.

---

[1]Heart System Research Center, Department of Biomedical Engineering, Technion–IIT, Haifa 32000, Israel

Analytical and Quantitative Cardiology
Edited by Sideman and Beyar, Plenum Press, New York, 1997

Table 1. The Cardionome: A One–Organ Component of the Physionome

Molecules	*Structure:*	proteins for channels, pumps, receptors, enzymes, junctions, contractile apparatus, binding sites.
	State:	conformational state, receptor occupancy.
	Kinetics:	activation energies for changes of state, diffusion, reaction, aggregation.
	Function:	transport, catalysis, signalling, energy transduction, regulation.
Organelle	*Structure:*	mitochondria, SR, Golgi, nucleus, gap junctions, T–system.
	State:	electrochemical potential, pH, pCa.
	Kinetics:	substrate and O_2 usage, ATP production.
	Functions:	sequestration reactions, microenvironment creation.
Cell	*Structure:*	cell, shape, size, arrangements of organelles.
	State:	membrane potassium, energy stores.
	Kinetics:	cellular function, rate of output of product.
	Functions:	ionic balance, action potential generation, calcium regulation, tension development, response to stretch.
Tissue	*Structure:*	cell arrangements, interstitial matrix, capillarity, fiber direction and cross connectivity, mechanical linkages (collagen to cytoskeleton), vascular arrangement.
	State:	material composition, mechanical properties.
	Kinetics:	blood–tissue exchange, deformation, excitatory spread.
	Functions:	solute exchanges between cells, blood–tissue exchanges, propagation of excitation, generating shortening stresses and strains.
Organ	*Structure:*	fiber arrangements, anisotropy, directed spread–of–excitation.
	State:	contraction, relaxation, inflow, outflow, innervation.
	Kinetics:	rate of deformation, ejection velocity, cardiac output, pressures (Coupling with body, e.g., output impedance).
	Function:	coordinated spread of excitation, cardiac contraction, volume ejection, responses to humoral agents and autonomic outflow, ANF production.

Reproduced with permission from *Molecular and Subcellular Cardiology* (S. Sideman, R. Beyar, editors), Plenum Publ. Corp., 1995, p. 331 [1].

Intensive research from different points of view of the various parameters of the cardiac physiology and pathophysiology is carried out all over the world. Practically all these studies concentrate on specific parameters which affect cardiac performance. While this approach is definitely commendable, and usually very instructive, it necessarily leaves out some important parameters which affect the cardiac function and the effects of the interactions between the parameters. For instance, it is easily conceived that mechanical contractions affect the blood flow in the coronary tree. It is less understood how the coronary blood flow affects cardiac mechanics, although pathological evidence is rampant.

Gaining insight into the various aspects of the cardionome listed in Table 1 requires utilizing many different models. Obviously, these models must each reflect their dependence on the other hierarchies of scale [1]. Thus, molecular level models of ionic channels, enzymes, or transporter require subcellular level feedback on the local concentrations of substrates, reaction products, and regulators. Cellular level models of excitation–contraction coupling require molecular biochemical information, as well as tissue level knowledge of channel conductances and ionic currents. Tissue level models for oxygen exchange and pH regulation with respect to solute exchanges must relate to the cellular level for the binding, buffering, and chemical reaction. Similarly, tissue and organ level models of cardiac mechanics require molecular level analysis to better explain the control mechanism of the contraction–relaxation phenomena. Organ level models of coronary blood flow and its transmural distribution require knowledge of intraorgan and intramural pressures, as well as information on perfusion pressures which are influenced by the state of vasoregulation throughout the body. The vasculature resistances influence the pressures available for coronary perfusion, and transcapillary transport which in turn influences the intramyocardial pressure, force generation and cardiac output [1].

Incorporating all the multilevel interactions and integrating them into a coherent picture is presently an insurmountable task. It requires the close interaction between scientists of different backgrounds collaborating to integrate knowledge of the many disciplines, from molecular and genetic cardiology to organ physiology, including engineering science, pharmacology and clinical expertise, so as to understand, control and modify cardiac performance and its ramifications. Whatever the approach, one must guarantee the close relevance of the analytical and experimental studies to the appropriate physiology and actual clinical applications. The many interacting parameters and the multifunctionality of the cardiac system, on the one hand, and the demand for relevancy to patients and clinical needs on the other hand, dictate maintaining a close bond between scientific know–how into clinical reality (Fig. 1).

The Henry Goldberg Workshops [2–10] set out in 1983 to enhance the study of these multiparameter interdisciplinary relationships. The interactions between mechanics, electrical activation, perfusion, metabolism, and imaging in the clinical environment are explored in [2]. The interactions of the cardiovascular system with some of its controls are described in [3]. The transformation of microscale myocardial function and electrical activity to overall electrical propagation and cardiac performance is given in [4], and parameters associated with ischemia are addressed in [5]. The effect of inhomogeneity of the cardiac muscle on its performance is detailed in [6]. Imaging modalities and their

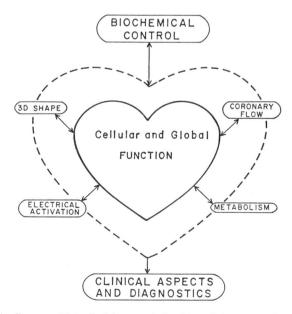

Figure 1. Schematic diagram of interdisciplinary relationships of the proposed center of excellence.

impact on cardiac diagnosis of global and regional performance is the focus of [7]. The exploration of the basic micro–level phenomena that affect the cardiac system, with a particular emphasis on electrical activation is described in [8]. Some of the basic interactions in the cellular and subcellular levels which affect the activation and performance of the cardiac system are highlighted in [9, 10].

The Technion's Heart System Research Center has developed integrated research projects addressing the interactions between the various parameters affecting cardiac function under different physiological and pathological conditions. Most of our earlier efforts were directed at system analysis of the interactions between the different observed and measurable parameters of the heart function. Like many other scientists, we have related measurable or estimated parameters to observed cardiac performance. But, unlike most others, we have tried to identify the effects of the interactions between the parameters on cardiac performance. By relating mechanics, circulation and hemodynamics, electrophysiology, biochemistry, metabolism, and energetics in normal and pathological hearts, we could gain better insight into cardiac function, including the roles of cellular, subcellular and molecular level control mechanisms which affect the global organ behavior.

The integrated approach of the Technion's Heart System Research Center relates physiology to physical laws, including transport phenomena and shape and structural considerations. Basic studies [11–17] related fiber structure and sarcomere dynamics to the normal [11–14] and pathological [16] global ventricular performance. The local perfusion within the myocardium was related to the local mechanical parameters [16] as well as to the instantaneous oxygen consumed [13] for the metabolic needs of cardiac function, yield–ing the local energetics and the temperature [24, 25] distribution in the healthy and infarcted hearts. An integrated, tissue–organ level model [26], which relates myocardial structure and mechanics to the coronary circulation and transcapillary mass transfer (briefly presented below) demonstrate the advantage and utility of this approach. Computer recon–struction of realistic 3D hearts based on tomographic data (MRI, Cine–CT), related cardiac shape to myocardial function and allowed the determination of regional local function [17–21]. The electrical characteristics of cardiac function and the excitation of the myocardium was related to the mechanical aspects of the heart, and arrhythmogenesis and fibrillation [22, 23].

The recent advances in ionic and molecular cardiac research have the led to better understanding of the control mechanisms at the cellular, subcellular and molecular levels, and allows to address these new frontiers in an integrated way so as to link these microscale phenomena coherently with global organ performance. The model, based on the molecular intracellular biochemical reactions is briefly presented below, and demonstrate the role of the intracellular control mechanism on the global organ function [27, 28].

EXAMPLES OF RECENT INTEGRATED INTERACTIVE MODELS

Mechanics, Blood Flow and Mass Transfer Interactions

Muscle mechanics, coronary flow and mass transport are three functionally related phenomena which strongly affect left ventricular (LV) performance. These are interactive phenomena, as the coronary flow [29–32] and fluid transport [30] affect LV mechanics and LV mechanics affects the coronary flow [34, 35] and interstitial fluid transport and increased coronary flow increases the myocardial oxygen consumption [36]. Past LV theoretical analyses have addressed these phenomena separately, and various LV mechanical models [37–41] coronary flow models [42, 43] and mass transport models [44] have been proposed. Some describe the effects of the LV mechanics on the coronary flow [15, 45], but are incapable of predicting the coupled inverse effects, i.e., the effects of the coronary flow on the LV mechanics [43, 44].

The new integrative and structural approach [26, 46, 47] allows to determine the global LV performance (muscle mechanics, coronary flow and mass transport) directly in terms of the prevailing physiological (muscle activity, composition and structure) and loading (preload, afterload) conditions. The principal advantages and significance of directly relating cause (myocardial activity and composition) and effect (muscle mechanics, coronary flow and mass transport), lies in the ability to investigate and predict the changes in global LV performance under various pathological conditions, e.g. coronary stenoses or myocardial edema.

The model has shown, in excellent agreement with the experimental findings [35, 48, 49], that the coronary flow is mainly affected by muscle contractility and perfusion pressure rather than by the LV pressure. Also, the interstitial fluid transport affects the LV mechanics and the coronary flow, determines the diastolic myocardial conditions, and explains the changes in LV compliance with changes in perfusion pressure [26] or the changes in LV performance due to blood osmotic transients [33]. Clearly, this integrative approach provides a better analytical tool for the analysis of the LV performance and function. The correspondence of the model prediction and reported experimental observations is partly demonstrated in Chapter 12.

Intracellular Control of Cardiac Function: From Molecule to Ventricle

Life and motion depend on the electromechanical coupling between electrical excitation and mechanical contraction of contractile proteins in the muscle cells. The generation of force by the muscle is determined by the contraction of the sarcomeres in each cell within the muscle tissue, and by the simultaneous interactions between the cells, which affect the propagation of the electrical stimulating wave, the propagation of the mechanical perturbation and the consequent contraction of the ventricles.

The dynamic control model of the intracellular excitation–contraction coupling in the intact cardiac cell [27, 51] is based on biochemical kinetics [53, 54] and on the regulation of the crossbridges cycling and recruitment by the calcium troponin–tropomyosin interactions [55, 56]. The analysis emphasizes the key role of the troponin regulatory proteins in regulating muscle activity [55, 57]. Crossbridge turnover from the weak to strong conformation requires ATP hydrolysis, and the generated pressure and energy consumption are determined by the amount of available crossbridges and the rate of crossbridge cycling. A positive feedback determines the affinity of troponin for calcium by the number of cycling crossbridges, the force–length relationship and the related Frank–Starling law. Calcium binding to troponin regulates crossbridge recruitment. A negative feedback relates the filaments' sliding velocity to the rate of crossbridges returning to the weak conformation, and provides the basis for Hill's equation for the force–velocity relationship and the generated power. These feedbacks determine the amount of bound calcium, the availability of crossbridges and the rate of crossbridge cycling. Consequently, the sarcomeres can adjust energy cost to mechanical constraints following stimulation.

The model was extended to multi–cell fibers [51] and the global LV performance [28, 52]. The utility of this intracellular control model is best demonstrated by evaluating the LV performance in comparison to Suga's [58, 59] time varying elastance model. The latter is essentially a linear, load independent, tool which describes the performance of the LV in the pressure–volume plane, and defines LV contractility based on the end–systolic pressure–volume relationship (ESPVR). However, *in vivo* studies [60] indicate that the

ESPVR is nonlinear and is affected by loading conditions. Furthermore, Sagawa *et al.* [59] have shown that the ESPVR is affected by the history of contraction or, by "short term memory" [61]. These characteristics contradict the assumption inherent in the time varying elastance model which considers the ESPVR to be the index of contractility. The studies of Hunter [62] and Burkhoff *et al.* [63] on isolated canine heart suggest that the elastance theory can not account for 1) the prolongation of the time to end–systole in ejecting beats as compared with isovolumic beats, 2) the decrease in the rate of relaxation in an ejecting beat, and 3) the increase in the end–systolic pressure of the ejecting beat relative to the isovolumic beat.

The performance of the cardiac fiber in the force–length plane, based on the intracellular control model [28] for isometric, isotonic and physiological contractions, is respresented by a unique curve. The results resemble the experimental data of Leach *et al.* [64], and are obtained by integrating the four–state excitation–contraction model [27, 51] with Beyar and Sideman's LV model [38, 65] to emulate the pressure–volume loops of the LV. The calculated instantaneous LV pressure–volume relationship resembles the experimental data of Sagawa *et al.* [66] and the time varying elastance concept. The analysis also yields the effect of various loading conditions on the work and rate of ATP consumption by the actomyosin ATPase.

The basic hypothesis underlining this model is that it is possible to describe the performances of the LV based on the intracellular control of contraction, i.e., calcium kinetics and crossbridge cycling. Specifically, it is suggested that: 1) The instantaneous pressure and volume are determined by a balance between the positive cooperative mechanism and the negative mechanical feedback mechanism; 2) the deviation of the ESPVR from linearity and the dependence of the ESPVR on the history of contraction and loading conditions can be determined by the model, which offers a simple approach for evaluating LV performance, requiring less PV loops to characterize the parameters of the feedback loops than are now needed to evaluate the ESPVR by the elastance model [59, 60]. The present method is based on the analysis of the instantaneous rate of pressure development during each contraction. This advantage makes the method feasible for clinical implementation.

The model describes the basic mechanical properties of the cardiac muscle: the force–length and the force–velocity relationship as a function of the activation level and mechanical loading conditions. It simulates the known mechanical phenomena of the cardiac muscle relating to one beat. It reproduces the control of relaxation, including load dependent relaxation [27, 51] and the conditions that cause calcium dependent relaxation [51]. Finally, it provides the molecular–cellular explanation for the elastance and related phenomena in the cardiac muscle and it enables to calculate the work and the energy consumption of the cardiac muscle. Clearly, this study of the electro–mechanical coupling in the myocardial cells enhances our fundamental understanding of the cardiac physiology and highlights the basic mechanism of cardiac performance.

The model noted here has the advantage of relating 'micro–scale', biochemically established, intracellular physiological characteristics (e.g. the sarcomere), to the instantaneous local and global 'macro–scale' function of the LV. This biochemically based intracellular model describes the basic mechanical properties of the cardiac muscle (e.g. the force–length and force–velocity relationships) at different activation levels and mechanical loading conditions. The model provides the molecular basis for the time–varying elastance concept and the instantaneous pressure–volume relationships during isovolumic contractions. Moreover, it describes the effect of ejection on the instantaneous pressure–volume relationship and explains the phenomena of the pressure deficit and shortening deactivation during ejection as well as the recent observation of the positive effect of the ejection on pressure development and on the systolic duration of the ejecting beat. As shown [28], the ESPVR is determined by the intracellular balance between the cooperativity mechanism and the mechanical feedback and is affected by the mechanical loading through these intracellular mechanisms.

CONCLUSION

The complexity of the cardiac system, as demonstrated in Table 1, precludes a single all encompassing model to describe cardiac performance. However, integrative multilevel models which account for some of the major parameters affecting cardiac performance have been shown here to be superior to single–level models with limited parameters.

DISCUSSION

Dr. S. Sideman: Another point to consider: We have recently proposed a model (Chapter 11) that showed a remarkable fit between the theoretical predictions and many reported experiments. The question: "how does such a relatively simple model fit such a wide range of data?" The answer is that if you have a good model and identify the major most effective parameters, you can have a relatively simple model that responds well to real life situations and corresponds to reliable experimental data. Do we need more models for similar answers?

Dr. Y. Rudy: Maybe one of the reasons that several models (rather than a unique model) provide acceptable descriptions of the system's behavior is the high level of redundancy and reserve that is built into the system. We are lucky it is designed that way, otherwise we would be walking a thin line between existence and non–existence. Examples: An action potential propagates in the heart (under normal conditions) generating five times the minimum charge needed for excitation (a safety factor of five); it is sufficient to open only 5% of available gap–junctions to insure conduction between cells (95% reserve); even more striking, action potential shortening by 50% (a protective response to ischemic insult) takes only 0.5% opening of I_K(ATP) channels. It seems that within this framework of large reserve, many models can work well.

The other issue that was raised was the ability to simulate phenomena starting from a genetic process all the way to the whole heart function. A beautiful example from cardiac electro–physiology is the long QT (LQT) syndrome. In this hereditary disorder, genotypic changes (i.e., mutations in genes that link to the sodium channel, I_{Na}, or to the potassium channel, I_{Kr}) were related to phenotypic changes (prolonged QT interval) in the ECG. In the case of I_{Na}, we have a good understanding of the entire process. The mutant I_{Na} is characterized by a non–absorbing inactivation state. That is, unlike the normal I_{Na} channel which basically opens once during the action potential (AP) and then inactivates, the mutant I_{Na} reopens to generate an inward current during the plateau, prolonging the AP. This, in turn,is reflected in a long QT interval in the ECG. So here is an example of a process that can be simulated starting from the genetic–based modifica–tion of the single ion–channel, which can then be introduced into a model of the AP, from which the ECG can be computed. This can work in the reverse direction as well, that is, the ECG can be used to detect functional modification of a particular channel (e.g., I_{Na}), identifying this channel as a target for clinical intervention (e.g., by drugs, or through genetic modification). At this stage, I do not feel that we are ready to build comprehensive models of the entire heart system with this level of vertical (from gene to function) integration. It is my opinion that we should be more modest and focus on specific processes that are well characterized experimentally at all levels, such as the LQT example.By constructing many examples of this type, we will acquire a better understanding of the entire system and will be better situated to address more comprehensive modeling challenges.

Dr. D. Noble: The question of redundancy is an extremely important point and it highlights one of the things that models can do beautifully well and which, at the moment, experiments have great difficulty with. Let me give an example.

There was in the 1980s a ferocious argument between the protagonists of two mechanisms of the natural pacemaker. The first was the i_f mechanism (hyperpolarizing–activated current mechanism) where one of my colleagues, Dario DiFrancesco, went for the view that this was the main contributor, generating maybe as much as 90% of the depolarizing current. The alternative hypothesis was the old g_K decay model, where the decay of a K conductance revealed a background conductance, which we call the background sodium current, $i_{b,Na}$, which leads to depolarization. This argument eventually resolved itself in a quantitative way. Both these mechanisms are present, the question is what are their respective contributions in normal circumstances. The redundancy is clearly there. We worked out that, in our models, around 20% of the depolarizing current might be i_f, while 80% might be $i_{b,Na}$. This leads to two very simple predictions: a drug that blocked i_f (and drug companies have produced such drugs) would be a relatively safe and limited cardiac slowing agent, whereas, if the figures I have just given are correct, then a blocker of $i_{b,Na}$ would be expected to be very dangerous. If you block a current that contributes up to 80% of the net depolarizing current then you might even stop the heart!

Yet this "back–of–envelope" prediction is completely wrong! When you do the simulations on the single sinus node cell models, what you find is that as you block one mechanism, the other takes over. We can't do this experimentally because there are no blockers of $i_{b,Na}$ available yet. So this is not only an example of redundancy but also of a question that only models are capable at present of answering. What happens if you block $i_{b,Na}$ progressively in any of the sinus node models currently available is that this produces a tiny amount (few mV) of hyperpolarization which, because the i_f activation curve is steep and the available current so very large compared to that required for pacemaker depolarization, kicks in a progressively larger amount of i_f. This effect is so strong that the reduction in sinus node frequency is in fact very moderate [*Noble et al. Role of the inward currents $i_{b,Na}$ and i_f in controlling and stabilizing pacemaker frequency of rabbit sino-atrial node cells. Proceedings of the Royal Society, 1992;B 250:199—207*]. This is an example of redundancy in which at least two systems are expressed, either of which may be adequate alone to ensure function, and which come together beautifully to ensure that one of the most important functions, the natural rhythm, is very strongly fail–safe.

Dr. J.B. Bassingthwaighte: There is a very powerful paper by John Platt [*Platt JR. Strong inference. Science 1964;146:347–353*]. He proposed that "thou shalt have an hypothesis" and then design an experiment to test that hypothesis. A model is a hypothesis that is explicit, quantitative and evaluatable. He went further. He said, "thou shalt have a second hypothesis." Now examine this issue because now you design an experiment that tests not just one hypothesis but must distinguish between two hypotheses. This forces a scientific advance. The result of the experiment either denies one or both of the hypotheses, and in either case it advances the science. That is Platt's contribution.

Dr. U. Dinnar: We have the Human model of Guyton in our laboratory. We use it sometimes for exercises and students they can operate the model. But it is very hard to understand the model or to understand the data because the data is presented by a bunch of numbers that nobody knows what to do with. A mathematical model is not a goal. A mathematical model is a tool, like a microscope or a pH meter. Sometimes it is good to look at a phenomena with a model, sometimes it is good to look with a microscope. It depends on what you want to achieve. If a mathematical model will tell you to look better into another phenomena with another tool, than you have a good model. The goal of the model is not to mimic and replace the real phenomena. It is a tool like any other tool and we should treat this as another tool.

Dr. J. Saffitz: I would like to comment on Dr. Beyar's point, which is a very important one: how will the new biology contribute to this effort? The molecular tools are sufficiently well developed so that the genome can be manipulated in very specific ways. The question is what happens when we do this. The extent to which one identifies a phenotype, in response to a genetic manipulation is a function of how carefully one looks. At this point we do not look very carefully because we have not developed the tools for doing these kind of analyses. In my view, the future, which I believe is a very bright one, is going to involve a combination of specific genetic manipulation and very careful physiological analysis in the whole animal, the whole organ, the whole cell, at any level you want. Analysis of effects of specific genetic manipulation within the milieu of the intact cell, tissue, organ, animal, is a very powerful strategy that we are just beginning to scratch the surface of. The opportunities for systems physiologists and molecular biologists to get together are extraordinary. To me, that is the link between the genome and the physiome.

Dr. Y. Lanir: Models represent the essence of the hypodeductive approach to scientific research. Yet, invariably, models only approximate the reality, and simplifications are an inherent part of each model. A good model retains the important (simplified) features most relevant to the hypotheses or questions asked. Hence, more specific and focussed questions lead to more powerful and realistic models. An overall comprehensive model of a physiological system must inevitably include a large number of simplifications. These reduce the model reliability.

Dr. H. Rockman: There are knockouts, receptors, integrins, transcriptional factors that have no phenotype and many are a total surprise. Everyone would have predicted that there would be an altered phenotype, and yet there is tremendous redundancy in pathways. Models are very important, but I do not know if people are thinking of these complex redundant pathways.

Dr. P. Hunter: I would like to comment on a role of modeling that has not yet been mentioned. The most important aspect of modeling is when it does not match things experimentally. When it does match the experiment, you think that is fine and good but probably a number of models can do that. When it does not match the experiment is when you really start learning because you go back and examine what aspects of your assumptions are wrong.

Also, just as the physiome project could enable models to be used by a wide range of scientists on a world wide collaborative effort, there is an equally important part of the physiome project that we have not talked about and that is the data–basing. It is very important that we establish data–bases that can be accessed by everybody and that there is a coordinated effort to build those data–bases in parallel with building the models.

Dr. A. Landesberg: Maybe we can compare the science of medicine, or physiology, to the science of physics. Modeling is a tool useful for expressing our understanding of the system, or as Dr. Bassingthwaighte has said, a tool for making predictions or studying a new theory. The purpose of the model is not to make quantitative data better understood, but rather to have a better physiological or physical understanding of the phenomena. For example, if you take a very simple phenomenon like the force–calcium relationship you can describe it by a model like the Hill equation. But then the question is, what are the parameters? What is the basic understanding you gain from this description? If I compare it to physics many years ago, when the apple fell down they measured the relationship between the velocity and the force. These were the genomes of that time. Then came Newton and made a model. The model was his equation which described a very simple system so it was a very simple model. But then came Einstein and said that the fact is not the true fact. Maybe that the genome that we have today will be changed in future years and there will be a new discovery that DNA has some sub–system that we are not aware of today. So the facts can also be changed, as well as the interpretation, because the logic of the model is our understanding the system. Einstein said that Newton's theory was not correct, and there is now another theory which is considered the best one. As I understand modeling, it is not only for obtaining the best quantitative study of the data; it is a tool for better understanding of physiology and for designing new experiments to answer questions or erase given assumptions or generate new questions. The idea of the genome, the physiome and modeling, in general, is to understand nature.

REFERENCES

1. Bassingthwaighte JB. Toward modeling the human physionome. In: Sideman S, Beyar R, eds. *Molecular and Subcellular Cardiology*. NY: Plenum Publ. Corp., 1995; 331–340.

2. Sideman S, Beyar R (Editors). *Simulation and Imaging of the Cardiac System – State of the Heart*. Proc 1st Henry Goldberg Workshop, Technion, Haifa, March 1984. Publ/Dordrecht/Boston: Martinus Nijhoff, 1985.

3. Sideman S, Beyar R (Editors). *Simulation and Control of the Cardiac System*. Parts I, II, III, Proc 2nd Henry Goldberg Workshop, Haifa, April 1985. Florida: CRC Press/Florida; 1987.

4. Sideman S, Beyar R (Editors). *Activation, Metabolism and Perfusion of the Heart. Simulation and Experimental Models*. Proc 3rd Henry Goldberg Workshop, Rutgers Univ, USA, April 1986. Dordrecht/Boston: Martinus Nijhoff Publ.; 1987.

5. Sideman S, Beyar R (Editors). *Analysis and Simulation of the Cardiac System – Ischemia*. Proc 4th Henry Goldberg Workshop, Tiberias, May 1987. Florida: CRC Press; 1989.

6. Sideman S, Beyar R (Editors). *Imaging, Analysis and Simulation of the Cardiac System*. Proc 5th Henry Goldberg Workshop, Cambridge, UK: Freund Publishing; 1990.

7. Sideman S, Beyar R (Editors). *Imaging, Measurements and Analysis of the Heart*. Proc 6th Henry Goldberg Workshop, Eilat, Dec. 1989. NY: Hemisphere Publ; 1991.

8. Sideman S, Beyar R, Kléber, A (Editors). *Cardiac Electrophysiology, Circulation and Transport*. Proc 7th Henry Goldberg Workshop, Gwatt, Switzerland, May, 1991. NY: Kluwer Publ; 1991.

9. Sideman S, Beyar R (Editors). *Interactive Phenomena in the Cardiac System*, Proc of the 8th Henry Goldberg Workshop, Bethesda, MD, 1992, NY: Plenum Publishing Corp; 1993.

10. Sideman S, Beyar R (Editors). *Molecular and Subcellular Cardiology: Effects on Structure and Function*, Proc. of the 9th Henry Goldberg Workshop, Haifa, Israel. NY: Plenum Publishing Corp.; 1995.

11. Beyar R, Sideman S. A model for left ventricular contraction combining the force length velocity relationship with the time varying elastance theory. *Biophys J* 45:1167–1177, 1984.

12. Beyar R, Sideman S. Computer study of the left ventricular performance based on its fiber structure, sarcomere dynamics, electrical activation propagation. *Circ Res* 55:358–374, 1984.

13. Beyar R, Sideman S. Left ventricular mechanics related to the distribution of oxygen demand throughout the wall. *Circ Res* 58:664–677, 1986.

14. Beyar R, Sideman S. Source parameters of the left ventricle related to the physiological characteristics of cardiac muscle. *Biophys J* 49:1185–1194, 1986.

15. Beyar R, Sideman S. Time dependent coronary blood flow distribution in the left ventricular wall. *Am J Physiol* 1987;252:H417–H433.

16. Beyar R, Sideman S. Mechanical pathophysiology of different heart diseases: A computerized analysis. *Med & Biol Eng & Comput* 28:237–248, 1990.

17. Lessick J, Sideman S, Azhari H, Marcus M, Grenadier E, Beyar R. Regional three–dimensional geometry and function of left ventricles with fibrous aneurysms: a cine–computed tomography study, *Circulation*, 84:1072–1086, 1991.

18. Azhari H, Beyar R, Grenadier E, Dinnar U, Sideman S. An analytical descriptor of 3–D geometry. Application to the analysis of the left ventricle shape contraction. *IEEE Trans Biomed Eng* 34:345–355, 1987.

19. Sideman S, Beyar R, Azhari H, Barta E, Adam D, Dinnar U. Three dimensional computer simulation of the cardiac system. *IEEE Proc* 76/6:708–719, 1988.

20. Azhari H, Sideman S, Weiss JL, Shapiro EP, Weisfeldt ML, Graves WL, Rogers WJ, Beyar R. Three–dimensional mapping of acute ischemic regions using MRI: Wall thickening versus motion analysis. *Am J Physiol (Heart Circ Physiol* 28), 259:H1492–H1503, 1990.

21. Halmann M, Sideman S, Dinnar U, Azhari H, Beyar R. Microcomputer–based system for reconstruction and 3D animation of the heart and its coronary arteries. *Computers in Cardiology* (Jerusalem, 1989), 16:29–31, 1990.

22. Barta E, Sideman S. 3–D simulation model for the electrical activity characteristics in ischemic heart. *Computers in Cardiology*, (Belgium, 1987). K.L. Ripley, Ed, Computer Society Press, Washington, D.C, pp. 495–498, 1988.

23. Barta E, Adam D, Salant E, Sideman S. 3–D ventricular myocardial electrical excitation: a minimal pathways model. *Annals Biomed Eng* 15:443–456, 1987.

24. Barta E, Sideman S, Beyar R. Spatial and temporal temperature distribution in the healthy and locally diseased wall of the heart. *Int J Heat Mass Transfer* 29:1253–1261, 1986.

25. Barta E, Sideman S, Beyar R. Temperature distribution within the left ventricular wall of the normal and infarcted heart. *Proc 8th Int Heat Transfer Conf,* San Francisco, 1986, Vol. 4, CL Tien, VP Casey, JK Farrell, Eds, Hemisphere Publ./New York, pp. 3073–3078, 1986.

26. Zinemanas D, Beyar R, Sideman S. An integrated model of left ventricular muscle mechanics, coronary flow and fluid and mass transport. *Am J Physiol* 268 (*Heart Circ Physiol* 37): H633–H645, 1995.

27. Landesberg A, Sideman S. Mechanical regulation in the cardiac muscle by coupling calcium binding to troponin–C and crossbridge cycling. A dynamic model. *Am J Physiol* 267 (*Heart Circ Physiol* 36): H779–H795, 1994.

28. Landesberg A. End–systolic pressure–volume relation based on the intracellular control of contraction. *Am J Physiol* 270: H338–H349, 1996.

29. Fukui A, Yamaguchi S, Tamada Y, Miyawaki H, Baniya G, Shirakabe M. Different effects of coronary perfusion pressure on diastolic properties of left and right ventricles (Abstract). *Circulation* 1991;84:I-45.

30. Kresh JY, Frash F, McVey M, Brockman SK, Noordergraaf A. Mechanical coupling of the myocardium with coronary circulation in the beating and arrested heart (Abstract). *Circulation* 1990; 84:II-45.

31. Laine GA, Granger HJ. Microvascular, interstitial and lymphatic interactions in normal heart. *Am J Physiol* 1985;249:H834–H842.

32. McCulloch AD, Hunter PJ, Smaill BH. Mechanical effects of coronary perfusion in the passive canine left ventricle. *Am J Physiol* 1992;262:H523–H530.

33. Anderson SE, Johnson JA. Tissue–fluid pressure in perfused rabbit hearts during osmotic transients. *Am J Physiol* 1987;252:H1127–H1137.

34. Kouwenhoven E, Vergroeses Y, Spaan JAE. Retrograde coronary flow is limited by time–varying elastance. *Am J Physiol* 1992;263:H484–H490.

35. Kresh JY. Myocardial modulation of coronary circulation (letter). *Am J Physiol* 1989;257: H1934–H1935.

36. Gregg DE. Effect of coronary perfusion pressure or coronary flow on oxygen usage of the myocardium. *Circ Res* 1963;13:497–500.

37. Arts T, Veenstra PC, Reneman RS. Transmural course of stress and sarcomere length in the left ventricle under normal hemodynamic circumstances. In: Baan J, Arntsenius AC, Yellin EL eds. *Cardiac Dynamics.* The Hague: Martinus Nijhoff, 1980; 115–122.

38. Beyar R, Sideman S. A computer study of the left ventricular performance based on fiber structure, sarcomere dynamics and transmural electrical propagation velocity. *Circ Res* 1984;55:358–375.

39. Chadwick RS. Mechanics of the left ventricle. *Biophys J* 1980;39:279–288.

40. Nevo E, Lanir Y. Structural finite deformation model of the left ventricle during diastole and systole. *J Biomech Eng Trans ASME* 1989;111:342–349.

41. Ohayon J, Chadwick RS. Effects of collagen microstructure in the mechanics of the left ventricle. *Biophys J* 1988;54: 1077–1088.

42. Kresh JY, Fox M, Brockman SK, Noordergraaf A. Model–based analysis of transmural vessel impedance and myocardial circulation dynamics. *Am J Physiol* 1990;258:H262–H276.

43. Beyar R, Camminker R, Manor D, Sideman S. Coronary flow patterns in normal and ischemic hearts: Transmyocardial and artery to vein distribution. *Ann Biomed Eng* 1993;21:001–024.

44. Bassingthwaighte JB, Goresky CA. Modeling in the analysis of solute and water exchange in the microvasculature. In: Renking EM, Michel CC, eds, *Handbook of Physiology,* Bethesda, MD: American Physiological Society, 1984; 549–626.

45. Arts T, Reneman RS. Interaction between intramyocardial pressure (IMP) and myocardial circulation. *J Biomed Eng* 1985;107:51–56.

46. Zinemanas D, Beyar R, Sideman S. Intramyocardial fluid transport effects on coronary flow and LV mechanics. In: Sideman S, Beyar R, eds. *Interactive Phenomena in the Cardiac System,* Proc. of the 8th Henry Goldberg Workshop, Bethesda, MD, 1992. NY: Plenum Publishing Corp., 1993; 219–231.

47. Zinemanas D, Beyar R, Sideman S. Relating mechanics, blood flow and mass transport in the cardiac muscle. *Int J Heat & Mass Transfer* 1994;37(1):191–205.

48. Krams R, Sipkema P, Zegers J, Westerhof N. Contractility is the main determinant of coronary systolic flow impediment. *Am J Physiol* 257: H1936–H1944, 1989.

49. Krams R, Sipkema P, Westerhof N. Coronary oscillatory flow amplitude is more affected by perfusion pressure than ventricular pressure. *Am J Physiol* 1990;258:H1889–H1898.

50. Olsson RA, Bunger R, Spaan JAE. Coronary circulation. In: Fozzard HA, ed, *The Heart and the*

Cardiovascular System, 2nd ed. NY: Raven Press, 1991; 1393–1425.

51.   Landesberg A, Sideman S. Calcium kinetic and mechanical regulation of the cardiac muscle. In: *Interactive Phenomena in the Cardiac System*, Proc. of the 8th Henry Goldberg Workshop. Sideman, S. and R. Beyar (Eds.), Bethesda, MD, 1992, Plenum Publishing Corp., NY, 1993, pp 59–77.

52.   Landesberg A, Beyar R, Sideman S. Time varying elastance and cardiac muscle energetics based on calcium kinetics and crossbridge cycling. *Computers in Cardiology*, London, September, 1993. *IEEE* supplement, 1993, pp. 373–376.

53.   Eisenberg E, Hill TL. Muscle contraction and free energy transduction in biological system. *Science* 227: 999–1006, 1985.

54.   Brenner B, Eisenberg E. The mechanism of muscle contraction. Biochemical, mechanical, and structural approaches to elucidate crossbridge action in muscle. *Basic Res. Cardiol.* 82(Suppl. 2): 2–16, 1987.

55.   Brenner B, Eisenberg E. Rate of force generation in muscle: correlation with actomyosin Atpase activity in solution. *Proc Natl Acad Sci* 1986; 83: 3542–3546.

56.   Chalovich JM, Eisenberg E. The effect of troponin – tropomyosin on the binding of heavy meromyosin to actin in the presence of ATP. *J Biol Chem* 261: 5088–5093, 1986.

57.   Ford EL. Mechanical manifestations of activation in cardiac muscle. *Circ Res* 68: 621–637, 1991.

58.   Suga H. Ventricular energetics. *Physiological Rev* 70: 247–277, 1990.

59.   Hofmann PA, Fuchs F. Effect of length and crossbridge attachment on Ca2+ binding to cardiac troponin–C. *Am J Physiol* 253: C90–C96, 1987.

60.   van der Velde ET, Burkhoff D, Steendijk P, Karsdon J, Sagawa K, Baan J. Nonlinearity and load sensitivity of end–systolic pressure–volume relation of canine left ventricle *in vivo*. *Circulation* 83: 315–327, 1993.

61.   Nwasokwa O, Sagawa K, Suga H. Sort–term memory in the in situ canine myocardium. *Am J Physiol* 247: H8–H16, 1984.

62.   Hunter WC. End–systolic pressure as a balance between opposing effects of ejection. *Circ Res* 64: 265–275, 1989.

63.   Burkhoff D, de Tombe PD, Hunter WC. Impact of ejection on magnitude and time course of ventricular pressure–volume capacity. *Am J Physiol* 265: H899–H909, 1993.

64.   Leach JK, Brady AJ, Skipper BH, Millar DL. Effect of active shortening on tension development of rabbit papillary muscle. *Am J Physiol* 238: H8–H13, 1980.

65.   Beyar R, Sideman S. Atrioventricular interaction: a computer study. *Am J Physiol* 252:H653–H665, 1987.

66.   Sagawa K, Suga H, Shoukas AA, Balkalar KM. End–systolic pressure–volume relationship: a new index of contractility. *Am J Cardiol* 40: 748–753, 1977.

CHAPTER 30

TECHNOLOGY VS PHYSIOLOGY: GENERAL DISCUSSION

Samuel Sideman, Moderator

Dr. S. Sideman: It is interesting to consider the interaction of physiology and technology. We are at a stage wherein technology is being used to manipulate physiology for information as well as for therapeutics. Obviously a lot of new techniques have saved a lot of lives, but so did modern biology and gene therapy, including biochemistry. I have the feeling that we need more manipulation of physiology by chemical as well as mechanical, physical, means.

Dr. M.S. Gotsman: Technology has outstripped our physiological knowledge. Consider the diseased arterial wall. We are uncertain of the molecular physiology of the intima and the media in the presence of atheroma. We understand normal arterial cellular function, but this is modified when the endothelium overlies pathological atheroma. We also create an injury model with balloons and stents and then ask the wall to respond normally to flow, and to continue with its normal processes of flow and antithrombosis. The injured arterial wall has an irregular surface, secretes growth factors and in particular platelet derived growth factor. Finally, the arterial wall has to heal and then to return to normal function.

  We have always understood how arteries dilate or contract, and their elastic and compliant components. Dr. Resnick's presentation (Chapter 13) adds to these features the molecular physiological mechanisms of cell modification, the secretion of paracrine and autocrine substances, the function of the receptors, intracellular transducers, DNA transcription, production of messenger RNA. We have learned a little about the response to injury and it would be important to identify the underlying mechanisms.

  We are spending millions of dollars on hundreds and thousands of patients without understanding the precise mechanism at the molecular level.

Dr. J. Saffitz: Another way of looking at technology vs physiology is to appreciate that sometimes physiology is directed by, or perhaps follows, technology. A good example is the basic research on the cell cycle relative to the smooth muscle cell. There was little interest in smooth muscle cell proliferation until, deriving from new technological advances, it became clear that restenosis was a serious problem . Now we have a very detailed, though not complete, understanding of some of the fundamental molecular mechanisms that determine whether a smooth muscle cell will remain withdrawn from the cell cycle or will enter the cell cycle. The more knowledge we have, the better opportunities we have to ultimately prevent the development of a disease. In another sense the technology is leading basic science to delve more fundamentally into processes that might eventually get ahead of the technology.

Dr. E. Ritman: Technology presents an opportunity for physiologists. For example, look at the stents. The stents are reducing the inevitable pulsatility. That might give us a lot of insight into changing a single factor that we otherwise have no control of. It is good that technology is ahead of physiology because it does allow us to do new experiments.

Dr. P. Hunter: There is also a continuing role for engineering in the issue of materials science. The prosthetic hip joint is a good precedent. It took 30 years of slow improvement in the technology to make hip joint prostheses better by the very careful study of the engineering materials and human tissue interface. I am very optimistic that we are making continued improvement in the use of technology and there is no reason to be pessimistic about it. My point is that while molecular biology has a tremendous amount to contribute, we should not downplay the role of engineering technology in improving materials science, for example, and improving the interfaces between engineering materials and tissue. The classic example is the continuing development of prosthetic hip joints which continue to get better, people survive with implanted hip joints longer because of a continuing improvement in the understanding of the interface between the engineering materials and the tissues that they are connected to.

Dr. S. Sideman: Technology is in fact pulling forward the science of physiology. New technological tools bring about better understanding and, sometimes, realization of new physiological phenomena. This is exactly what we are doing here. We are in a sense running ahead of physiology by measuring, quantifying, and analyzing the various aspects of the cardiac system. However, technology can also modify physiology. Balloons and stents are one example. If you could, by introducing some kind of a fluid into the artery, affect a desired chemical reaction or gene expression, then of course you have technology modifying physiology.

Dr. M. Morad: One of the things that has fascinated me, for somebody who does not work in this field, is the incredible influence of shear stress on vascular proliferation or gene expression. The heart must also see a lot of shear stress. But the heart does not seem to have the problem of proliferation against the continuous dynamic pounding it receives. Why is that?

Dr. R. Beyar: Muscle fibers do not see the shear stress. Mostly, they see normal stresses, like wall tension. Extensive work has been done on the mechanism of hypertrophy. What is the stimulus for hypertrophy? If you suddenly increase load, it increases the wall stress and the stress along the fiber direction. Some of it is shear stress, which may also affect the collagen arrangement of fibers. I believe that stress is a major player in remodeling dynamic structures, as well as static structures like bone.

Dr. A. McColloch: In experiments in my laboratory, where we expose cardiac cells in culture to strain, the biaxial strain does affect the gene and protein expression of cardiac cells in culture. We have mostly studied the cardiac fibroblast, but there are reports by other groups on the myocyte. In doing these studies and listening to the very beautiful work that has been done on endothelial cell shear stress, I have become aware that the *in vitro* models are very poor approximations to the *in vivo* situation. There may be almost as many responses that have been measured *in vitro* in say, the endothelial cell, that are at odds with *in vivo* behavior, as those that are consistent with it. Therefore, the most important technology for physiology at this time is the transgenic animal. That brings a new engineering challenge of developing the experimental techniques to make measurements in experimental animals, which we are currently used to make in patients.

Dr. S. Sideman: Does anyone want to give the famous "I have a dream" speech? What would be the ultimate? what would be the ideal?

Dr. A. McCulloch: You wait long enough, that would be transgenic rats. I do not think that is very far off.

Dr. H. ter Keurs: My dream is to develop a diet that would eliminate and prevent atherosclerosis. All of us would be out of work, but all of us are still creative so we could look for a new problem to tackle.

Dr. M. Morad: Since we are dreaming, there is something that I have been very fascinated with besides the transgenic and knockout mice. It is the stem cell technology. The stem cell technology combined with knockout genes, which some laboratories are now attempting, promises to be a great breakthrough. First of all, the technique will not be as expensive as the transgenic animals, and you will not have the problem of lethal mutations that one is confronted with in whole animal work.

Dr. S. Sideman: I would like to bring up interaction between artificial matter and the living tissue, and the problem of the human variability in response to external factors. The issue is the compatibility of the normal tissues to a foreign body. Every patient behaves differently. There is a large variability in the response of patients to the implantation of an artificial organ into the body. As far as I know, this is, to this day, a major obstacle in applying and using artificial hearts. There are other parameters involved, but this one seems to be the major one.

My question to experts in stents and implantation: is there a variability between people that can negate the application of artificial stents? There seems to be a common denominator which makes stents a success, in spite of the variability.

Dr. R. Beyar: There is great variability between patients. That is why 20–30% of patients who receive stents in lesions that look similar will have restenosis, i.e., they will have a lumen dimension at 6 months which is less than 50% of the original dimension. The other 70–80% of the patients will not show restenosis. There is a group of patients who have a larger proliferative response. The reason may be multi–factorial: there is variability in the disease, in the disease process, and in the response to injury.

Dr. U. Dinnar: All the people who received artificial hearts died due to thrombus formation. Its an engineering problem. It all had to do with flow and shear stress and formation of thrombus.

Dr. S. Sideman: In a round–about way, yes, assuming that you can control the biochemical initiation of this phenomena. The problem is first biochemistry and then the creation of clots which are of course affected by the blood flow. This is very different in each individual, so it is not just engineering.

Dr. H. Strauss: One other issue that has not been addressed at all here is the long–term sequela. The history in coronary artery surgery suggest that the average life time of a bypass procedure is about 7 years due to progression of atherosclerosis. In the angioplasty field, everyone currently is focusing on the acute proliferative response in the early 6 months period, but there may be similar processes occurring, such as acceleration of atherosclerosis, in these patients, perhaps modified by stents, occurring 5–10 years after the angioplasty has been performed. It would be appropriate to think about the progress that has been made in the study of patients with coronary artery disease and bypass grafts, and start setting up some prospective trials to evaluate and follow these patients, to see what can be done to minimize the progression of atherosclerosis in this group of patients. The data on coronary disease and the patients with bypass grafts suggest that they have a more aggressive form of atherosclerosis. Whatever the cause, this group of patients may be potentially a very vulnerable group for developing complications some 5–10 years out and it is time to think about this problem now because the number of angioplasty procedures is going to continue to grow.

Dr. R. Beyar: A five year follow–up of stenting has shown that 40% need revascularization at five years, mostly due to progression of new lesions rather than the old treated lesions. So the atherosclerotic disease continues to progress. One of the major challenges is to stop or delay the progress of this disease.

Dr. M.S. Gotsman: If I had a dream I would like to prevent coronary atherosclerosis. We have two different kinds of diseases: one is atheroma progression and the other is the ruptured plaque. Both are influenced and developed as a consequence of risk factors. But when we manipulate the risk factors, this in itself produces side–effects. At present we are dealing with the third–wave patients. The first–wave involved treatment of patients with coronary atherosclerosis before the development of bypass surgery. The second–wave was the introduction of the bypass and second and third bypasses. The third–wave was the use of interventional procedures in patients returning after their first or second bypass operation. Nevertheless, the future is very bright: we have new methods of invasive cardiology with improved balloons, drills, cutting devices, lasers, and stents. Coronary artery surgery has also improved in the era of minimally invasive surgery and the use of multiple arterial grafts. We have learned to control risk factors and reduce the rate of progression of the disease. However, ventricular dysfunction is the tragic consequence of arterial obstruction. Chemical lysis or mechanical reperfusion aim at restoring normal coronary artery blood flow thereby protecting the myocardium. Ventricular dysfunction continues to develop, so that patients develop heart failure, and after medical treatment fails, need cardiac transplantation or the insertion of artificial hearts.

CLOSURE

This is a story about a poor student who tutors for his livelihood. He is going out for his next assignment. It is cold and snowing. When he puts on his galoshes, he notes that one has a big hole in the toe. As he leaves the rich student's house, he is ashamed of his obvious poverty and throws his galoshes on the snow bank... He watches as the snow slowly covers the disappearing galoshes, but for the black hole which keeps glaring at him...

We all face this hole that does not get covered, and good science is made of trying to cover these holes in our knowledge. We are all entitled to be satisfied with the 10th Henry Goldberg workshop and the nine previous ones which covered a fair number of holes. We believe that these workshops have had some important impact on international cooperation. The need for database and the smooth transfer of data, specifically good experimental data, and new theoretical concepts, is very acute to many of us. The Henry Goldberg Workshops, and similar types of meetings, enabled one to avail himself to data in different laboratories around the globe, and this is an important achievement. Another achievement is the development of close cooperation between different scientists and institutes. Not least important, we have succeeded to develop personal friendships and learn from each other. We have seen some beautiful presentations here which clearly indicate that the science of cardiology marches on and I am proud that we all are part of it.

Thank you for coming to this workshop and for being outstanding contributors to the science of the heart. I hope we shall have a chance to meet again, whether under this or a different umbrella. Let's keep pursuing our goals of an enlightened understanding of the cardiac system. Progress has been remarkable and all of you have demonstrated outstanding progress. Thank you all for being part of the Henry Goldberg Family.

S. Sideman
Haifa, December, 1996

THE EDITORS

Samuel Sideman, D.Sc., R.J. Matas/Winnipeg Professor of Biomedical Engineering, has Chaired the Department of Biomedical Engineering, and Directed the Julius Silver Institute of Biomedical Engineering, for some 15 years. He founded and directed the Heart System Research Center of the Technion–Israel Institute of Technology unti 1995.

Born in Israel (1929), he received his B.Sc. and D.Sc. from the Technion and his M.Ch.E. from the Polytechnical Institute of Brooklyn. On the faculty of the Technion since 1957, he served as Dean of Faculty, Dean of Students, and Chairman of the Department of Chemical Engineering. He was a Visiting Professor at the University of Houston and CCNY, a Distinguished Visiting Professor at Rutgers University, NJ, and is a Visiting Professor of Surgery (Bioengineering) at the University of Medicine and Dentistry, New Jersey (UMDNJ), USA.

His interests include transport phenomena, with particular emphasis on the analysis and simulation of the cardiac system. He has authored and co–authored over 250 scientific publications and co–edited 15 books. He received of a number of professional awards and citations, President of the Assembly for International Heat Transfer Conferences, and is on the editorial board of some major scientific journals. He is a Senior Member of a number of professional societies, Fellow of the American Institute of Chemical Engineering and the New York Academy of Science. Fellow of the Council on Circulation of the AHA, Honorary Fellow of the International Centre for Heat and Mass Transfer, Honorary Fellow of the Israeli Institute of Chemical Engineers, and has recently been awarded an Honorary D.Sc. from the Academy of Science of the Republic of Belarus.

Rafael Beyar, M.D., D.Sc., is a Professor in the Department of Biomedical Engineering and is Head of the Heart System Research Center at the Technion, and Director of the Division of Invasive Cardiology, Rambam Medical Center.

Born in Israel (1952), he received his M.D. from Tel Aviv University and obtained his D.Sc. in Biomedical Engineering from the Technion–Israel Institute of Technology. In the Julius Silver Institute, Department of Biomedical Engineering, Technion–IIT since 1984, he was (1985 to 1987) at the Division of Cardiology, Johns Hopkins University Hospital, Baltimore. He was a Visiting Professor of Medicine and a Visiting Scientist to Alberta at the University of Calgary (1991–1992).

His interests include modeling, simulation of the cardiovascular system, 3D analysis of ventricular function, MRI, coronary flow, interventional cardiology, CPR and cardiac assist. He is a member of medical and engineering societies, and a recipient of a number of institutional and national excellence awards. He has authored and co–authored over 100 scientific publications and is editor of ten volumes dealing with imaging, analysis, simulation and control of the cardiac system and interventional cardiology.

LIST OF CONTRIBUTORS

Dan Adam, Ph.D., Heart System Research Center, The Julius Silver Institute, Department of Biomedical Engineering, Technion–IIT, Haifa, 32000, Israel

Dan Admon, M.D., Cardiology Department, Hadassah University Hospital, P.O. Box 12000, Jerusalem 91120, Israel

Norman R. Alpert, Ph.D., Department of Molecular Physiology and Biophysics, University of Vermont College of Medicine, Burlington, VT, USA

Keith R. Anderson, M.Sc., Division of Vascular Biology, Pathology Department, Brigham and Women's Hospital, 221 Longwood Ave., Boston, MA 02115, USA

Theo Arts, Ph.D., Department of Biophysics, Cardiovascular Research Institute Maastricht, University of Limburg, P.O. Box 616, 6200 MD Maastricht, the Netherlands

Leon Axel, M.D., Ph.D., Department of Radiology, Hospital of the University of Pennsylvania, 308 Stemmler, 36th & Hamilton Walk, Philadelphia, PA 19104–6086, USA

Haim Azhari, D.Sc., Heart System Research Center, The Julius Silver Institute, Department of Biomedical Engineering, Technion–IIT, Haifa, 32000, Israel

James B. Bassingthwaighte, M.D., Ph.D., Center for Bioengineering, University of Washington, WD–12, Seattle, WA 98195, USA

Patricia E. Beighley, Ph.D., Mayo Clinic, Department of Physiology and Biophysics, Alfred Bldg. 2–409, 200 First Street SW, Rochester, MN 55905 USA

Shlomo A. Ben–Haim, M.D., D.Sc., Cardiovascular System Laboratory, The Bruce Rappaport Faculty of Medicine, Technion–IIT, Haifa, Israel and Harvard–Thorndike Electrophysiology Institute and Arrhythmia Service, Beth Israel Hospital, Boston, MA 02215, USA

Rafael Beyar, M.D., D.Sc., Heart System Research Center, The Julius Silver Institute, Department of Biomedical Engineering, Technion–IIT, Haifa, 32000, Israel

Pablo Burstein, M.Sc., Heart System Research Center, The Julius Silver Institute, Department of Biomedical Engineering, Technion–IIT, Haifa, 32000, Israel

Robert C. Castellino, M.D. Student, Department of Cell Biology, Duke University, Box 3845, Durham, NC 27710, USA

Frederick Ch'en, Balliol College, University of Oxford, Oxford, OX1 3PT, UK

Kieran Clarke, Ph.D., Department of Biochemistry, University of Oxford, Oxford, OX1 3PT, UK

Lars Cleemann, Ph.D., Department of Pharmacology, Georgetown University Medical Center, Washington, DC, 20007, USA

Michael V. Cohen, M.D., Departments of Physiology and Medicine, University of South Alabama, College of Medicine, Mobile, AL 36688, USA

Tucker Collins, M.D., Division of Vascular Biology, Pathology Department, Brigham and Women's Hospital, 221 Longwood Ave., Boston, MA 02115, USA

Forbes C. Dewey, Ph.D., The Fluid Mechanics Laboratory, Massachusetts Institute of Technology (MIT), Cambridge, MA 02139, USA

Uri Dinnar, D.Sc., Department of Biomedical Engineering, Technion–IIT, Haifa 32000, Israel

Giancarlo Dimassa, B.A., Department of Pharmacology, Georgetown University Medical Center, Washington, DC, 20007, USA

James M. Downey, Ph.D., Departments of Physiology and Medicine, University of South Alabama, College of Medicine, Mobile, AL 36688, USA

Michael Eldar, M.D., Neufeld Cardiac Research Institute, Chaim Sheba Medical Center, Tel Aviv University, Tel Hashomer 52621, Israel

Moshe Y. Flugelman, M.D., Department of Cardiology, Lady Davis Carmel Medical Center and the Bruce Rappaport School of Medicine, Technion, IIT, Haifa, Israel

Lior Gepstein, M.D., Cardiovascular System Laboratory, The Bruce Rappaport Faculty of Medicine, Technion–IIT, Haifa, Israel

Michael A. Gimbrone, Jr., M.D., Division of Vascular Biology, Pathology Department, Brigham and Women's Hospital, 221 Longwood Ave., Boston, MA 02115, USA

Jeffrey J. Goldberger, M.D., Neufeld Cardiac Research Institute, Chaim Sheba Medical Center, Tel Aviv University, Tel Hashomer 52621, Israel

Mervyn S. Gotsman, M.D., F.R.C.P., F.A.C.C., Cardiology Department, Hadassah University Hospital, P.O. Box 12000, Jerusalem 91120, Israel

Arnold J. Greenspon, M.D., Neufeld Cardiac Research Institute, Chaim Sheba Medical Center, Tel Aviv University, Tel Hashomer 52621, Israel

David A. Halon, M.B., Ch.B., Department of Cardiology, Lady Davis Carmel Medical Center and the Bruce Rappaport School of Medicine, Technion, IIT, Haifa, Israel

Peter J. Hunter, D.Sc., School of Engineering, The University of Auckland, Private Bag 92019, Auckland, New Zealand

Ronen Jaffe, M.D., Department of Cardiology, Lady Davis Carmel Medical Center and the Bruce Rappaport School of Medicine, Technion, IIT, Haifa, Israel

Steven M. Jorgensen, M.D., Ph.D., Mayo Clinic, Department of Physiology and Biophysics, Alfred Bldg. 2–409, 200 First Street SW, Rochester, MN 55905 USA

Prof. Dr. Med. H. Kammermeier, Institute of Physiology, Faculty of Medicine, RWTH, Pauwelsstrasse 30, D 52057, Aachen, Germany

Gad Keren, M.D., Department of Cardiology, Tel Aviv Medical Center, Tel Aviv University, Tel Aviv, Israel

Levon M. Khachigian, Ph.D., Center for Thrombosis and Vascular Research, University of New South Wales, Sydney NSW 2052, Australia

Amir Landesberg, M.D., D.Sc., Department of Biomedical Engineering, Technion–IIT, Haifa 32000, Israel

Ann A. Lee, Ph.D., Department of Bioengineering and Institute for Biomedical Engineering, University of California San Diego, La Jolla, CA, USA

Basil S. Lewis, M.D., F.R.C.P., Department of Cardiology, Lady Davis Carmel Medical Center and the Bruce Rappaport School of Medicine, Technion, IIT, Haifa, Israel

Chaim Lotan, M.D., F.A.C.C., Cardiology Department, Hadassah University Hospital, P.O. Box 12000, Jerusalem 91120, Israel

Andrew D. McCulloch, Ph.D., Department of Bioengineering and Institute for Biomedical Engineering, University of California San Diego, La Jolla, CA, USA

Masahito Miura, The University of Calgary, 1667 Health Sciences Center, 3330 Hospital Drive N.W., Calgary, Alberta T2N 4N1, Canada

Martin Morad, Ph.D., Department of Pharmacology, Georgetown University Medical Center, Washington, DC, 20007, USA

Michael J. Morales, Ph.D., Department of Pharmacology, Duke University, Box 3845, Durham, NC 27710, USA

Morris Mosseri, M.D., F.A.C.C., Cardiology Department, Hadassah University Hospital, P.O. Box 12000, Jerusalem 91120, Israel

Louis A. Mulieri, Ph.D., Department of Molecular Physiology and Biophysics, University of Vermont College of Medicine, Burlington, VT, USA

Hisham Nassar, M.D., Cardiology Department, Hadassah University Hospital, P.O. Box 12000, Jerusalem 91120, Israel

Denis Noble, Ph.D., F.R.S., F.R.C.P., Department of Biochemistry, University of Oxford, Oxford, OX1 3PT, UK

Dan G. Ohad, D.V.M., Neufeld Cardiac Research Institute, Chaim Sheba Medical Center, Tel Aviv University, Tel Hashomer 52621, Israel

Nitzan Resnick, Ph.D., Department of Morphological Sciences, Rappaport Family Institute for Research in the Medical Sciences, Bruce Rappaport Faculty of Medicine, Technion–IIT, Haifa, 31096 Israel

Erik L. Ritman, M.D., Ph.D., Mayo Clinic, Department of Physiology and Biophysics, Alfred Bldg. 2–409, 200 First Street SW, Rochester, MN 55905 USA

Howard A. Rockman, M.D., Department of Medicine, Basic Science Building, 0613B, UCSD School of Medicine, La Jolla, CA 92093, USA

Yoseph Rozenman, M.D., F.A.C.C., Cardiology Department, Hadassah University Hospital, P.O. Box 12000, Jerusalem 91120, Israel

Yoram Rudy, Ph.D., The Cardiac Bioelectricity Research and Training Center, Department of Biomedical Engineering, Case Western Reserve University, Cleveland, Ohio 44106–7207, USA

Jeffrey E. Saffitz, M.D., Ph.D., Department of Pathology, Washington University School of Medicine, 660 South Euclid Ave., St. Louis, MO 63110, USA

Edward P. Shapiro, M.D., Division of Cardiology, School of Medicine, Johns Hopkins University, Baltimore MD, USA

Robin M. Shaw, Ph.D., The Cardiac Bioelectricity Research and Training Center, Department of Biomedical Engineering, Case Western Reserve University, Cleveland, Ohio 44106–7207, USA

Samuel Sideman, D.Sc., D.Sc. (Hon.), Heart System Research Center, The Julius Silver Institute, Department of Biomedical Engineering, Technion–IIT, Haifa, 32000, Israel

Pieter Sipkema, Ph.D., Laboratory for Physiology, Institute for Cardiovascular Research (ICaR–VU), Van der Boechorst straat 7, 1081 BT Amsterdam, The Netherlands

Harold C. Strauss, M.D., Department of Medicine, Duke University, Box 3845, Durham, NC 27710, USA

Bruno D.M.Y. Stuyvers, Ph.D., The University of Calgary, 1667 Health Sciences Center, 3330 Hospital Drive N.W., Calgary, Alberta T2N 4N1, Canada

Yuichiro J. Suzuki, Ph.D., Department of Pharmacology Georgetown University Medical Center, Washington, DC, 20007, USA

Randall L. Rasmusson, Ph.D., Department of Biomedical Engineering, Room 136, School of Engineering, Box 90281, Duke University, Durham, NC 27710, USA

Zeev Rotstein, M.D., Neufeld Cardiac Research Institute, Chaim Sheba Medical Center, Tel Aviv University, Tel Hashomer 52621, Israel

Henk E.D.J. ter Keurs, M.D., Ph.D., The University of Calgary, 1667 Health Sciences Center, 3330 Hospital Drive N.W., Calgary, Alberta T2N 4N1, Canada

Paul J. Thomas, Ph.D., Mayo Clinic, Department of Physiology and Biophysics, Alfred Bldg. 2–409, 200 First Street SW, Rochester, MN 55905 USA

Richard Vaughan–Jones, Ph.D., Department of Physiology, University of Oxford, Oxford, OX1 3PT, UK

Martijn A. Vis, Ph.D., Laboratory for Physiology, Institute for Cardiovascular Research (ICaR–VU), Van der Boechorst straat 7, 1081 BT Amsterdam, The Netherlands

Shimin Wang, M.D., Ph.D., Department of Medicine, Duke University, Box 3845, Durham, NC 27710, USA

James L. Weiss, M.D., Division of Cardiology, School of Medicine, Johns Hopkins University, Baltimore MD, USA

Nicolaas Westerhof, Ph.D., Laboratory for Physiology, Institute for Cardiovascular Research (ICaR–VU), Van der Boechorst straat 7, 1081 BT Amsterdam, The Netherlands

Hava Yahav, M.Sc., Department of Morphological Sciences, Rappaport Family Institute for Research in the Medical Sciences, Bruce Rappaport Faculty of Medicine, Technion–IIT, Haifa, 31096 Israel

INDEX

ATE DUE

To renew